THE COMPLETE BOOK OF

TAI CHI CHUAN

A COMPREHENSIVE GUIDE TO THE PRINCIPLES AND PRACTICE

By the same author

The Art of Chi Kung
The Complete Book of Zen
The Art of Shaolin Kung Fu
Chi Kung for Health and Vitality

For Mr. Wong's web site, please visit
http://shaolin-wahnam.tripod.com

THE COMPLETE BOOK OF TAI CHI CHUAN

A COMPREHENSIVE GUIDE TO THE PRINCIPLES AND PRACTICE

WONG KIEW KIT

TUTTLE Publishing

Tokyo | Rutland, Vermont | Singapore

Disclaimer: Please note that the publisher and author(s) of this instructional book are NOT RESPONSIBLE in any manner whatsoever for any injury that may result from practicing the techniques and/or following the instructions given within. Martial arts training can be dangerous—both to you and to others—if not practiced safely. If you're in doubt as to how to proceed or whether your practice is safe, consult with a trained martial arts teacher before beginning. Since the physical activities described herein may be too strenuous in nature for some readers, it is also essential that a physician be consulted prior to training.

Published by Tuttle Publishing, an imprint of Periplus Editions (HK) Ltd.

Published in 2001 by Vermilion,
20 Vauxhall Bridge Road, London SW1V 2SA

www.tuttlepublishing.com

ISBN 978-0-8048-3440-7

First Edition

24 23 22 21 15 14 13 12 2110TP

Printed in the Singapore

Distributed by:
North America, Latin America & Europe
Tuttle Publishing
364 Innovation Drive
North Clarendon, VT. 05759-9436 U.S.A.
Tel: 1 (802) 773-8930
Fax: 1 (802) 773-6993
info@tuttlepublishing.com
www.tuttlepublishing.com

Japan
Tuttle Publishing
Yaekari Building, 3rd Floor
5-4-12 Osaki, Shinagawa-ku
Tokyo 141 0032
Tel: (81) 3 5437-0171
Fax: (81) 3 5437-0755
sales@tuttle.co.jp
www.tuttle.co.jp

Asia Pacific
Berkeley Books Pte. Ltd.
3 Kallang Sector #04-01
Singapore 349278
Tel: (65) 6741 2178
Fax: (65) 6741 2179
inquiries@periplus.com.sg
www.tuttlepublishing.com

Indonesia
PT Java Books Indonesia
Jl. Rawa Gelam IV No. 9
Kawasan Industri Pulogadung
Jakarta 13930
Tel: (62) 21 4682-1088
Fax: (62) 21 461-0206
cs@javabooks.co.id

Contents

List of Illustrations

Dedication

This book is dedicated to all great teachers of Tai Chi Chuan, present and past, whose dedication to the art has helped to bring tremendous benefits to all people irrespective of race, culture and religion.

Preface

Tai Chi Chuan, or Taijiquan in Romanized Chinese, is a wonderful art, but more than 90 per cent of those who practise it gain less than 10 per cent of its potential benefits! This book will not only justify this claim, but will also provide the information you need to gain the remaining 90 per cent of the benefits. Although it is written from personal experience, much of the information given is derived from the writings of the greatest masters of the art, mainly in classical Chinese, which have been cherished by Tai Chi Chuan practitioners throughout the ages.

For those who are unfamiliar with Tai Chi Chuan, it is a time-tested art which gently exercises the body, the energy flow and the mind, and can be used for health, longevity, self-defence, mental freshness and spiritual development, irrespective of your race, culture or religion. It has been described both as poetry in motion and, erroneously, as shadow boxing and slow calisthenics. 'Poetry in motion' is an apt description of the beauty and grace of Tai Chi Chuan, but the terms 'shadow boxing' and 'slow calisthenics' reveal a lack of understanding of its depth and dimension.

This book, as its title suggests, gives a complete explanation of Tai Chi Chuan, from the most basic to the most advanced levels. It has something for everybody interested in the art, or in their own or others' well-being. This is what Tai Chi Chuan aims at, including the attainment of grace and balance, the promotion of physical and emotional health and the development of internal force or energy flow – for which Tai Chi Chuan is well known but little understood. It shows how to apply Tai Chi Chuan for combat, especially how to use an opponent's strength against him- or herself, and compares the various styles which have evolved to meet different needs. It will also help you understand how the early masters employed Tai Chi Chuan for spiritual cultivation.

Yet, despite its extensive and often deep coverage, no prior knowledge of Tai Chi Chuan is required. If you want to enjoy its wonderful benefits, however, you must practise it correctly and consistently; no amount of reading can make you a competent Tai Chi Chuan practitioner. This book provides invaluable information, culled from the accumulated wisdom of the greatest Tai Chi Chuan masters, but unless you put it into practice it will remain simply theoretical knowledge, giving you perhaps some reading pleasure. You may be able to discuss Tai Chi Chuan intelligently with your friends, and even offer good advice to some practitioners, but you yourself are unlikely to acquire the type of radiant health, graceful agility and mental clarity that such advice is intended to accomplish.

Apart from some advanced training, such as that involving energy and mind control which requires a master's personal guidance, the book is written as a self-teaching manual. But as many fine movements cannot easily be learnt from a book, however clear its presentation, it is advisable for beginners to seek personal instruction from a competent teacher. It is a common mistake for students to rush their learning; if there is one golden rule on which all masters would agree, it is to practise the correct methods patiently. All the established methods have passed the test of time; if a particular method is said by many masters to produce certain effects, it means that thousands of people who followed that method have experienced the effects. If you fail to do so, it is usually because you have not practised sufficiently or correctly.

Nevertheless, practising patiently does not mean following a method blindly. If a student who has patiently practised Tai Chi Chuan for many years still remains sickly, weak, emotionally unstable or mentally dull, then he or she has not been judicious or wise. Such a person should either turn to something else, or seek more information from masters or books to improve his or her practice. Generally, people who have correctly practised an established method for a year should reap the benefits that method is reputed to bring.

This book offers many of the established methods taught by some of the greatest Tai Chi Chuan masters in history. Besides explaining in detail the fundamental techniques common to all styles, and the Simplified Tai Chi set which has helped literally millions of the Chinese population to remain healthy and sane despite the traumatic effects of numerous wars and three revolutions in recent times, it presents all the various styles of Tai Chi Chuan in the way in which their best-known masters taught and demonstrated them.

Since Tai Chi Chuan is a very effective martial art, combat applications are treated in detail, and martial artists can discover the Tai Chi Chuan tactics for remaining unhurt even if one loses a fight – in many other martial systems getting hurt is inevitable even for the victor. There are also numerous exercises to put principles like 'soft overcoming hard' and 'flowing with the opponent's momentum' into practice.

Virtually all the great masters have stressed that the significance of Tai Chi Chuan lies in its internal aspects and not its external form; most Tai

Chi students know that this is an internal art but few understand what this really means and fewer still can experience its internal aspects. This book aims to help students overcome this problem: by explaining the relevant principles as well as providing suitable exercises, it shows you how to realize the Tai Chi Chuan tenet that every movement of this internal art is a training of energy and mind.

Although Tai Chi Chuan has a rich philosophy, usually recorded in poetic language, and some examples are found in this book, it is geared towards practical use in combat and, more significantly, in our daily life. In other words, if you have practised Tai Chi Chuan for 20 years, but cannot yet defend yourself when an assailant attacks you, or are still prone to anger or nervousness, or lack the energy to run and jump irrespective of how old you are, you have wasted your time. This book explains why and how Tai Chi Chuan enhances your health, work and play.

Many people, especially in the West, are surprised to discover that Tai Chi Chuan is a martial art; they are even more surprised to learn that it was originally devised for religious cultivation, irrespective of one's spiritual conviction or lack of it. This book traces its Taoist connection, and shows how an aspirant can practise Tai Chi Chuan for spiritual development.

My original idea for the title of this book was *The Wonders of Taijiquan*, for it was the desire to share the wonderful benefits of this art that prompted me to write this book. But my capable editor at Element Books, Julia McCutchen, having the readers' interest in mind, suggested *The Complete Book of Tai Chi Chuan*, which I must admit is better. I would like to comment briefly on the word 'complete'. The book is complete in the sense that it presents every aspect of Tai Chi Chuan a student might wish to know about, including little-known but interesting snippets such as why the stances in one Wu style are higher than those of another, or how the flowing movements in all Tai Chi Chuan styles are linked to Lao Tzu's teaching in the *Tao Te Ching*. Even the question of knee injury, which appears to be a contemporary serious problem among many Tai Chi practitioners in America, is discussed. But it does not mean that all the important information about Tai Chi Chuan is found here in its entirety. There is so much wisdom in Tai Chi Chuan that volumes could be written on the material contained in each chapter.

For me personally, the writing of this book is both an unexpected accomplishment and a rewarding learning process. I never thought of writing a book on Tai Chi Chuan, and for a long time I even resisted teaching Tai Chi Chuan despite many requests and despite knowing that it has many wonderful benefits. The reason was that I thought I would do better to stick to teaching aspiring students Shaolin Kungfu, as that was the best system I could offer them. Although I have learnt Tai Chi Chuan for more than 20 years, my training is mainly in the Shaolin arts. I have been privileged to learn from distinguished Shaolin masters with a succession line extending directly back to the famous Shaolin Monastery, and I cherish the belief that a good teacher should always give his best to his students.

However, a few years ago when I was teaching Shaolin Chi Kung to students who were also Tai Chi Chuan teachers, and therefore incidentally imparted some Tai Chi Chuan principles and methods to them, I came to realize that my reason for teaching only Shaolin Kungfu – the fact that it was what I am best at – was only valid from my own perspective. From the students' perspective, Tai Chi Chuan would be more beneficial, because, apart from the fact that their circumstances were more conducive to Tai Chi Chuan practice, not many people actually have the endurance and discipline needed for Shaolin Kungfu training. And when I noticed that 90 per cent of those practising Tai Chi Chuan were gaining less than 10 per cent of its potential benefits, mainly because they lacked the kind of knowledge that was once regarded as top secret in the martial arts field, the desire to write a book and share this knowledge took shape.

In conclusion I wish to thank my disciple Cheong Huat Seng for taking the photographs on which the illustrations are based, and my disciple Goh Kok Hin and my son Wong Chun Nga for acting as my opponents in them. I would also like to thank my editor Julia McCutchen at Element Books, my literary agent Doreen Montgomery at Robert Crew Ltd, and their efficient assistants for their help and support.

Wong Kiew Kit
Kedah, Malaysia

1

Tai Chi Chuan as a Martial Art

The Aims and Benefits of Practising Tai Chi Chuan

A typical Tai Chi Chuan master frequently exhibits many of the qualities of a model martial artist: while confident of his martial skills, he is soft-spoken, humble, tolerant and at peace with himself and with others.

A Concise and Comprehensive Martial Art

Tai Chi Chuan, or Taijiquan as it is spelt in Romanized Chinese, is one of the most wonderful martial arts in the world. This chapter explains why; so if you are not getting the best from your Tai Chi practice you will at least know what you are lacking. Other chapters show how you can derive the full benefits from Tai Chi Chuan.

Some people may be unaware that it is actually a martial art at all, yet it is extremely effective for combat, from the viewpoint of technique as well as force. The amazing thing about Tai Chi Chuan is that to defend yourself against almost any form of physical aggression, you need to know only a few fighting patterns!

You do not have to learn a mass of martial art patterns because past masters have reduced a wide variety of fighting techniques to about 20 Tai Chi Chuan patterns which you can use to meet almost any attack. It is a concise, comprehensive fighting system which covers all four of the main categories of attack – hitting, kicking, throwing or gripping.

Because of the nature of many other martial arts, their exponents often have difficulty if opponents use attacks that fall outside the categories in which their respective arts specialize. For example, Karate specializes in hitting, so a Karate exponent meeting someone who uses Taekwondo or Siamese Boxing, which specialize in kicking, would be handicapped, because the Karate repertoire does not include many kicking techniques. If a Taekwondo exponent meets a Judo expert, the former would have difficulty overcoming the latter's throws, because in Taekwondo, throws are seldom used. Conversely, the Judo expert would be hard pressed to defend against Taekwondo kicks or Karate punches, because the normal Judo training provides little practice against such combat situations. One way to prepare yourself to handle any fighting situation is to learn all these different martial arts. A better alternative is to learn Tai Chi Chuan; it not only saves time and effort, it also gives advantages not found in these other martial arts.

Besides the conciseness of the fighting techniques, there is also the advantage of better control of force. A Tai Chi Chuan master can cause devastating injury to his opponent without leaving any outward marks, whereas the injuries caused in most other martial arts are often a reminder of how gruesome fighting is, and how brutal some martial artists can be. The Tai Chi Chuan masters would not usually hurt their opponents, however, first because their training is such that they tend to be very calm rather than violent in a fight, and secondly because they can demonstrate their superiority in a gracious way which is not readily available in most other martial arts. They can, for example, throw their opponents several feet, thereby making their victory quite clear, yet without hurting them. In some martial arts, where the urge to win has been over-emphasized and aggressive emotion blindly aroused, the exponents may have to break their opponent's bones or smash their heads before victory is conceded.

The Mechanics and Psychology of Different Arts

Unbelievable violence and hostility are found in some systems, even in sparring between fellow students. It is not uncommon to find instructors themselves yelling 'Go for him! Kill! Kill!' at their students. It is hardly surprising that such students come out of their training sessions with bruises and pains in their bodies, and arrogance and hatred in their hearts. Such unacceptable behaviour is not found in Tai Chi Chuan training, not because Tai Chi Chuan practitioners are necessarily morally superior, but because the nature of the training is such that a calm disposition and a feeling for one's sparring partners are developed intrinsically, and harbouring selfish, aggressive attitudes would work against the practitioners themselves.

An investigation into the mechanics and psychology of the training methods of the different martial arts reveals their different effects. In other arts, mechanical strength and speed are necessary in sparring. When one student punches or kicks another, if the defender does not block or avoid the attack in time, the fast, direct momentum of the attacking technique is such that it is very difficult for the attacker to hold back the punch or kick. When the partner is hit, therefore, it can be very painful. The basic strategy in these arts is to strike the opponent as hard and as fast as possible, with little or no concern for one's own defence. Both sides concentrate on attack, usually hurting each other, and the more one is hit, the more one wants to get even. This desire for vengeance is accentuated by a stoic philosophy which teaches that in combat, one's sole aim is to strike down one's opponent, irrespective of who he or she is – a philosophy going back to a time when a warrior took a misplaced pride in killing without question whoever his lord had instructed him to kill, even if the victim was his own father.

The mechanics and psychology of Tai Chi Chuan are totally different. Because the basic combat strategy is to flow with one's opponent's movements rather than going against them, a Tai Chi Chuan exponent must be relaxed and calm in combat in order to use the skills and techniques effectively. As the striking force is derived from internal energy flow and not from mechanical momentum, one can exert force at the point of contact. This means that if one accidentally hits a sparring partner, it will not hurt because one will not back up the hit with force.

Moreover, the approach to sparring in Tai Chi Chuan is different from that in other aggressive martial arts. Instead of exchanging blows, Tai Chi Chuan students develop sparring skills in a specially devised art known as Pushing Hands, in which their arms are in gentle contact with one another in a rhythmic motion. The aim is to sense the other's weakness, such as an unguarded opening or a moment of imbalance, so that one exponent can push the other off without causing any hurt. It is significant that in Pushing Hands, one not only flows with one's partner's movements, but also with his or her feelings! If one senses that one's partner feels hesitant, anxious or distracted, for example, one exploits the opportunity and throws the other person off. Pushing Hands will be explained later.

The philosophy of Tai Chi Chuan originated not with warlords whose aim was to kill, but with Taoist masters whose aim was to prolong life and attain immortality. This difference in philosophy and history has led to a difference in the basic psychology of the art's exponents. Taoism is well known for its love of freedom, its disregard for mundane trifles, and its penchant for joviality. Translated into Tai Chi Chuan, it manifests as a carefree, joyful and spontaneous attitude in solo practice as well as in sparring with partners.

Internal Force, Not Brute Strength

The approach to force development in Tai Chi Chuan is internal, with the emphasis on mind power and intrinsic energy flow. Thus, if you practise Tai Chi Chuan, your force training does not require you to hit sandbags, lift dumb-bells, jab your fingers into granules, strike your shins against poles, or do any of the tough and painful conditioning that leaves calluses on your hands and feet. Yet the force developed, if you know how to make use of cosmic energy, is greater than all the sandbags and dumb-bells put together.

In external force training, the force developed is usually localized and specific. For example, if you strike your palms against sandbags or kick your shins against poles in your training, the force you will develop will be localized at your palms and shins. Its use is also usually specific – having powerful palm strikes and shin kicks. But in the internal force training of Tai Chi Chuan, the force developed is usually versatile and capable of varied uses. If you enhance your mind power through meditation and your intrinsic energy through Chi Kung practice, you can not only develop a clear mind to observe your opponent's moves calmly and be able to channel your intrinsic energy to your palms or legs for powerful strikes, but also increase your mental focus and clarity of thought, as well as facilitating harmonious energy flow for better physical and emotional health. Moreover, you also have the advantage of convenience: if you adopt internal force training, you need not worry about carrying your sandbags and dumb-bells with you whenever you travel. Numerous methods of internal force training will be described later.

Many people believe that in Judo brute strength is not necessarily a winning factor. A classic illustration of Judo shows a small girl using a little finger to push a gigantic sumo wrestler, who is already off balance, to fall backwards. In real life, however, a sumo wrestler is unlikely to be caught off balance in such a position. Even if he were, all he, or anybody else for that matter, would have to do to save himself would be to take a step backwards to regain balance. The truth is that it needs a lot of strength, in Judo or any other art, to throw even an ordinary person down – unless that person is naive enough to be caught in a falling position.

Tai Chi Chuan rather than Judo is the art that best demonstrates that brute strength is not necessary in fighting. A fragile-looking girl who is expert in Tai Chi Chuan can not only effectively defend herself against a strong man, but also cause him serious injury, including pushing him onto the ground. She still needs a lot of strength, but not necessarily of the brute or mechanical kind.

An Art of Convenience and Culture

If you are one of those people who like martial arts but dislike the inconvenience of changing into and then out of special training clothing every time you begin and complete your practice, Tai Chi Chuan is an excellent choice, because it does not require any special dress for serious training. If you are caught in a fight and want to use your martial arts techniques without tearing your clothes, you can avoid having to ask your opponent to wait while you change into your martial arts attire!

Moreover, unlike many other martial arts, in Tai Chi Chuan you do not normally perspire a lot, despite the great benefits you can derive from it. You can, for example, have a morning walk in a park wearing your business suit, practise your Tai Chi Chuan without attracting the embarrassing attention from uninvited spectators which is often accorded to other martial arts, and then go straight to your office. Tai Chi Chuan can even be practised within the confined space of your office or bedroom. It is difficult to find another martial art that is so convenient.

In Chinese culture an ideal person is accomplished in both the scholarly and the martial arts, expressed in a poetic saying as *wen wu shuang quan*. Confucius himself, the patriarch of the gentry, whom many people mistakenly think of as an old bookworm, was actually an expert in archery and swordsmanship. Many great generals were also poets and writers. Tai Chi Chuan satisfies this ideal, and is thus often regarded as a scholar's martial art. Its popularity comes from both sides. Many scholars prefer Tai Chi Chuan because its training methods are graceful and gentle, and the art itself emphasizes features already found in and highly valued by scholars, such as clarity of thought, a relaxed disposition, and an abhorrence of brutality. On the other hand, Tai Chi Chuan practitioners, probably more than those of other martial arts, are also attracted to literature and other cultural pastimes like painting, music and chess because the concept of yin-yang in Tai Chi Chuan (which will be explained in detail in the next chapter) opens vistas of Chinese philosophy and literature. Moreover, its feeling of relaxation and spontaneity, compared with the tense, competitive attitude found in most other martial arts, encourages participation in these pastimes.

The Richness of Tai Chi Chuan Theory

Tai Chi Chuan has a very rich body of theory, which touches on various aspects of the art and is frequently recorded in poetic language. This embodiment of theoretical knowledge not only summarizes effective techniques of fighting and force training, many of its principles can be applied to daily living. One good example is the following four-fold principle in force training: differentiate the real and the apparent, regulate breathing, use mind rather than brute strength, be calm and relaxed in your action.

Even a brief explanation of this principle can reveal the depth of Tai Chi Chuan theory. In most other martial arts, force training is simplistic and mechanical. If a practitioner of these arts wishes to increase his or her punching power or stamina, for example, it usually requires nothing much more than punching sandbags and skipping over a rope. In Tai Chi Chuan force training, however, punching sandbags, skipping and running are discouraged because not only are these methods crude, they actually diminish the fighting ability of the Tai Chi Chuan exponent. These crude methods give an apparent, not a real, improvement in punching power and stamina.

Punching sandbags hardens the fist, which is quite different from increasing power. A hardened fist covered with calluses may lessen the pain you feel when you smash your fist against a brick, but it does not necessarily increase your power. Any increase in power is not the result of your fist's repeated contact with the sandbag, but of the action of your repeated punching. Hence, if you just punch into the air repeatedly, instead of into a sandbag (which actually discourages you from punching hard, as it causes you pain), the increase in your punching power will be greater and faster. The failure of many martial artists to appreciate this is an example of not differentiating the real from the apparent. The power you gain from such punching practice is mechanical, and depends upon how fast your momentum is – and how well your knuckles escape from cracking. A better alternative is to use internal force, which resembles a form of electricity; your punch is therefore not a bony hammer but a connecting bridge channelling the internal force from you into the opponent. If you co-ordinate your breathing, use your mind, and remain calm and relaxed, you will not only increase the internal force in your punch, but also enhance other aspects of your fighting.

Similarly, Tai Chi Chuan masters consider skipping over a rope or running on a machine a crude method of increasing stamina. Like punching a sandbag, it shows an inability to differentiate the real from the apparent. The increase in stamina is apparent, not real, because you will end up panting for breath if you allow the increase in your need for air which results from your increased activity to regulate your rate of breathing, instead of your trained mind. Your heart will also be working harder, and your blood rushing unnaturally, which is not only stressful and impairs your ability to think clearly and react spontaneously in combat, but may in the long run unfavourably affect your health in ways you may not be able to envisage. Tai Chi Chuan methods of force training overcome all these setbacks, and they will be explained in Chapter 6.

Tai Chi Chuan in Health, Character Development and Philosophy

Tai Chi Chuan is not only an efficient fighting art; it is also effective for curing and preventing organic and psychotic illness like hypertension, rheumatism, asthma, gastritis, insomnia, migraine, depression and nervousness – the very same diseases that conventional medicine considers incurable. If practised properly it can prevent or relieve knee injury, which the American Academy of Orthopedic Surgeons reported in 1989 as the largest category of all injuries in the United States. Furthermore, it provides a gentle system of exercise for promoting health and vitality. In other words, you do not need to be sick or have someone attack you to enjoy the wonderful benefits of Tai Chi Chuan. If you feel you have no time to exercise, or working out in a gym is too demanding, practising Tai Chi Chuan is a good answer to your problem. Just 15 minutes a day in the comfort of your home can provide you with all the exercise you need but can find neither the time nor the energy for. The benefits are not just physical; the meditative aspect of Tai Chi Chuan and its emphasis on relaxed movement contribute to serenity of mind and clarity of thought.

While many martial arts tend to make their practitioners belligerent and aggressive, Tai Chi Chuan helps its adepts to become calm and composed. This comes about not through moralizing by instructors, but through the nature of Tai Chi Chuan practice itself. It is more suitable than most other martial arts for character development, as the very nature of its training, with its emphasis on gracefulness, gentleness and harmonious energy flow, is intrinsic to the development of mental freshness and cosmic harmony. A typical Tai Chi Chuan master frequently exhibits many qualities of a model martial artist: while confident of his martial skills, he is soft-spoken, humble, tolerant and at peace with himself and with others.

But Tai Chi Chuan is not just a martial art; it is deeply rooted in Chinese philosophy and Taoist wisdom. The term 'Tai Chi', which literally means 'the grand ultimate', and figuratively 'the cosmos', originated from the *Yi Jing* (*I Ching*), the *Book of Change*. At the start of the classic *Treatise on Tai Chi Chuan* which we shall study in detail later, the great master Wang Zong Yue said that 'Tai Chi is born from the Void. It generates movement and stillness, and is the mother of yin and yang. When moved, it separates; when still, it unites.' It is amazing how close this philosophy is to that of modern physics concerning the universe and the atom.

If you have read this far, I hope I have impressed you with the wonders of Tai Chi Chuan. Some of you may find it hard to believe that these benefits are possible. This is understandable because only a few people have had access to the knowledge this book will share. There are various reasons for this, including a tendency on the part of past masters to withhold their secrets and a communication gap between the East and the West. You should not, however, accept anything in this book on faith alone, but practise it for some time, preferably with the help of competent instructors, then evaluate the teaching to the best of your understanding and experience.

2

The Concept of Yin-yang in Tai Chi Chuan

What You May Have Missed in Your Tai Chi Class

In many ways, Tai Chi Chuan is all about yin-yang. If there is only yin and no yang, or vice versa, then that is not Tai Chi Chuan.

The Philosophy of Yin-yang

Have you ever wondered why Tai Chi Chuan is called Tai Chi Chuan, why this effective martial art is widely practised for health, why we normally perform its movements slowly, and why many students gain such a small portion of the tremendous benefits that can be derived from it? An understanding of yin-yang will provide us with answers to these and other questions.

Yin-yang is probably the most widely used Chinese concept in the English language; it is also one of the most misunderstood – even among Chinese! Many scholars, for example, give the impression that yin and yang, representing the positive and the negative or the male and female principles, are the two primordial forces operating the universe, or the two fundamental ingredients that make up the whole cosmos. This interpretation is quite wrong, despite its popularity among otherwise authoritative figures. Yin and yang by themselves are neither forces nor ingredients; they are symbols and may have different meanings in different contexts. So at times they may *symbolize* forces or ingredients, cosmic or otherwise, but they do not always do so.

While its manifestations are many and often profound, in its simplest form the concept of yin and yang refers to the two opposing yet complementary aspects of everything in the universe, be it an object, a process or an idea. For example, if we talk about looking up at the sky, 'up' and 'sky' become meaningful only when we relate them to their corresponding aspects of 'down' and 'earth'. We usually do this unconsciously, because we have become so familiar with these terms, but we do it none the less. In other words, 'up' and 'sky', and 'down' and 'earth' are two opposing yet complementary aspects, which give meaning to each other. If there were no 'down' and 'earth', there would be no 'up' and 'sky', and vice versa. If we were deep in outer space, 'up' and 'sky', or 'down' and 'earth', would be meaningless. One of the two aspects is designated as yin, and the other aspect as yang. In this example, 'up' and 'sky' are conventionally referred to as yang, and 'down' and 'earth' as yin.

Now let us look at the sky, which is yang when compared to the earth, on its own. If it is overcast and comparatively dark, we may refer to it as yin compared to other times, when it is bright and sunny. However, if we compare this overcast sky with the way it is at night, then it is yang, as it is brighter than the night sky, even though it is dark when compared to sunnier days. Hence, we can see that yin and yang, as manifested by 'dark' and 'bright' here, are relative as well as complementary.

Yin and yang are two aspects of one unity or holism. This unity is usually expressed in a diagram known as the Tai Chi symbol (see *figure 2.1*). Tai Chi is usually translated as the cosmos. Notice that the symbol is perfectly symmetrical from all angles. This superbly symbolizes the opposing yet complementary aspects of yin-yang. Notice also that yin begins when yang is at its maximum, and vice versa.

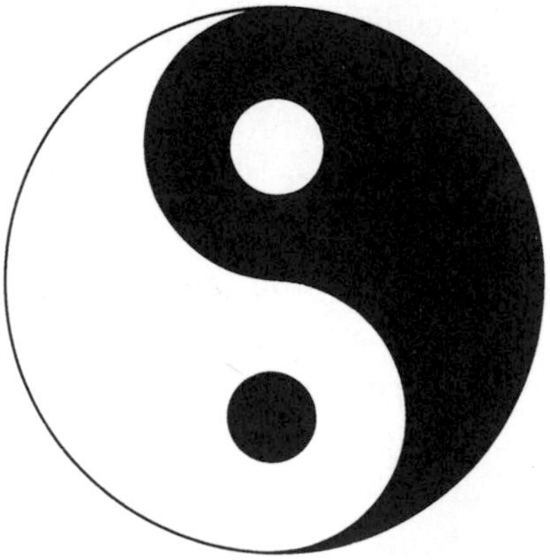

Fig 2.1 The Tai Chi symbol

The concept of yin-yang and its Tai Chi symbol are used in many other disciplines besides martial arts. They are particularly significant in medicine, alchemy, divination, astrology, geomancy and Taoist philosophy. In Chinese medical thinking, for example, we often hear that yin-yang harmony is essential for health. Like a mathematical formula, this is a concise but great principle that can manifest in countless situations in health and medicine. The Tai Chi symbol is the main motif in Taoist illustration, symbolizing, among other things, the physical as well as the spiritual in Taoist philosophy.

Yin-yang in Tai Chi Form and Force Training

The name 'Tai Chi Chuan' is derived from this concept of yin-yang as expressed in the Tai Chi symbol. Yin-yang is manifested in all the four aspects or dimensions of Tai Chi Chuan, namely form, force training, application and theory.

When Zhang San Feng modified Shaolin Kungfu into Wudang Long Fist, which later became Tai Chi Chuan, he elaborated on the soft, circular movements of the fighting art so as to harmonize the comparatively hard Shaolin forms. Notice, for example, how the 'hard' attack of the Shaolin pattern A Black Tiger Steals the Heart, *figure 2.2a*, has evolved into the comparatively 'soft' punch of the Tai Chi pattern Move–Intercept–Punch, *figure 2.2b*; and how the diagonal, straight block of the Shaolin A Beauty Looks at a Mirror, *figure 2.2c*, has developed into the circumferential movement of the Tai Chi Ward-off, *figure 2.2d*.

Hence, we generally find Tai Chi Chuan movements graceful and gentle, distinctly different from the fast, forceful movements of Shaolin Kungfu. Tai Chi Chuan students also normally perform their movements slowly, as it is easier to develop the flow of internal energy with slow movements, but when they have become skilful in doing this, the movements can, and should, be fast and forceful, thus completing the harmonious cycle of yin (slow and gentle) and yang (fast and forceful).

At the time that Chen Wang Ting was developing a philosophy for Tai Chi Chuan, most of the other martial arts emphasized hard, external methods in their training, like punching sandbags, carrying weights and striking poles. Chen Wang Ting emphasized soft, internal methods, like circular movements and energy flow, to balance what he regarded as excessive hard training.

In the hard, external method used to develop Shaolin Iron Palm for example, exponents strike their palms regularly and consistently on a sandbag in a daily routine for many months or years. In the soft, internal method to develop Tai Chi Palm, exponents use graceful movements to generate a flow of internal energy to their palms. In this method, it is necessary to practise appropriate breathing co-ordination and visualization: merely performing the external movements will have hardly any significant effect.

This method of developing powerful Tai Chi Palm illustrates the concept of yin-yang – a reminder that the best results are obtained when yin and yang are in harmony. Here, the yang aspect is manifested in the external, circular hand movements, and the yin aspect in the breathing co-ordination and visualization. An exponent can still develop a great deal of force by means of breathing and mind alone, but the result is better if appropriate hand movements are also used. The approach here is soft and internal, but when the exponent has acquired the force, the application can be hard and external.

However, many Tai Chi Chuan students have nowadays gone to the other extreme, thinking that hard, external training and application are alien to Tai Chi Chuan. An appreciation of the yin-yang principle helps to overcome this superficial view and provide the necessary insight to more effective training.

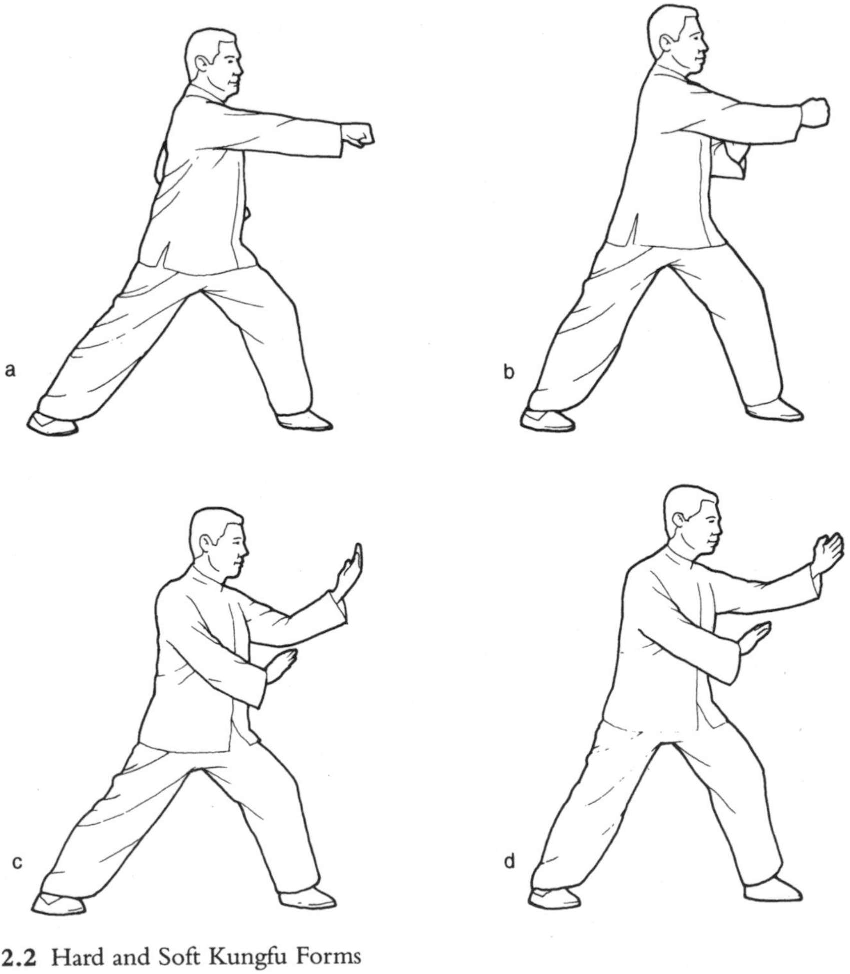

Fig 2.2 Hard and Soft Kungfu Forms

Yin-yang in Tai Chi Chuan Application

Some martial artists stress only the fighting aspect of their arts, often sacrificing their health for a better fighting ability, developing toughened hands and feet that have lost much of their original sensitivity, and sustaining insidious bodily injuries that often go untended. But more serious even than this physical injury is the emotional and spiritual damage they do. They can sometimes be aggressive and brutal, easily becoming irritated when accidentally hit by their partners during practice, and even taking sadistic pride in punishing their fellow students during sparring.

Tai Chi Chuan masters regard such unhealthy practices and attitudes as excessive yang, ie over-emphasis of the yang aspect of fighting at the expense of the yin aspect of health. To remedy this imbalance, while maintaining the excellent function of the system as a fighting art, they place more emphasis on its health aspect, practising Tai Chi Chuan for preventing illness, enhancing vitality and promoting longevity. Indeed, it is a superb system for relieving degenerative and psychiatric illnesses like asthma, arthritis, rheumatism, gastritis, depression and nervousness, which conventional medicine and psychiatry often prove inadequate to help.

Again, many students and instructors today have overdone the emphasis on health, with the result that their practice of Tai Chi Chuan is also imbalanced. Most Tai Chi Chuan students do not know how to apply their art to defending themselves, even against simple attacks like a straightforward punch and kick. Some I have spoken to were actually surprised to discover that it is a martial art. Not one of the more than a dozen English Tai Chi Chuan books I found in a recent survey provides any substantial information on the martial aspects of the system, although most of those written in Chinese describe it as a martial art.

Of those practitioners who do know that Tai Chi Chuan is basically a martial art, many insist that they practise it for health and not for fighting, without reflecting that practising a martial art without understanding its martial function is to miss its essence. Such an excess of yin, like the excess of yang explained earlier, is contradictory to the spirit of Tai Chi Chuan.

What many Tai Chi Chuan enthusiasts do not realize is that its best health benefits are derived from practising it as a martial art, even if they do not want to use it for fighting. If you practise Tai Chi Chuan as a form of gentle exercise, as many people do, the benefits will be minimal, probably less than you would normally derive from most physical exercises like gymnastics, aerobics or swimming. But if you practise it as it should be practised – as a martial art, in the way all the great Tai Chi Chuan masters in the past practised it – the benefits are tremendous. For example, you will be free from physical and emotional illness, have abundant stamina and energy, be calm and clear even under trying circumstances – and all these benefits will be enhanced as you age! Why this is so, and how you should train to derive these benefits, will be explained later in the book. Here suffice it to say that the yin-yang concept is significant; it reminds us of the yin-yang balance of Tai Chi Chuan in its health and martial aspects, as well as in the guiding principles of the training methods to derive these benefits.

Let us examine how this concept is applied in Tai Chi Chuan for combat. An important Tai Chi Chuan principle is: 'If my opponent does not move, I do not move; if my opponent moves, I move faster.' An example of its application is as follows. My opponent gets ready to attack me. Instead of moving my hands and feet about aimlessly, as some novices may do, I remain fairly still, to assess the other person and to focus my mind and energy. As soon as my opponent moves to attack me, however, perhaps by giving me a straight punch or a side kick, I move in faster to frustrate the attack before it is even half complete, and to counterattack, perhaps by deflecting the punch or kick and striking simultaneously with my other palm. This is a Tai Chi pattern known as Green Dragon Emits Pearl, also called Twist Knee Throw Step.

The strategy in the above example involves stillness and motion, which are represented by yin and yang. Symbolically it may be expressed as follows: 'If yin, more yin; if yang, more yang.' Obviously, this strategy can only be used by someone who is competent. If, while your opponent is preparing to attack, you become impatient instead of remaining still, then you do not have sufficient yin to implement this strategy; and if, when the opponent attacks, you react too slowly, then you do not have sufficient yang.

Instead of using more yin against the opponent's yin, and more yang against the opponent's yang, the Tai Chi Chuan exponent may apply a different strategy, that of using yin against the opponent's yang, and yang against the opponent's yin. Symbolically, it is expressed as: 'If yang, use yin; if yin, use yang.' A whole class of combat situations where this strategy may be employed can be summed up by a tactical principle known as 'circular against straight; straight against circular,' where circular is symbolized by yin, and straight by yang, as shown in *figure 2.3*.

In *figure 2.3a*, the opponent attacks with a powerful straight punch. The exponent deflects it with a circular arm movement – 'circular against straight' – and counters with a palm strike *(figure 2.3b)*. Both the opponent's and the exponent's patterns here are the same as those described in the previous example, but here the exponent's emphasis is on circular movement rather than speed.

The opponent takes a small step back; pushes aside the exponent's arms by 'threading' up his left arm *(figure 2.3c)*, and counters with a circular side kick to the exponent's ribs *(figure 2.3d)*. Without having to block this circular kick, the exponent moves his right leg a small step diagonally to the right and executes a left thrust kick to the opponent's thigh, instead of at his genitals, to avoid hurting him seriously, using 'straight against circular' *(figure 2.3e)*.

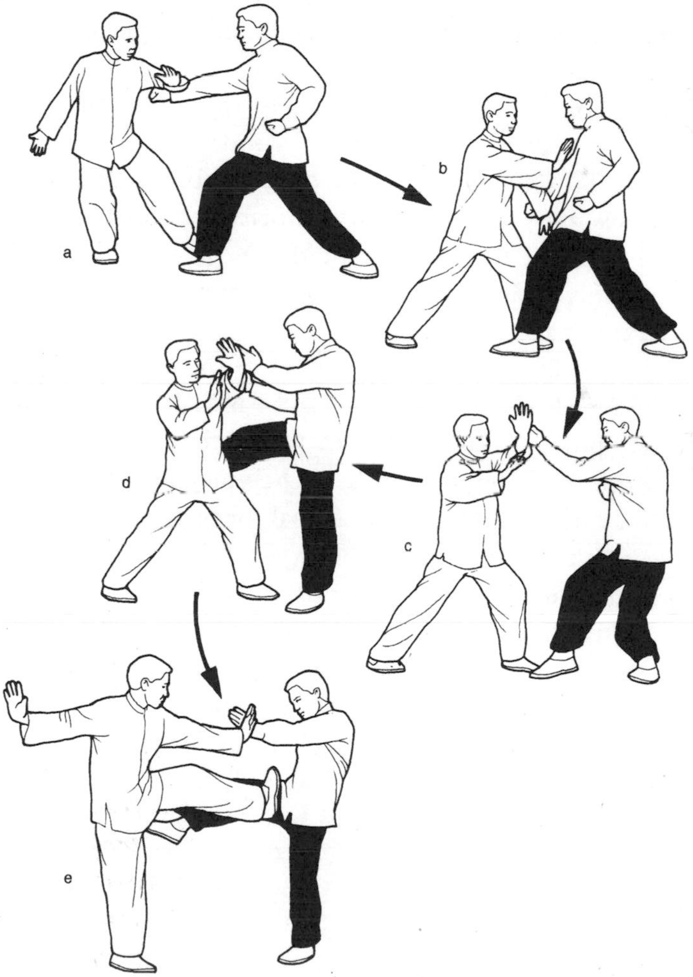

Fig 2.3 Yin-yang of circular and straight

Yin-yang in Tai Chi Philosophy

The yin-yang concept constitutes the basis of Tai Chi Chuan philosophy. The fundamental Tai Chi Chuan set, from which many other sets derive, is sometimes called the 13 Techniques of Tai Chi. These 13 Techniques are the eight fundamental Tai Chi hand movements of warding off, rolling back, pressing, pushing, spreading, taking, elbowing and leaning, and the five fundamental leg movements of moving forward, moving back, moving to the left, moving to the right, and remaining in the centre. These 13 fundamental techniques will be explained in some detail later.

The eight hand movements and the five leg movements derive their inspiration from the concepts of the Eight Trigrams, or *bagua* (*pakua*), and of the Five Elemental Processes, or *wuxing* (*wu hsing*), in Taoist philosophy. *Bagua* and *wuxing* are closely related, and the principle of yin-yang is the basis of their operation.

Bagua symbolizes the eight archetypal forms of the universe, which are represented by heaven, earth, thunder, wind, water, fire, mountain and swamp. We must remember that these are symbols, not absolute objects; heaven, for example, may stand for authority and power. The *bagua* concept is the basis for the working of the *Yi Jing* (*I Ching*), the *Book of Change*, not only in divination but also in various fields like military strategy, government and economics.

Wuxing is the Five Elemental Processes of the universe, which are represented by metal, water, wood, fire and earth. It is important to realize that they are processes, and not elements, as they are often described by Western scholars. Water and fire as archetypical processes in *wuxing* are different from water and fire as archetypal forms in *bagua*. Again, we must remember that the terms are symbolic; water as a process, for example, may represent training methods that promote health.

An understanding of the concepts of *bagua* and *wuxing* is very helpful, but not essential, in practising Tai Chi Chuan for health or fighting. But if we aim at the highest level, where our practice leads to philosophical insight and spiritual development, such an understanding is vital.

Bagua and *wuxing* in Tai Chi Chuan will be discussed in some detail in a later chapter. Meanwhile, let us briefly examine how the yin-yang concept helps us to understand Tai Chi Chuan theory at a more physical or practical level. It is evident in fundamental Tai Chi Chuan precepts like 'stillness and motion', 'mind and body', 'skill and application'. In these precepts, stillness, mind and skill are conventionally represented by yin, whereas motion, body and application are represented by yang.

Understanding yin-yang harmony enables us to appreciate that both stillness and motion are important. In the previous section, we saw how the concept of stillness and motion is used in actual combat. It is also used in the theory that governs combat. For example, Tai Chi Chuan exponents who only know how to move about without being able to be still and observe their opponents, or who can only stand their ground without knowing how to move in swiftly when an opportunity arises, are not efficient fighters. They fail to apply yin-yang harmony.

This yin-yang concept is of course also used in other areas. In practice, for example, if a student merely performs Tai Chi movements, like practising a routine Tai Chi set, without putting some time and effort into the stillness of Tai Chi Chuan, like stance training or sitting meditation, he or she is unlikely to gain the best results because the practice is incomplete.

Similarly, good Tai Chi practitioners employ both mind and body in combat as well as in their daily work and play. If their Tai Chi Chuan practice has given them fit, healthy bodies, but they still have dull minds, then their training is incomplete. They may likewise be very skilful in performing Tai Chi Chuan, but if they remain clumsy in their work and play, then they have failed in the yin-yang principle of skill and application.

Hence, a good understanding of yin-yang enables us to gain a better appreciation and greater benefits from Tai Chi Chuan. In many ways, Tai Chi Chuan is all about yin-yang. If there is only yin and no yang, or vice versa, then that is not Tai Chi Chuan. For example, if we just practise Tai Chi Chuan form, but never develop Tai Chi Chuan force, then we are not practising the art completely, for there is only yin but no yang. At best, we perform a sort of graceful dance, and we will achieve little, even if we practise for a lifetime. If we practise Tai Chi Chuan for health but do not know how to apply it to self-defence, or if we only use it for fighting but derive no benefit from its health aspects, then our training lacks this yin-yang harmony.

Tai Chi Chuan is a wonderful art, providing us with vitality, the ability to defend ourselves, emotional stability, mental freshness and a healthy, long life. At its highest level, if we are ready, it helps us to transcend the physical and attain the Taoist quest for immortality. Understanding the concept of yin-yang gives us a glimpse of such wonders.

3

The Historical Development of the Various Styles

Health, Combat and Spiritual Joy in Tai Chi Chuan

There are three characteristic stages in its 'development', which are best represented by Wudang Tai Chi Chuan, Chen-style Tai Chi Chuan and Yang-style Tai Chi Chuan.

The Earliest References to Tai Chi

If you are puzzled by the many styles of Tai Chi Chuan, as many students are, this chapter will explain how the root of Tai Chi Chuan grew into a sturdy tree with all these different branches. You will also appreciate the differences as well as the similarities between the various styles, which will be described in greater detail in later chapters, and their typical Tai Chi sets presented, as taught by their best known masters.

As we have seen the term 'tai chi' means 'the cosmos', and is derived from the *Yi Jing* (*I Ching*), or the *Book of Change*. It is closely connected with Taoist philosophy. But no one is sure of the origin of Tai Chi Chuan, although a number of theories have been postulated. Records show that in the Tang Dynasty (618–906) a hermit named Xu Xuan Ping practised an art known as the 37 Patterns of Tai Chi. It was also called *Changquan* or Long Fist, after the Long River – the name the Chinese give to their longest river, Yangtze Kiang – because its performance should be long and continuous like a river. At about the same time on Wudang Mountain a Taoist priest named Li Dao Zi practised an art called Primordial Long Fist, which was similar to the 37 Patterns of Tai Chi.

The earliest known use of the term 'Tai Chi Chuan' was found in a classical text called *The Method to Attain Enlightenment through Observing the Scripture* (*Guan Jing Wu Hui Fa*), which was written by Cheng Ling Xi who lived in the Later Liang Dynasty (907–23). Cheng Ling Xi studied under Han Gong Yue, who called his art 14 Patterns of Tai Chi Training.

Zhang San Feng and the Origin of Tai Chi Chuan

The most popular theory of the origin of Tai Chi Chuan, however, concerns the Taoist priest Zhang San Feng (pronounced – and sometimes spelt – as Chang San Foong), who lived towards the end of the Song Dynasty in the 13th century. After graduating from the famous Shaolin Monastery, the fountainhead of Shaolin Kungfu, Chi Kung and Zen, Zhang San Feng continued his martial arts practice and spiritual development in the Purple Summit Temple on Wudang Mountain, which is one of the most important of the sacred mountains of Taoism.

One day Zhang San Feng witnessed a fight between a snake and a crane (some documents say a sparrow), and this inspired him to modify his comparatively hard Shaolin Kungfu into a softer style which was then known as Wudang 32-Pattern Long Fist. This later developed into Tai Chi Chuan. Zhang San Feng was the first master to discard external training methods like hitting sandbags, jabbing palms into granules and practising with weights, and to emphasize internal methods like breath control, *chi* channelling and visualization. He is thus regarded as the first patriarch of internal kungfu, which includes Tai Chi Chuan, Pakua Kungfu and Hsing Yi Kungfu. Most Tai Chi schools today honour Zhang San Feng as the founder of Tai Chi Chuan. The notable exception is Chen-style Tai Chi Chuan, for reasons which will be explained later.

The following 'Song of Silent Sitting', taken from *The Secret of Training the Internal Elixir in the Tai Chi Art*, which was said to have been written by Zhang San Feng, shows that the original aim of Tai Chi Chuan was spiritual fulfilment.

Sitting silently, practise meditation;
The impulse is at *yuanguan*.
Continuously and gently regulate your breathing;
One yin and one yang brewing in the internal cauldron.
Nature must be enlightened, life be preserved.
Don't rush, let the fire burn slowly.
Close your eyes and look at your heart of life,
Let tranquillity and spontaneity be the source.
In a hundred days you will see a result:
A drop of elixir rises from *kan*,

The Yellow Woman is the matchmaker in between,
Both the baby and the red lady are perfect.
The beauty is boundless and inexplicable,
All over the body vital energy arises.
Who can know such a marvellous experience?
It's like a dumb person having a beautiful dream.
Swiftly take in the primordial essence;
The elixir breaks through the three obstacles,
Rising from *dantian* to the top at *niyuan*,
Then submerging into *zhongyuan*.
Water and fire combine to form real mercury,
Without *wu* and *ji* there is no elixir.
Let the mind be still, and life be strong,
The spirit radiates throughout 3,000 worlds.
Golden cockerel crows beneath the shadowless tree,
The red lotus blossoms in the middle of night.
Winter comes the sun shines again,
A thunderous roar shatters heaven and earth.
Dragons call, tigers play,
Heavenly music fills the sky in full harmony.
In nebulous mixture everything is empty,
The infinite phenomena are all here.
Marvellous in its mystery, mysterious in its marvel.
The circulation of the stream breaks through the three obstacles;
All phenomena are born in the union of heaven and earth.
Drink the dew of nature, sweet like honey,
Saints are buddhas, buddhas are saints.
When ultimate reality reveals dualism disappears,
Now I realize all religions are the same!
Eat when hungry, sleep when tired,
Offer a joss stick and practise meditation.
The great Tao is just before your eyes,
If you are deluded, you'll miss the chance.
Once you've lost your human form you may have to wait for
a million aeons.
The uninformed dream of going to heaven,
The blind go into a deep forest to practise.
The ultimate secret is marvellous beyond the profane,
Letting out the ultimate secret is a heavy sin.
The four true principles you have to cultivate,

Breaking the gate of mystery to reach the marvellous.
Cultivate day and night without break,
Get a master early to develop your elixir.
There are people who know that real mercury
Is the elixir of longevity and immortality.
Cultivate each day, be more determined each day;
Do not regard spiritual cultivation as just an *ad hoc* task.
To succeed one must cultivate for three years, nine years,
Before a pearl of elixir can be obtained.
If you want to know who composed this song,
It's by the Taoist Priest of Purity and Void, the Saint San Feng.[1]

Purposely written concisely in symbolic language to prevent the arcane knowledge from being revealed to the uninitiated, this song provides both the philosophy and the method to attain the highest goal in Tai Chi Chuan, Taoism or any spiritual discipline. Spiritual development in Tai Chi Chuan will be explained in more detail in Chapter 21.

Yuanguan, dantian, niyuan and *zhongyuan* are various energy fields in the body. *Kan* refers to the abdomen; *wu* and *ji* refer to the circulation of vital energy round the body in a Chi Kung art known as The Small Universe. Yellow woman, baby, red lady, dragons, tigers and golden cockerel are symbolic terms describing the application of mind and energy in harmonious unity to produce a pearl of elixir or an internal illumination. Shadowless tree is an allusion to Hui Neng's 'Bodhi is not a tree', which is a Zen way of saying that ultimate reality is formless; the four true principles are the Four Noble Truths, which form the basis of the Buddha's teaching. These two references, as well as other concepts in the song, reflect the Shaolin teaching of Zhang San Feng.

The evidence for the existence of Zhang San Feng is impressive, although some scholars say that he was a myth. Erected on Wudang Mountain are two huge stone tablets honouring him as a Taoist saint, one decreed by the Ming emperor Seng Zu, and the other by the Ming emperor Ying Zong. The *Imperial History of the Ming Dynasty* recorded that Zhang San Feng was born in 1247, learned Taoism from a Taoist master called Fire Dragon at Nanshan Mountain in Shenxi, cultivated his spiritual development for nine years at Wudang Mountain, was known by the honorific title of 'the Saint of Infinite Spiritual Attainment', and was the first patriarch of internal martial arts. *The Records of the Great Summit of Eternal Peace Mountain* mentions that he studied the yin-yang of the cosmos, observed the source of the longevity of tortoises and cranes, and attained remarkable results. *Collections of Clouds and Water* describes him as carrying his lute and sword on his back, singing Taoist songs, working in the mountains, and studying the marvellous secrets of the cosmos.[2]

Early Tai Chi Chuan Masters

Zhang San Feng's successor was the Taoist priest Taiyi Zhenren, who was well known for his Wudang sword. By the end of the Ming Dynasty this Wudang Kungfu, which was originally taught to Taoist priests at the Purple Summit Temple, had spread to secular disciples. The Taoist priest Ma Yun Cheng transmitted the art to his famous secular disciple, Wang Zong Yue, who called this Wudang art Tai Chi Chuan, and whose *Treatise on Tai Chi Chuan* has remained a classic to this day.

Two more of Ma Yun Cheng's celebrated disciples were Mi Deng Xia and Guo Ji Yuan, who were popularly known as 'the two saints'. There is some indication that they taught Wudang Kungfu to Dong Hai Chuan the founder of Pakua Kungfu. If this is true, then Tai Chi Chuan and Pakua Kungfu (or *Baguazhang* in Romanized Chinese) originated from the same source, Wudang Kungfu.

Wang Zong Yue transmitted the art to another famous secular master, Zhang Song Xi, who in turn taught Dan Si Nan. Dan's disciple was Wang Zheng Nan, who specifically referred to Wudang Kungfu as an internal art, distinguishing it from Shaolin Kungfu which he referred to as external. It is reputed that Wang Zong Yue or Zhang Song Xi taught the Wudang art to the Chen family at Chen Jia Gou, or the Chen Family Settlement, in Wen District of Henan Province, where the art was known as Tai Chi Chuan. However, the Chen family, the originators of Chen-style Tai Chi Chuan, maintain that Tai Chi Chuan was developed in the 17th century by their 9th generation ancestor, Chen Wang Ting, a general of the Ming Dynasty, and that Wang Zong Yue actually learnt it from the Chen family.

Chen Wang Ting and Chen-style Tai Chi Chuan

When the Ming Dynasty was replaced by the Qing Dynasty, Chen Wang Ting retired to the Chen Family Settlement to pass his time in studying literature and martial arts, subsequently developing Tai Chi Chuan.

It is not clear where Chen Wang Ting originally learnt his martial arts, but there are two popular theories to explain how Chen-style Tai Chi Chuan developed. The first is that Wang Zong Yue's Wudang Kungfu, or

Wudang Tai Chi Chuan as it is commonly known now, is the foundation upon which it is based, because Wang Zong Yue stayed in the Chen Family Settlement for many years and his *Treatise on Tai Chi Chuan* describes the philosophy and techniques of Tai Chi Chuan superbly. The second theory is that Chen Wang Ting learnt his art in the army as a legacy from Qi Ji Guang, the great 16th century Ming general who repulsed the Japanese naval invasion, because Qi's masterpiece, *The Classic of Kungfu*, provides the fundamental principles of Chen-style Tai Chi Chuan.

Some people suggest that Chen Wang Ting might have been influenced by Shaolin Kungfu directly, as the Chen Family Settlement is not far from the Shaolin Monastery in the same province, and virtually all Tai Chi patterns and principles, except those touching on Taoist philosophy, are also found in Shaolin Kungfu.

Tai Chi Chuan students can derive a great deal of inspiration from the following poem by Chen Wang Ting, who demonstrated the spirit of an unbeatable warrior even though his beloved country had been defeated. This poem also records the process by which he developed Tai Chi Chuan. The *Classic of the Yellow Palace* which he mentions below is an important Taoist work on Chi Kung and spiritual cultivation.

Sighing for past times when I was strong and sharp,
Sweeping away dangerous obstacles without fears.
My gratitude to the emperor for his kindness,
Allowing me to live till my ripe old years.
Now I only have the *Classic of the Yellow Palace* to accompany me.
In times of leisure I invent martial arts,
In times of activity I farm the fields,
And teach children and grandchildren to be strong and healthy to meet life's expediencies.
My imperial pension has long been used up,
I must work hard to repay my debts.
Never indulge in vainglory,
Humble and tolerant one should always be.
Everyone says I am sad,
Everyone says I have gone mad.
I have heard this time and again,
But it does not move me.
I smile at countless people struggling to remain ahead in their profane activities;

They do not understand the inner peace of non-greed for wealth
and fame.
Let your emotion be calm like evening water,
Let your endurance be like mountains and streams.
Success makes no difference;
Failure too makes no difference,
Who is happy like a carefree saint?
I am happy like a carefree saint.[3]

It is not certain whether Chen Wang Ting invented Tai Chi Chuan, but it is clear that he contributed greatly to its philosophy and in his time the term Tai Chi Chuan became established; before then it was usually called Wudang Kungfu.

The Old, the New, the Small and the Big

Tai Chi Chuan was originally taught only to members of the Chen family. By the 18th century two sub-styles had emerged: the Old Form represented by Chen Chang Xin (1771–1853), and the New Form represented by Chen You Ben. After learning the New Form from Chen You Ben, his disciple Chen Jing Ping (1795–1868) further modified it by adding small circular movements to the patterns. Hence, Chen Jing Ping's sub-style is known as the Small Form. Later he moved to a nearby urban centre called Zhao Bao, where he taught Tai Chi Chuan to students outside the Chen family. His Small Form is therefore also known as the Zhao Bao Form.

These three forms are not three different styles, but three variations of the same Chen-style Tai Chi Chuan. In the Old Form the movements 'lead from the body to the arms'. For example, if you want to execute a punch, you first adjust your stance, then move your body accordingly, and subsequently let your rotating body flow into your arm with a continuous movement, starting in the legs and developing into the punch. The Old Form is therefore characterized by big movements, with the emphasis on developing force.

In the New Form the movements 'lead from the arms to the body'. So when executing a punch, you do not initially move your legs and body, but your arm. You finish your punch by moving your body according to the punching momentum. The New Form uses fewer movements than the Old Form and is therefore faster; it is intended for combat. It should be noted that this slight body movement following the momentum of the punch is not intended to add body-weight to the punch, as is common in some external martial art, but to promote a better flow of internal force.

In the Small Form, this body movement is not necessary; it is replaced by a circular thrust of the punching arm, which produces what is known as spiral force. Thus, the combat effectiveness of Tai Chi Chuan is further enhanced in the Small Form: not only is it forceful, because less movement is involved, it is also faster, conserves energy and maintains better balance.

Tai Chi Chuan masters advise that beginners should start with the Old Form, which provides the basic mechanics. At the intermediate stage, when students have developed internal force by practising the Old Form, and understand its execution, they can proceed to the New Form for combat application. At a later stage, they can employ the Small Form for enhanced force, speed and balance.

There is also a fourth form, the Big Form, which was developed later in Yang-style Tai Chi Chuan.

Yang Lu Chan and Yang-style Tai Chi Chuan

There is an interesting story which describes the emergence of Yang-style Tai Chi Chuan. Yang Lu Chan (1799–1872) sold all his property and worked as a servant in Chen Chang Xin's family in order to 'steal' Chen-style Tai Chi Chuan by learning it in secret. He was so successful that not only did no one notice him, but he also attained a high standard.

One day a kungfu expert came to challenge the master, Chen Chang Xin. His son and best disciple took the challenge but was badly defeated. The challenger asked to meet the master. Chen's students told him that the master was away. But the challenger was determined to meet the master; he put up in a local hotel and came back every three days to seek him. This went on for a few months. The Chen family was desperate; there was no way, it seemed, that they could overcome this embarrassing situation.

One day, the challenger came and said as usual, 'I would like to meet Sifu Chen Chang Xin, and request him to teach me some fighting techniques.' This was the conventional way of saying, 'I am here for a friendly challenge.'

'I'm sorry, Sifu, our master has not returned from his trip,' one of the senior students said.

'Then, I'll come again in three days' time.'

But before the challenger walked away as usual, a servant came forward and to everybody's surprise said:

'Sir, I have also practised some Chen-style Tai Chi Chuan. I am not very good at it and would be honoured if you would kindly teach me.' This was a polite, conventional way of saying, 'I accept your friendly challenge.' The servant, of course, was Yang Lu Chan.

They were even more surprised when Yang Lu Chan, using genuine Chen-style Tai Chi Chuan, defeated the challenger. But defeating a challenger was one thing; upholding the Chen family discipline was another. 'Stealing' a secret martial art was an extremely grave offence, punishable by death. So Yang Lu Chan knelt before the master, in front of all his students who had gathered in the family hall to see him disciplined. After prostrating thrice and offering tea to the master, Yang Lu Chan solemnly said: 'Sir, I have committed a grave offence in stealing your secret martial art. I know the consequences, and am ready to accept your punishment.'

The atmosphere was tense. Would the master impose the death sentence? Everyone was grateful to Yang Lu Chan for defeating the challenger, but the master had to set an example by upholding discipline. What would he do now?

Chen Chang Xin sipped his tea thoughtfully. Then he said, 'What offence? What punishment? It is an offence only if an outsider steals our art. But you are not an outsider. By accepting your tea and drinking it, I have accepted you as my disciple. We are proud of you as a new member of the Chen-style Tai Chi Chuan, for you have saved us from shame and will bring honour to us.'

It is unlikely that this story is true, but Yang Lu Chan did bring much honour to Chen-style Tai Chi Chuan. Before settling down in Beijing to teach Tai Chi Chuan, he travelled the country challenging other kungfu masters in friendly matches, and he always won. He was nicknamed 'Yang the Ever Victorious'. He was the first outsider to break the tradition of restricting Chen-style Tai Chi Chuan to Chen family members only, one generation before Chen Jing Ping taught it to outsiders at Zhao Bao.

The Wu and the Sun Styles

Yang Lu Chan passed his knowledge on to Wu Yu Xiang (1813–1880) and to his sons Yang Ban Hou (1837–1890) and Yang Jian Hou (1839–1917). Wu Yu Xiang later also learnt from Chen Jing Ping, and in turn taught Yang Ban Hou. The style of Wu Yu Xiang's Tai Chi Chuan,

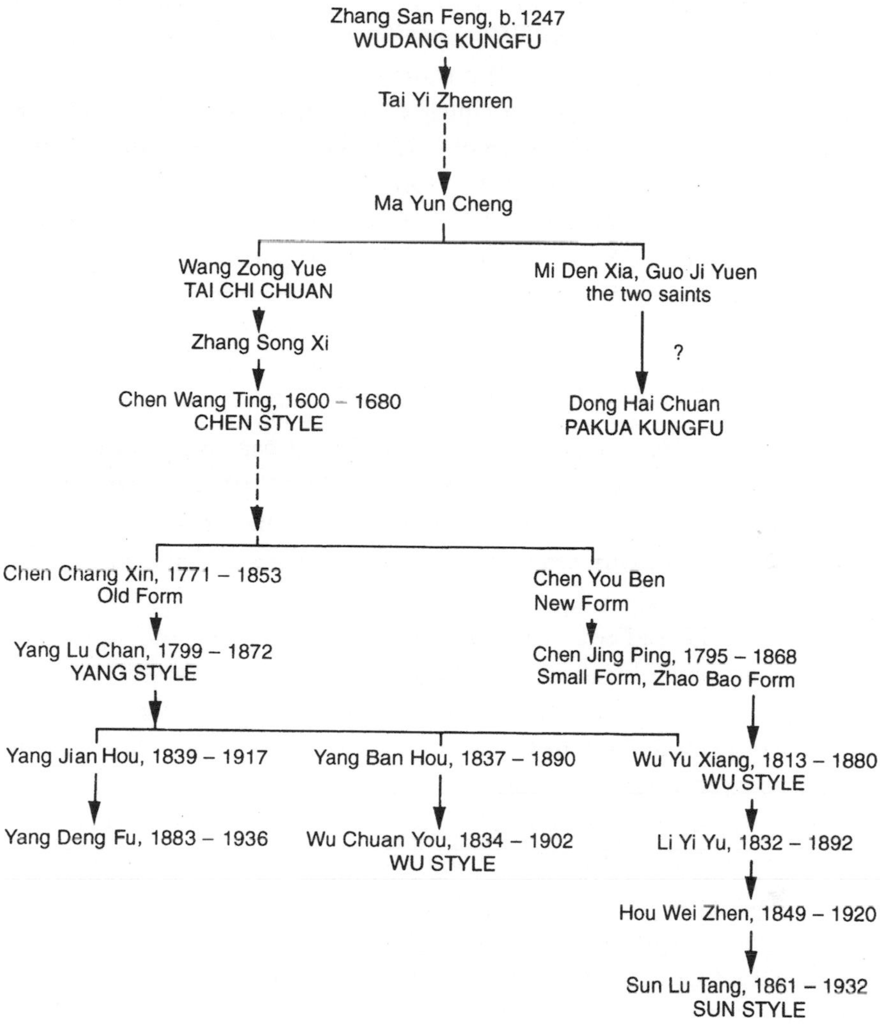

Fig 3.1 The 'family tree' of Tai Chi Chuan

which is a combination of the Old Form of Yang Lu Chan, and the New Form of Chen Jing Ping, is known as Wu-style Tai Chi Chuan.

Yang Ban Hou's most accomplished disciple was Wu Chuan You (1834–1902), who later developed another Wu-style Tai Chi Chuan. The 'Wu' of Wu Chuan You is pronounced slightly differently from the 'Wu' of Wu Yu Xiang (the first is pronounced in the second tone, the second in the third tone). Although they are written with totally different Chinese characters the similarity in their pronunciation and the fact that they are written the same in English can cause confusion for many Westerners. So if you practise Wu-style Tai Chi Chuan, you may like to find out which one of the two Wu styles yours actually is.

Another of Wu Yu Xiang's disciples, Li Yi Yu (1832–1892), taught the Small Form to Hao Wei Zhen (1849–1920). Hao Wei Zhen's disciple was the well-known Sun Lu Tang (1861–1932), who was accomplished in all three schools of internal kungfu, namely Hsing Yi Kungfu, Pakua Kungfu and Tai Chi Chuan. His style of Tai Chi Chuan is known as Sun-style Tai Chi Chuan.

The Three Stages of Tai Chi Chuan

The most popularly practised style of Tai Chi Chuan today is the Yang. Yang Lu Chan's grandson, Yang Deng Fu (1883–1936), enlarged and made smoother the movements of the Old Form patterns he had learnt from his father so as to promote the health aspect of Tai Chi Chuan. Hence, the Yang style of Tai Chi Chuan he developed is sometimes called the Big Form. He did away with jumping, foot-stamping, straight punches and other forceful, aggressive actions which are more appropriate for combat. He also performed the patterns slowly, gently and gracefully, almost transforming Tai Chi Chuan into an exquisite dance, although he himself was a formidable fighter.

While this development of Tai Chi Chuan over three generations from the martial art of Yang Lu Chan to the health exercise of Yang Deng Fu has many good points – for example it makes it easier for elderly or less able people who may find the original martial style too vigorous – it is not without its drawbacks. The most serious, in my opinion, is that it has lost its martial aspect to such an extent that the term Tai Chi Chuan becomes meaningless. The term is a shortened form of *Tai Chi quanfa* (pronounced 'T'aiji ch'uan-fa'). *Tai Chi*, as we know, means the cosmos, and *quanfa* means the art of the fist, or martial art. Indeed, some people who practise the art only for health, perhaps embarrassed by this loss of its essence, refer to their practice as Tai Chi, and not Tai Chi Chuan.

If they practise Tai Chi without the martial aspect, however, they are unlikely even to obtain the full health benefits, such as being fit and agile, calm and mentally fresh, full of vitality and stamina, because these are derived from practices that aim to turn practitioners into top-class martial artists. In other words, if you practise Tai Chi Chuan purely as a gentle health exercise, you may have a general feeling of well-being, but you are unlikely to develop the speed of a deer, the calmness of a crane, the patience of an ox, the courage of a tiger or the longevity of a tortoise – all features that a martial artist can expect to attain. On the other hand, if you practise Tai Chi Chuan as it is taught by the masters, you can achieve all these qualities.

If we examine the historical development of Tai Chi Chuan from the time of Zhang San Feng to the present day, we can see that as it progresses in time, it retrogresses in quality. There are three characteristic stages in its 'development', which are best represented by Wudang Tai Chi Chuan, Chen-style Tai Chi Chuan and Yang-style Tai Chi Chuan. The aim of Wudang Tai Chi Chuan is grand and lofty; it is nothing short of merging into the cosmos. By the time of Chen-style Tai Chi Chuan, the primary aim has shifted from spiritual cultivation to excellence in combat. But by the time of Yang-style Tai Chi Chuan, the martial dimension has almost disappeared; most students of Tai Chi Chuan today practise it for health, many are quite unaware that it is a martial art, and hardly any know that it is also a way of spiritual cultivation.

This representation is not intended to suggest that Wudang Tai Chi Chuan is superior. Any style of Tai Chi Chuan, if practised correctly, can lead to the highest achievement, and any style, if practised without an understanding of its deeper meaning and dimension, can degenerate into a dancelike exercise. The present situation of Tai Chi Chuan is precarious: when people who have only attended a few weekend courses begin to teach the art, when instructors themselves lack the energy to jump up onto a chair or run after a bus, it is hardly surprising that it can become degraded until it is merely a demonstrative form – what masters refer to as 'flowery fists and embroidered kicks'. The aim of this book is to present the philosophy and methods of Tai Chi Chuan as taught by its greatest masters, so that aspiring practitioners can achieve their objectives according to the level or stage of attainment they choose.

4

Advice from the Great Masters

Achieving Better Results in a Shorter Time

What better way is there to equip ourselves with the appropriate knowledge of any art than to learn from the masters themselves?

What better way is there to equip ourselves with the appropriate knowledge of any art than to learn from the masters themselves? Some of the most important advice recorded by Tai Chi Chuan masters still in existence is in the 'Song of Secrets for Training in the 13 Techniques' of Wu Yu Xiang (1813–80), the 'Five Characters Formula' of Li Yi Yu (1832–92), and the 'Ten Important Points of Tai Chi Chuan' of Yang Deng Fu (1883–36).

The 'Song of Secrets for Training'

The 'Song of Secrets for Training in the 13 Techniques' is in the form of a poem. As usual, much of its poetry is lost in translation, although the meaning remains. Wu Yu Xiang, who combined the Old Form of Yang Lu Chan and the New Form of Chen Jing Ping, is the founder of Wu-style Tai Chi Chuan. Here is his advice:

Don't underestimate the thirteen techniques,
The source of life is at the waist.
Pay attention to 'apparent' and 'solid',
Without hindrance *chi* flows with grace.
Stillness in movement, movement in stillness,
Adjust according to what the situation is.
Every technique must be guided by will,
Combat efficiency will be achieved with ease.
All the time pay attention to your waist,
The abdomen is charged with *chi* and might.

The spine is straight and full of spirit,
The whole body is relaxed with head upright.
Be attentive to details in every move,
Spontaneous let your movements be.
A teacher's guidance is needed to enter the way,
When accomplished, unrestricted by rules is he.
What is so difficult about the form?
Mind and energy are the king.
What is the aim of Tai Chi Chuan practice?
Health and vitality and eternal spring.[1]

As is the case with all 'songs of secrets', Wu Yu Xiang's advice is expressed concisely. The following is only a brief introductory commentary on his advice; all the points made by the master will be explained in more detail elsewhere in this book.

Tai Chi Chuan is often known as the 13 Techniques. Its focus is not the hands or legs but the waist. Moreover, the ability to differentiate between 'apparent' and 'solid' constitutes a fundamental lesson in Tai Chi Chuan; if you fail to realize this, your movements are likely to be clumsy and a skilful opponent can exploit this weakness.

In Tai Chi Chuan, internal energy flow is essential, and it can be achieved only if you are relaxed. This explains why Tai Chi Chuan is usually practised in a slow, graceful manner. However, merely performing the movements slowly and gracefully is insufficient; without internal *chi* flow, it degenerates into a gentle dance.

When applying Tai Chi Chuan in combat, you must be calm yet alert: your form is still, but your chi is moving inside you. When you move, your movement is very swift, but your mind is still. You must adjust yourself according to the ever-changing combat situation, including the harmonious interaction of stillness and movement. All your techniques must be directed by your mind, which means that all your movements serve predetermined purposes, and are executed as fast as the mind wills them. In this way you will always be effective in combat.

The importance of the waist is again emphasized. There is a saying in Tai Chi Chuan that all movements start from the waist. The movements must be backed by power, and it is derived from the energy accumulated at the abdomen. The head and body must be upright and relaxed, and attention should be paid to every movement. But, when one has become familiar through practice, then all movements become spontaneous.

A teacher's guidance is necessary to initiate a beginner into the art.

Initially, you should closely follow the rules made by past masters, but when you have become accomplished you need not be restricted by them.

Some students may feel that to perform Tai Chi Chuan correctly in every detail is difficult, but more important than correct form are the mind and energy aspects of the training. Even if you carry out the forms of Tai Chi Chuan perfectly, without mind control to channel your internal energy, you will achieve no more than mediocre results, no matter how long you practise. Why do we practise Tai Chi Chuan? It is to attain health, vitality and longevity.

The Five Characters Formula

Many people are aware that Tai Chi Chuan is an internal art, but few really understand what it means, and fewer still know how to realize this internal aspect. The Five Characters Formula advocated by the master Li Yi Yu shows how this internal aspect can be accomplished.

The following is my translation of the original Chinese text. You should appreciate that while both Chinese and English are beautiful languages, they are linguistically different; so if you find some of the expressions or vocabulary odd, it is because as far as possible I have attempted a literal translation so as to maintain the original flavour. The original Chinese version is poetic and meaningful.

> The Five Characters Formula refers to mind tranquil, body agile, energy full, force complete, and spirit focused.
>
> One, it is called mind tranquil. If the mind is not tranquil, it means the mind is not concentrated. Whenever one moves – forward, back, left and right – there is no focussed direction. Initially, your movements are not spontaneous. You have to pay careful attention to your opponent's movements. Follow his movements closely; if he extends, you contract; if he does not retreat, you do not advance; do not move of your own accord. If he uses strength, you also use strength; if he does not use strength, you also do not use strength. Your movement must be led by your mind. You must be mindful all the time; wherever you change your movement, there your mind is. Experience that there is no obstruction. If you train in this way, after a year or six months you can apply this skill to your opponent. You use your will-power, not your strength. Eventually you control your opponent, you are not controlled by your opponent.

Two, it is called body agile. If your body movement is sluggish, you cannot move as efficiently as you wish; hence it is necessary for your body to be agile. Whenever you move, your movement must not be hesitant. My opponent's strength merely brushes my skin, but my will-power has penetrated into his bones. Your two hands are in combination linked by continuous *chi* flow. When an opponent attacks on your right, you make your right side 'apparent' and attack him with your left. Your *chi* flow is like a wheel; every part of your body must be well co-ordinated. Any part that is not co-ordinated is unfocussed and has no power. Its weakness lies at the waist and legs. First, let your mind lead your body, following your opponent's movement not your own. If you move of your own accord, you will be awkward; if you move with your opponent, you will be smooth. When you are able to flow with your opponent, your hands must be sensitive; assess correctly whether the opponent's strength is big or small, rough or fine; gauge without mistake the extent of the opponent's advance. Irrespective of moving forward or back you flow exactly with your opponent. The longer you train, the better is your skill.

Three, it is called energy full. If your *chi* is diffused and slow, your movement will be disorderly. The purpose is to cultivate energy so that it flows in the spine, and to attain breath harmony so that every part of the body is connected. Breathing in represents storing and accumulation; breathing out represents expansion and assertion. Breathing in symbolizes the ability to uphold and sustain (figuratively meaning to bear responsibilities); breathing out symbolizes the ability to sink and let go (figuratively meaning to tolerate and forgive). Use will, not brute strength, to lead energy.

Four, it is called force complete. All the force of the body is developed into one unity, and you must differentiate between 'apparent' and 'solid'. When executing force, there must be a source. Force starts from the heel, controlled by the waist, materialized at the hand, and executed from the spine, with full mindfulness. When my opponent is about to execute his force, my force is already in contact with his force. It should be timely, neither too early nor too late, coming out like a gushing stream. Moving forward or back, there is not the slightest trace of disorder. Even when you are in a disadvantageous position, you are able to overcome it. Prepare first, then inflict; this will result in success according to your intention. This is called using the opponent's strength

> against him, using four *tahils* [a Chinese weight measurement, equal to about an ounce] against a thousand *katies* [about a thousand pounds].
>
> Five, it is called spirit focused. All the preparation for the earlier four points can be summarized as spirit focussed. When spirit, or *shen*, is focussed, energy or *chi* can be concentrated and cultivated; cultivation of energy, in return, can nourish spirit. Hence, focussing spirit can lead to abundant energy, mental freshness, coordinated movement, and the ability to differentiate between 'apparent' and 'solid'. Being 'apparent' does not mean there is no strength; it means that the application of energy is flexible; being 'solid' does not mean that it is immovably solid; it means that the mind is focussed there. It is important that the movement of your chest and waist is not from the outside. Strength is borrowed from your opponent, energy is executed from your spine. Executing energy from the spine means that energy is sunk below, the shoulder blades are withdrawn towards the spine, with focus at the waist. When energy flows thus from top to below, it is called 'closed'. When energy flows from the waist to the spine, spreads to the shoulders, and reaches the hands and fingers, it is called 'open'. 'Closed' is receiving, 'open' is releasing. If you understand 'open' and 'closed', you understand yin-yang. When you have reached this stage, you will be more and more skilful each day until eventually you will attain the stage where you will achieve whatever your mind desires; there will then be nothing that you cannot achieve.[2]

This masterpiece is expressed in simple language, but many students may still not understand it because of their unfamiliarity with the terms and concepts used. Why is it, for example, that 'if you move of your own accord, you will be awkward; if you move with your opponent, you will be smooth'. How is it that 'energy flows from the waist to the spine, spreads to the shoulders, and reaches the hands and fingers'? Do not worry if you find this passage difficult to comprehend at present; your understanding will increase as you read more.

Meanwhile, it is helpful to know that all the crucial lessons of Tai Chi Chuan training can be summarized into five areas:

- mind – as in being mindful of the opponent's movements
- body or form – to flow with the opponent's form
- vital energy or *chi* – diffused all over the body

- internal force – controlled at the waist
- spirit or *shen* – as a general preparation for the above four

Four of the five areas are concerned with internal training; even in the sole external area, body or form, a great deal of internal work is needed to develop the skill to flow with the opponent's form. Hence, if you have spent 20 years practising only Tai Chi form and nothing else, at best you will have achieved only 25 per cent of what Tai Chi Chuan can offer you. And when you read the master's advice on form, and become aware that you know neither how to differentiate between 'apparent' and 'solid' nor how to assess the opponent's advance, neither how to let your mind lead your body nor how to co-ordinate your movement with flowing chi, it is doubtful whether you will have gained even that much. Understanding and then experiencing the benefits of the inner areas of training, all of which will be explained in this book, will increase the amount of potential benefit available to you.

The Ten Important Points of Tai Chi Chuan

Although form (*xing*) is the least important of the three fundamental elements of Tai Chi Chuan – the others being energy (*chi*) and spirit (*shen*) – to beginners it is the most immediate. Only when you can perform Tai Chi Chuan form properly, can you fruitfully venture into the elements of energy and spirit. Hence, Yang Deng Fu's Ten Important Points of Tai Chi Chuan, which devote much attention to form training, are probably the most helpful to students who are still at the beginners' level, irrespective of when they first started Tai Chi Chuan.

Yang Deng Fu was the master responsible for transforming the vigorous Chen-style Tai Chi Chuan into the gentle and graceful Yang style which is widely practised today. Let us look at his Ten Important Points of Tai Chi Chuan in his own words.

1. ***Shen* Rising to the Top.** To enable *shen* or spirit to rise to the top of the head, the head must be upright. Do not use strength; although your head can be upright if you use strength, blood and *chi* cannot flow smoothly. So although there is the will to let *shen* rise to the top, if it is forced, there is no *shen* rising and you will not attain mental freshness.

2. **Lower the Chest, Raise the Back.** Lower the chest means the chest is drawn in to enable *chi* to sink down to the *dan tian* (or the

abdominal energy field about 3 inches below the navel). Do not extend your chest; if you do so, *chi* will rush to your chest resulting in 'top heavy, bottom light', and your heels will 'float' up. Raising the back means *chi* focussing on your back. If you lower your chest, you will naturally raise your back. If you can raise your back, you can bring internal force from your back into play, enabling you to be victorious in combat.

3 **Loosen the Waist.** The waist is the controlling part of the torso. Loosening your waist enables your feet to be strong so that your stance is stable. All the variations and interactions of 'apparent' and 'real' are executed from the waist. Thus, there is the saying: 'The will of life has its source at the waist.' Those who fail to acquire power in their combat should remedy the situation at the waist.

4 **Differentiate between 'Apparent' and 'Solid'.** Differentiating between 'apparent' and 'solid' is the first fundamental of Tai Chi Chuan. If the whole body-weight is over the right leg, the right leg is 'solid' and the left leg is 'apparent'; if the whole body-weight is over the left leg, the left leg is 'solid' and the right leg is 'apparent'. When 'apparent' and 'solid' can be differentiated, movement becomes agile, as if effortless. If they are not differentiated, leg movements become heavy, and stances are unstable and can be easily exploited by the opponent.

5 **Sink Shoulders, Drop Elbows.** Sinking shoulders means that both the shoulders are relaxed and dropped down naturally. If the shoulders are not sunk but raised, then *chi* rises and the whole body will lack strength. Dropping elbows means that both the elbows are relaxed and dropped naturally. If the elbows are raised, the shoulders will not sink. Then the flow of *chi* will not be far reaching; this weakness is similar to the weakness in external kungfu known as 'interrupted strength'.

6 **Use Will, Not Strength.** The Tai Chi Chuan philosophy says: 'All this means use will and do not use strength.' When you practise Tai Chi Chuan, your whole body must be relaxed; there must not be the slightest tension retained amidst muscles, bones and blood flow, resulting in self-restriction. After you have attained complete relaxation, you are able to be flexible and versatile in circular movements according to your wish. Some people may wonder: How can we develop strength if we do not use strength? This is because our body

possesses meridians, just as the earth possesses channels. If the channels are not blocked, water flows smoothly. Similarly, if the meridians are not blocked, *chi* flows harmoniously. If the whole body is tensed with strength, *chi* and blood flow are blocked, and movements become awkward. Even if you pull a hair, the whole body moves. (This means that as every part of the body is interconnected by meridians, every part of the body affects every other part.) If you do not use strength but will, wherever your will directs *chi* will arrive. Hence you must have your *chi* and blood flowing smoothly every day all over your body, without interruption at any time. Persistent practice will develop true inner force. Thus in Tai Chi Chuan philosophy it is said: 'Be extremely soft and gentle, then be extremely hard and forceful.' The arm of a Tai Chi Chuan expert is like iron in cotton wool, extremely powerful and stable. For those who are trained in external martial art, they are powerful when they use strength, but light and floating when they do not use strength. This shows that their strength is external and floating on the surface. Using strength without using will easily results in instability, which is not a complete art.

7 **Co-ordination between Top and Bottom.** The meaning of co-ordination between top and bottom is revealed in the Tai Chi Chuan philosophy: 'Its root is in the feet, executed from the legs, controlled by the waist, materialized in the hands and fingers.' From the feet to the legs to the waist, the action is completed 'in one *chi*' (which is a kungfu term meaning 'continuously and spontaneously without any interruption within the time of one comfortable breath'). Hand movement, waist movement, leg movement, as well as 'eye-alertness' movement are all in one unified movement; only this can be said to be top and bottom co-ordinated; if there is one movement lacking, if there is any interruption, the unified movement is disorderly.

8 **Internal and External Unity.** The training of Tai Chi Chuan is in the mind; thus 'the mind is the commander, the body is the agent'. When the mind is trained, movements and actions become naturally light and agile. Tai Chi Chuan patterns are none other than movements of 'apparent' and 'real', opening and closing. By opening is meant not only that hands and legs are extended, but also that the mind and will are extended; by closing is meant not only that the hands and legs are brought back, but also that the mind and will are brought back (meaning focussed). If the internal and the external can

be united into one *chi* (or body of energy), it means there is no separateness in the cosmos.

9 **Continuity Without Break.** In external martial arts, power is the result of post-natal (or artificial, as opposed to natural) tension; thus, there is beginning and completion, continuity and interruption. When old strength is spent and new strength has not been generated, this is the instant that is easiest for the opponent to exploit. In Tai Chi Chuan, will and not strength is used; from beginning to end it is continuous, without any break; after each cycle it starts again, circulating without end. The original treatise mentions that it is like the continuous waves of Long River [Yangtze Kiang, the longest river in China]. It is also mentioned that application of force in Tai Chi Chuan is like weaving silk (long and continuous), which expresses its accumulation and continuity in one *chi* (meaning that internal force is channelled continuously, regulated by appropriate breathing).

10 **Seeking Stillness in Movement.** External martial arts stress running and jumping swiftly as desirable abilities; much strength is expended, thus the exponents pant for breath after training. In Tai Chi Chuan stillness directs movement. When a Tai Chi Chuan exponent moves, he is like being in stillness. Thus while practising Tai Chi Chuan, the slower the movement is, the better. When movement is slow, breathing becomes deep and long, *chi* is sunk down to the *dan tian* (abdominal energy field), and naturally there is no setback from blood and *chi* flow being swollen (ie blocked). Students should pay careful attention to this advice and experience its effect; then they can appreciate the purpose of Tai Chi Chuan.[3]

These points are invaluable not only to students but also to advanced exponents.

It is obvious from the advice of all three of the great masters quoted above, that the primary aim of Tai Chi Chuan is combat efficiency (although Wu Yu Xiang concludes his advice by saying that the aim of practising Tai Chi Chuan is 'to attain health, vitality and longevity'). All the points highlighted in their advice are concerned with making the Tai Chi Chuan exponent a better fighter: for example, the differentiation between 'apparent' and 'solid', the accumulation of *chi* in the abdomen, and the rising of *shen* or spirit to the head are aimed at giving exponents poise, internal force and mental freshness so that they can fight well. These qualities, derived from practising Tai Chi Chuan as a martial art, are of course also beneficial in daily life. But if students or instructors adopt the attitude that their practice or teaching of Tai Chi Chuan is only for health and never for combat, then they may neglect those training methods which are aimed at developing these qualities, in the belief that they are irrelevant to their purpose; hence they will miss the very qualities that encourage health, vitality and longevity.

Many students tend to overdo the second of Yang Deng Fu's points, 'lower the chest, raise the back', with the result that they close the chest so much that natural breathing is affected, and they hunch the back. The purpose of 'lowering the chest, raising the back' is to let *chi* sink down to the abdominal energy field, and not to cramp the heart or suffocate the lungs! Commenting on this point, the modern Tai Chi master Cheng Man Ching says, 'Depress the chest means that one must not stick out the chest, but also not allow it to cave in. Rather, the chest should be relaxed. Only this is the correct method.'[4]

5

Fundamental Hand Movements and Footwork

Acquiring Balance and Gracefulness in Tai Chi Movements

Experience has shown that delaying the practice of a Tai Chi set in order to spend more time on these basic hand and leg movements usually results in the student progressing faster in the long run.

The 13 Techniques of Tai Chi

In classical literature, Tai Chi Chuan is sometimes referred to as the 13 Techniques of Tai Chi. These do not refer to 13 prototype patterns, as is often assumed, but to eight fundamental hand movements and five fundamental leg movements which are sometimes symbolized by *bagua* or the Eight Trigrams and *wuxing* or the Five Elemental Processes.

The eight fundamental hand movements in the 13 Techniques are:

- *peng* or warding off
- *lu* or rolling back
- *qi* (pronounced 'ch'i') or pressing
- *an* or pushing
- *lie* (pronounced 'liat') or spreading
- *cai* (pronounced 'chai') or taking
- *zhou* or elbowing
- *kao* or leaning

The five fundamental leg movements are:

- *jin* or moving forward
- *tui* or moving back
- *ku*, or moving to the left

- *pan* or moving to the right
- *ding* or remaining at the centre

These techniques are explained in this chapter. The sequence in which they are dealt with is different from the above lists; this is to enable you to progress methodologically. As the exercises in this chapter form the foundation of Tai Chi Chuan training, it is worth practising them patiently and conscientiously; experience has shown that delaying the practice of a Tai Chi set in order to spend more time on these basic hand and leg movements usually results in the student progressing faster in the long run.

It is not easy for beginners to learn any martial art from a book; it is even harder to learn internal arts like Tai Chi Chuan, where subtle factors like poise and balance, visualization and energy control are more important than mere physical action. Hence, although this book is written as a self-teaching manual, I would strongly advise you to seek personal supervision by a competent instructor.

The Secret of Tai Chi Internal Force

Chinese martial arts masters of all schools have advised that 'before you begin to learn techniques, you must develop force'. The most basic way to develop force is stance training – standing in a particular stance for a period of time which may range from a few minutes to an hour or more. It is a common misconception that stance training is important only in Shaolin Kungfu, where it is commonly known as *zuo ma*, which means 'sitting on a horse' because the most important stance in Shaolin Kungfu is the Horseriding Stance. Stance training is just as important in Tai Chi Chuan, as well as in the two other famous styles of internal kungfu, Pakua Kungfu and Hsing Yi Kungfu where it is known as *zhan zhuang*, which means 'standing in a stance'. But do not be misled into thinking that the main purpose of *zhan zhuang* is just to develop strong, stable stances. Much more important is the development of internal force, without which Tai Chi Chuan, Pakua Kungfu and Hsing Yi Kungfu cannot be called internal arts.

The most important stance for developing internal force in Tai Chi Chuan is the Three-circle Stance. Indeed it is so commonly used in Tai Chi Chuan that it is often called the Tai Chi Stance. *Tai Chi* means 'the grand ultimate' and some students may have heard of the expression: 'From the infinite ultimate or the void is born the grand ultimate or the cosmos.' We will start our internal force training with an exercise which reflects this.

Stand upright with your feet fairly close together and your arms hanging naturally at your sides *(figure 5.1 a)*. Your mouth should be slightly open, as if you are smiling. Gently close your eyes, clear your mind of all thoughts, and be totally relaxed. This is known as the *Wuji Zhuang*, or the Infinite Ultimate Stance. Remain in it for a few minutes.

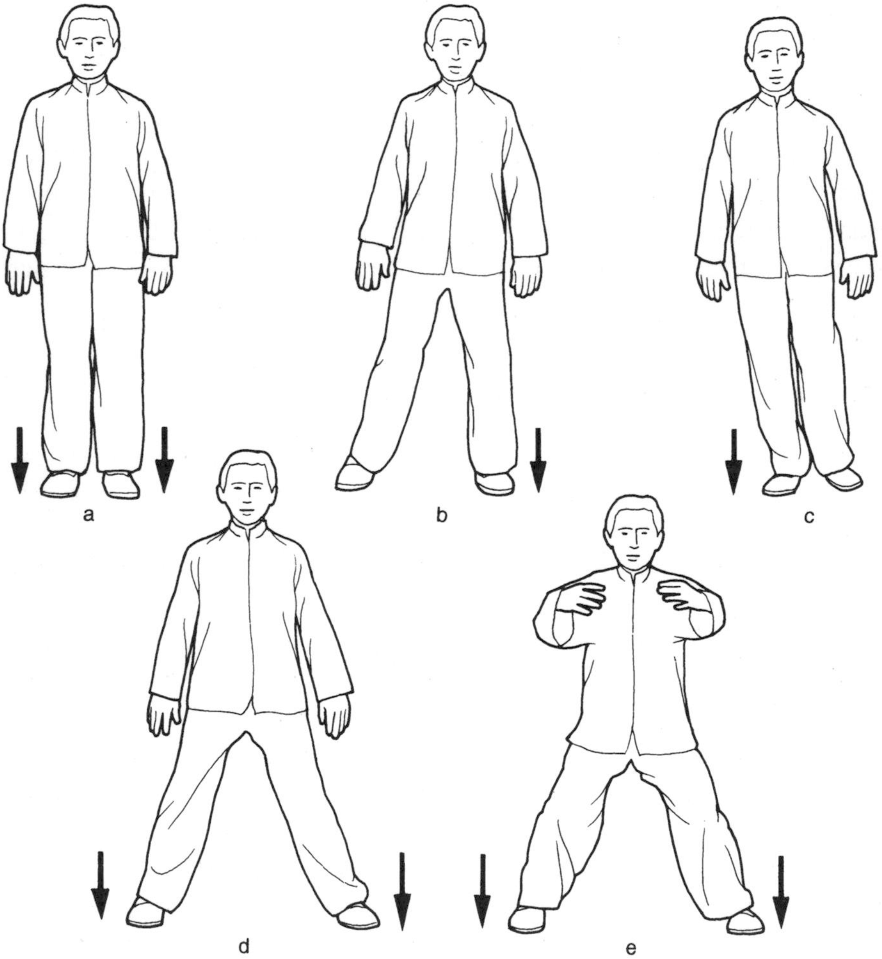

Fig 5.1 From the Infinite Ultimate Stance to the Tai Chi Stance

The crucial point of this training is not just standing upright, which is merely the external form. The greatest benefit is derived from the deep relaxation and sense of inner peace this stance training develops. At a later stage, you may feel internal force flowing inside your body; at an advanced stage you may feel your own vital energy merge with the cosmic energy of the universe, the experience of which is reflected in the name of the stance – the Infinite Ultimate Stance.

After standing for a few minutes in the Infinite Ultimate Stance, proceed to the Three-circle or Tai Chi Stance. Without moving your feet, transfer your body-weight to your left leg. With your left leg, which is now known as the 'solid' leg supporting your body-weight, move your right leg, known as the 'apparent' leg in this case, about a foot to your right *(figure 5.1b)*. Then gradually transfer your weight from your left leg to your right, which becomes the 'solid' leg, and move your left leg, the 'apparent' leg, close to your right, *(figure 5.1c)*. With your body-weight now over your right 'solid' leg, move your left 'apparent' leg about two feet to your left *(figure 5.1d)*. Distribute your body-weight evenly over both legs so that both are 'solid'. Your feet should be about 2 feet, or one and a half shoulder-widths, apart, and your toes pointed inwards very slightly.

Bend your knees so that they are above your toes. Make sure your body is upright and relaxed. Then raise both arms in front of you to about chest level, with your elbows bent so that your arms form a circle in front of you *(figure 5.1e)*. Hold the fingers of both hands in such a way that the thumb and index fingers form two arcs which if continued would form a circle in front of your chest. 'Hook' in your bent knees as if you were holding a ball with your thighs and knees. You are now holding three imaginary balls: a small one with your palms, a bigger one with your arms, and a third one with your thighs and knees.

This is known as the Goat-riding Stance, but the special form of the stance, with the arms held up in front in a circle as if holding a huge ball, is known as the Three-circle or Tai Chi Stance.

Make sure that your shoulders and elbows are dropped naturally. Have your lips slightly open as if smiling, close your eyes gently, very gently focus your mind on your abdomen, and then clear it of all thoughts. Remain perfectly still and relaxed in this stance for about five minutes.

At the end of this stance training, return to the *Wuji* or Infinite Ultimate Stance, and remain still for a few more minutes. Then gently focus your internal force at your abdominal *dan tian*, or the energy field about 3 inches below your navel, for a minute or two. Rub your palms together to warm them, place them on your eyes and dab your eyes a few times as you open them. Walk about briskly to complete this very important exercise.

Practise every day and gradually – I repeat, gradually – increase the time until you can stand in the Tai Chi Stance for at least half an hour. This will take at least a few months of daily practice. After a few months, if you have been training correctly and consistently, you will feel your internal force swelling inside your body, and flowing to your arms and legs. Sometimes it will be so powerful that your palms, arms or other parts of your body may vibrate vigorously. If this happens, it is important that you do not tense any part of your body; just relax and enjoy the spontaneous vibration. If, for any reason, you wish to stop the vibration, gently think of your *dan tian*, and the internal force will be stored at the abdominal energy field. The vibration of internal force as the result of prolonged stillness is a manifestation of the often stated but little understood principle that 'extreme stillness generates movement', expressed symbolically as: 'When yin has reached its maximum, yang is born.'

This training is an example of the expression '*Wuji* creates *tai chi,* and *tai chi* returns to *wuji*', or 'The infinite ultimate creates the cosmos, and the cosmos returns to the infinite ultimate.' At the beginning the infinite ultimate is void and nebulous; then because of the operation of yin-yang, form or substance appears as the phenomenal cosmos. Eventually the cosmos returns to its primordial state of the nebulous and void. This happens at the infinitesimal scale of the sub-atomic particle in an instant, as well as the infinite scale of galaxies in terms of aeons. As the body is a miniature cosmos, this cosmic transformation also occurs inside it, generating a tremendous amount of internal force.

Developing Poise and Balance

In addition to training in stillness, which is the yin aspect of Tai Chi Chuan, we must also have training in movement, which is the yang aspect. Start with the Tai Chi Stance *(figure 5.2 a)* and transfer your body-weight to your right 'solid' leg, moving your left 'apparent' leg a small step towards your right, with the left toes merely touching the ground and the right leg still supporting the body-weight. Simultaneously rotate your waist and bend both knees slightly so that you turn to your left *(figure 5.2 b)*. It is important that you rotate your waist, rather than turning your body. If you turn your body without rotating your waist, you interrupt the flow of energy from your *dan tian,* but if your rotate your waist, your body will turn naturally, and your energy flow will be spontaneous. Feel this internal flow of energy as you rotate your waist.

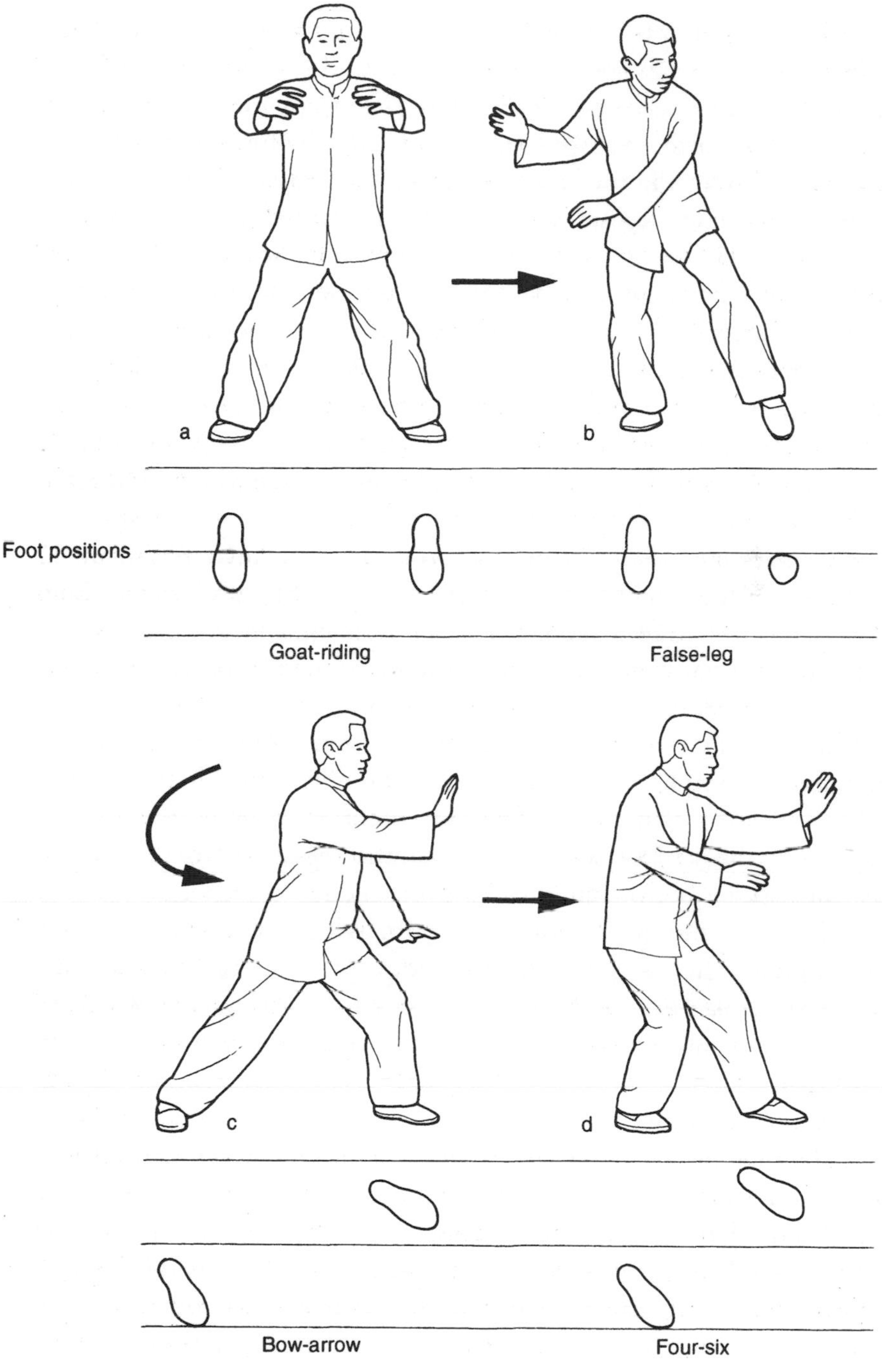

Fig 5.2 Bow-arrow and Four-six stances (left)

With your right 'solid' leg still supporting your weight, glide your left 'apparent' leg about 2½ feet or about two shoulder-widths forward (this is the left side of your previous Tai Chi Stance) to move into what is called a left Bow-arrow Stance *(figure 5.2 c)*, with the front (left) leg bent, representing a bow, the toes pointing about 45° diagonally to the right, and the back (right) leg straight, representing an arrow, with the foot turned about 45° to the left from its position in the earlier Tai Chi Stances. Your movement should be such that should your left leg step on something slippery, you will not fall because it is an 'apparent' leg, and you are supported by your right 'solid' leg. When you are certain that your left leg is on firm ground, gradually transfer half your weight to it, so that you stand solidly on both legs. Your feet should be 'hooked in' so that if you were to draw a line between your heels, each foot would make a 45° angle with it.

Simultaneously make an anti-clockwise circle with your right hand and strike out your right palm at chest level, but with your right elbow slightly bent, not fully extended. At the same time make a clockwise circle with your left hand, completing the movement near your front left knee. This pattern is called Green Dragon Shoots out Pearl.

We may classify foot movements as gross or fine. The gross movement in the above example is turning from the Tai Chi Stance leftwards into the left Bow-arrow Stance. The fine movements are rotating the waist to the left side, the start of which generates the movement of the whole body, shifting the body slightly backwards, gliding the left foot forward into the correct position, transferring your weight as you rotate your knees, adjusting the position of the back foot and focusing your centre of gravity at your *dan tian* or abdominal energy field. An understanding of the fine movements is necessary for good balance, which is particularly important in Tai Chi Chuan, and for generating a spiral force, which starts from the back heel.

To continue to the next stance, momentarily transfer your body-weight to your front (left) leg then to your back (right) leg and move your left leg about 1 foot back, still keeping it in front of your right. Next transfer about 40 per cent of your weight to your left leg; bend both legs, your back leg slightly more than your front, and focus your centre of gravity at your *dan tian*. This stand is called a Stream-character Stance, also known as Four-six Stance because your front leg supports about 40 per cent of your weight, and your back leg about 60 per cent. Hold your hands as shown in *figure 5.2d*. This pattern, built on the Four-six Stance, is called Playing the Lute.

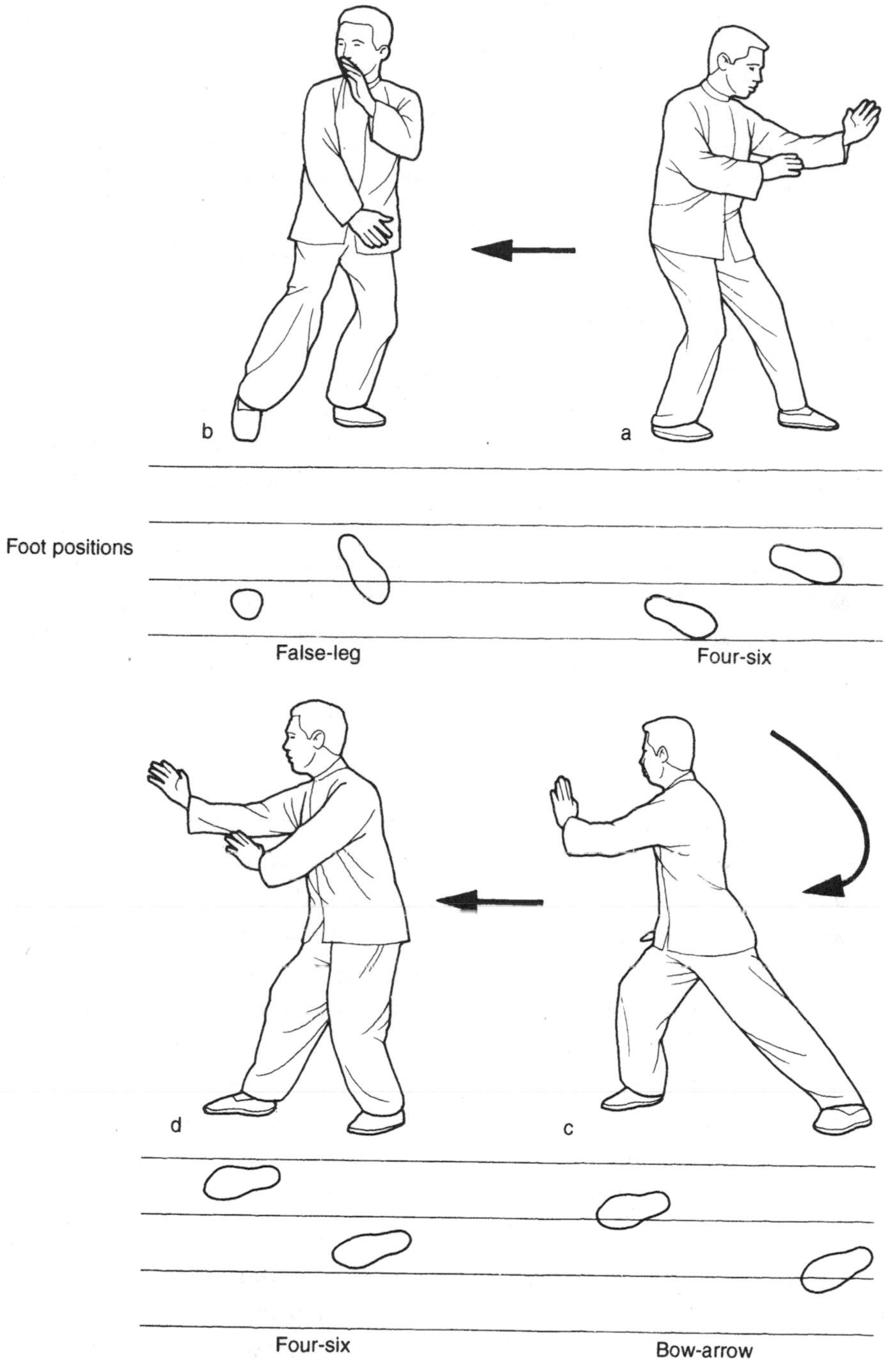

Fig 5.3 Bow-arrow and Four-six Stances (right)

Now turn around and repeat these two patterns on the reverse side as follows. From the Playing the Lute pattern *figure 5.3a*, transfer your weight to your right leg, and using your left heel as a pivot, rotate your waist and your left foot to your right so that your body makes a right about turn. This turn should be led by the rotation of your waist. Then transfer your weight to your left leg, which is now the 'solid' back leg, with your right toes merely touching the ground *(figure 5.3b)*. Simultaneously rotate your left hand in a clockwise direction and your right hand in an anti-clockwise direction.

Continue the rotation of your hands. Move your right foot forward to a right Bow-arrow Stance, rotating your waist appropriately as you do so, so that as you stabilize into the stance, your weight is distributed evenly over both legs, and your centre of gravity is located at your *dan tian (figure 5.3c)*.

Simultaneously with your foot movement, conclude the clockwise circle of your left hand and anti-clockwise circle of your right hand, with your left palm striking out in front with your left elbow slightly bent, and your right palm placed near your right knee.

Next, momentarily transfer your weight to your right leg, then to your left leg, and move your right leg about 1 foot back to take up a right Four-six Stance. Simultaneously place both hands in the position shown in *figure 5.3d*. Your centre of gravity should be at your *dan tian*.

Now place your body-weight on your left (back) leg, and with your waist as the source of movement, rotate your right foot slightly to your left. Transfer your weight to your right leg, and by rotating your waist turn to your left *(figure 5.4a)*. Lift your left leg, with your left knee held high up, your left foot protecting your groin and your left toes pointing down. Simultaneously cross your palms in front of your face *(figure 5.4b)*. Kick out your left foot with your heel as the striking point and spread out both hands in a pattern called Cross-hands Thrust-kick *(figure 5.4c)*. Then immediately bring it back to its original position protecting your groin, but hold your hands in the position shown in *figure 5.4d*. This pattern is called Golden Cockerel Stands Solitary. The stance that supports both this Golden Cockerel pattern and the Thrust-kick pattern is called a Single-leg Stance.

Next, lower your left leg to the ground about 2 feet to your left, and gracefully transfer your weight from your right leg to your left. Lift your right leg and stand on your left leg alone. Cross your palms in front of your face *(figure 5.4e)*. Kick out your right heel and spread your palms *(figure 5.4f)*. Immediately bring your right leg back to the pre-kick

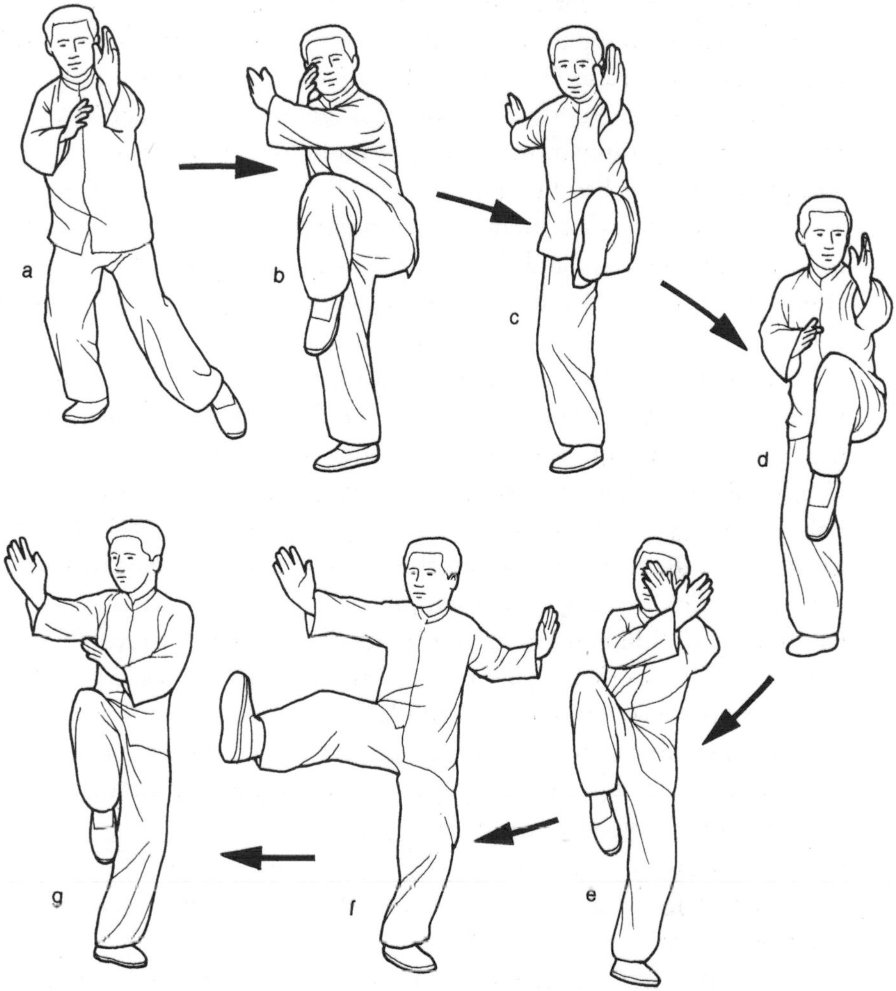

Fig 5.4 Single-leg Stances

position with the foot protecting your groin *(figure 5.4g)*. These are the reverse of the Cross-hands Thrust-kick and Golden Cockerel Stands Solitary patterns mentioned in the previous paragraph.

From this left Single-leg Stance, gracefully lower your right leg onto the ground in front of you about 2 feet diagonally to your right, to form a right Four-six Stance. Lift your hands as shown in *figure 5.5a*. This pattern, known as Lifting Up Hands, is a popular poise pattern in Tai Chi Chuan, ie exponents pose like this in combat while awaiting attack or defence.

Transfer your weight to your back (left) leg and move your right leg slightly back, with the toes pointed and merely touching the ground in a momentary right False-leg Stance carrying a ball of *chi (figure 5.5b)*. Move the right 'apparent' leg forward about 2 ½ feet to form a right Bow-arrow Stance; simultaneously move your right hand forward and up to eye-level, and place your left hand near your right elbow as shown in *figure 5.5c* in a *peng* or warding off technique. Your weight should now be distributed evenly over both legs, and your centre of gravity should be at your *dan tian*. The positions of the feet in these various steps are shown in *figure 5.6*.

Transferring your weight to your left leg, take your right foot back and place it momentarily near your left *(figure 5.5d)*, with your arms following the rotation of your waist – the source of your movement. Continuing the rotation of your waist, place your right leg about 2 ½ feet behind you, and transfer your weight to it so that it is now the 'solid' leg *(figure 5.5e)*. Remember to adjust the angle of your left foot so that your left toes, which pointed to your left just before this movement, now point to your right. Still continuing the rotating movement, move your body forward, without moving your foot positions, to a left Bow-arrow Stance, and distribute your weight over both legs. Simultaneously move your left hand forward and up to eye-level, and place your right hand near to your left elbow in a *peng* technique *(figure 5.5f)*. All these movements should be done smoothly without any break; and when you change the direction of movement, such as changing from moving back to moving forward, the change should be in the form of a curve, as in a figure of eight, and not angular.

To complete the exercise, transfer your weight to your back (right) leg and move your left leg a few inches to your right with your left toes pointing forward. Then transfer your weight to your left leg, and bring your right leg forward close to and alongside your left to stand upright with your feet close together and toes pointing forward. Your bodyweight should now be evenly distributed between both legs.

At the same time bring both arms, with the palms facing up, above your head *(figure 5.5g)*, simultaneously breathing in gently. Then with both palms facing the ground, lower them until your arms hang naturally at your sides, gently breathing out in the process, *(figures 5.5h and i)*. While you raise your arms above your head and simultaneously breathe in, visualize good cosmic energy from the universe flowing into you; and while you lower your arms and simultaneously breathe out, visualize the cosmic energy flowing to and accumulating at your *dan tian* or

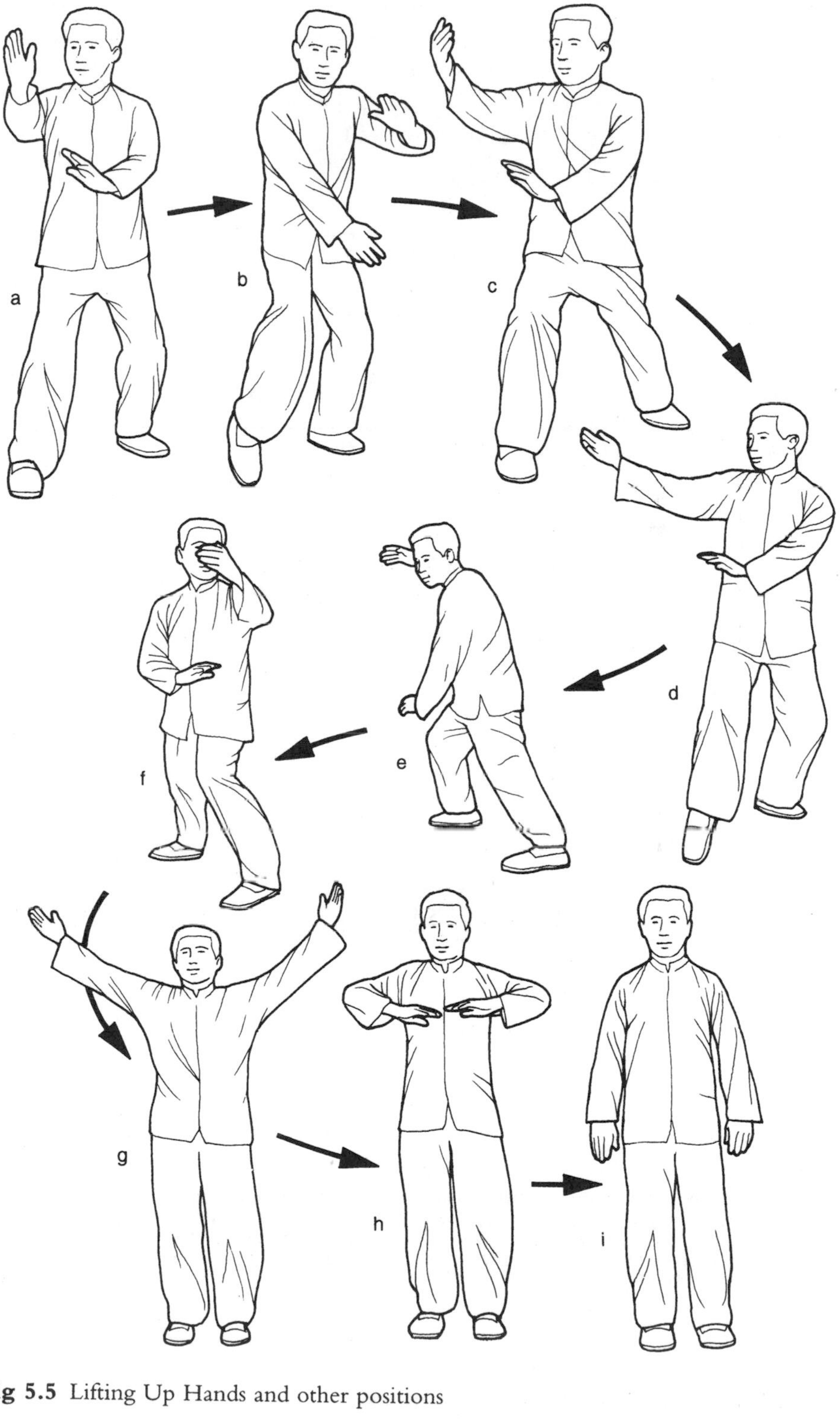

Fig 5.5 Lifting Up Hands and other positions

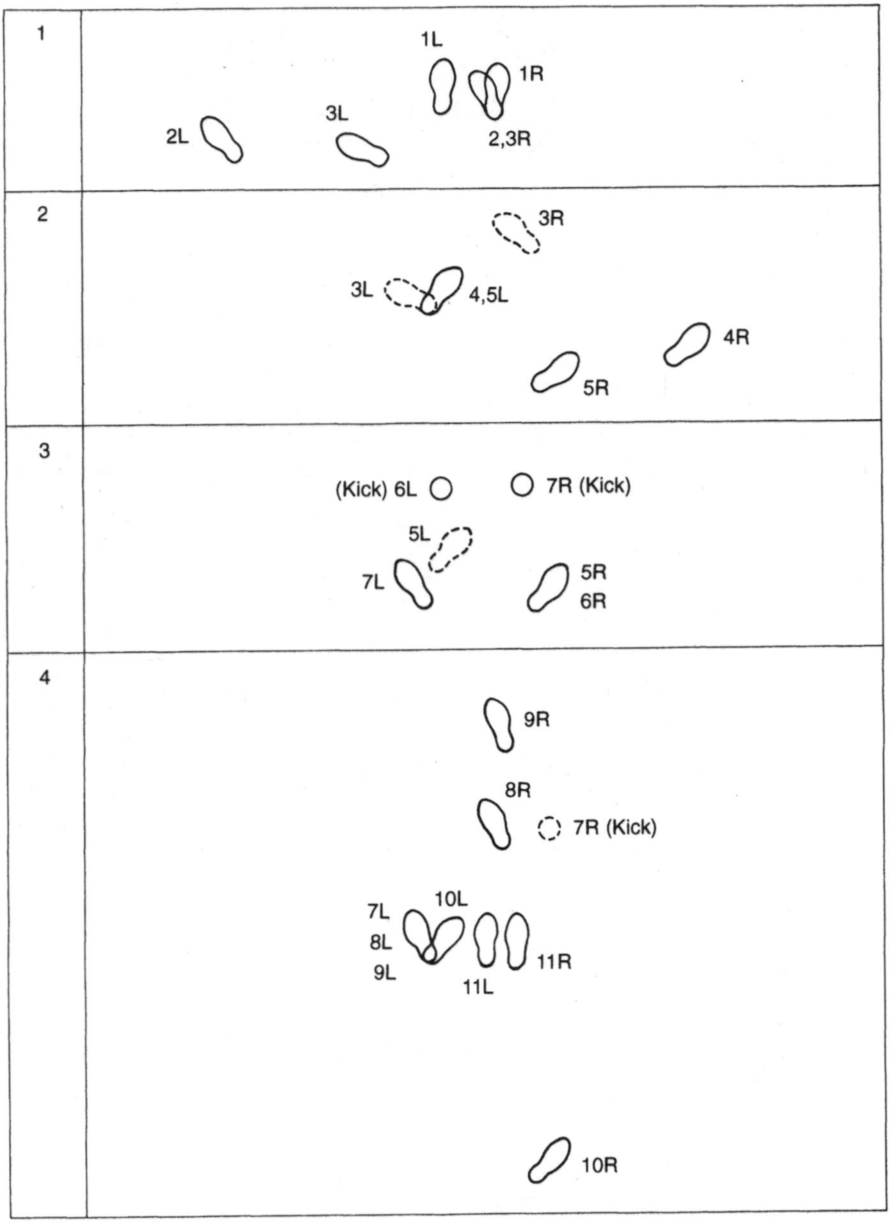

Note: To avoid crowding, each pnase is shown separately. In reality, however, each succeeding phase is superimposed upon the previous one, so that foot position number 11, for example, is at the same place as foot position number 1. The foot positions are drawn from the performer's, not the observer's perspective.
L = Left, R = Right.

Fig 5.6 Foot positions for the leg movements

abdominal energy field. The movement, breathing and visualization must be co-ordinated and performed gently; any forced action may result in unwanted side-effects. This technique, which is often used to complete a training programme in Tai Chi Chuan as well as in other styles of kungfu, is known as Energy Accumulating at Energy Field.

Gently close your eyes, clear your mind of all thoughts, relax totally and remain in this Infinite Ultimate Stance for a few minutes. End the exercise by rubbing your palms together, then dab your eyes with them as you open your eyes. Massage your face and head, loosen your body and walk about briskly.

This short routine provides good training for the five basic Tai Chi Chuan leg movements and the four basic stances. The five basic leg movements are *jin,* or moving forward; *tui,* or moving back; *ku,* or moving to the left; *pan,* or moving to the right; and *ding,* or remaining at the centre. The four basic stances in Tai Chi Chuan are the Goat-riding or Tai Chi Stance; the Bow-arrow Stance; the Four-six Stance; and the Single-leg Stance. *Figure 5.6* shows the foot positions for the leg movements, and *figure 5.7* shows the foot positions for the major stances.

This routine, with its emphasis on movement and the training of balance and poise, starts with the cosmos or grand ultimate, and ends with

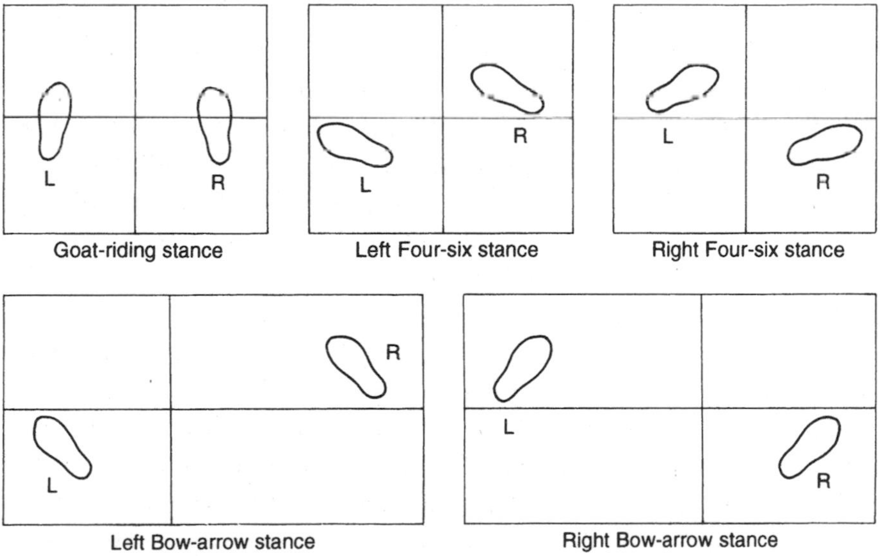

Note: The foot positions here are drawn from the performer's perspective, whereas in Figures 5.2 and 5.3 the positions are shown from the observer's perspective.
+ = body's centre of gravity; L = Left; R = Right.

Fig 5.7 Foot positions for the major stances

the void or infinite ultimate. It complements the earlier exercise, which emphasized stillness and the development of internal force, which proceeds from the void to the cosmos. In Tai Chi Chuan terms, it is 'From *wuji* is born *tai chi*; and *tai chi* returns to *wuji*.' If you recall the principle of yin-yang explained in Chapter 2, you should practise both the quiescent and the dynamic aspects, or both the yin and the yang , if you want the best from your Tai Chi Chuan.

The Four Primary Hand Techniques

There are eight basic Tai Chi hand movements, which are divided into primary and secondary techniques.

The procedure for practising the four primary hand movements is as follows. Start from an Infinite Ultimate (*Wuji*) Stance *(figure 5.8a)*. Transfer your body-weight to your right leg, then move your left leg a little to your left, transferring your body-weight to it, to stand in a False-leg Stance with your right toes merely touching the ground, and rotate your waist toward your right *(figure 5.8b)*. Your palms should be in front of your abdomen as if holding a ball of *chi*, with your right palm below your left.

Then move your right leg forward to a right Bow-arrow Stance. Remember to initiate your movement from your waist, differentiate between 'apparent' and 'solid', and adjust the foot positions accordingly. Simultaneously move your right arm forward to about 2 feet in front of your face, with your right palm turning in, and your left palm near your right elbow, which should be slightly bent *(figures 5.8c and d)*. Your hand movements should also be initiated by the rotation of your waist. This technique is called *peng*, or warding off, and is the same as the one we used when we learnt the basic leg movements.

Then, starting from your waist, bring back your body and lower it over your left leg. Do not move your feet but bend both knees, with your back knee bent more than your front one. Simultaneously draw back your palms from the front to the left of your waist, with your right palm facing down and left palm facing up, rotating your waist from right to left in the process *(figure 5.8e)*. This technique is called *lu*, or rolling back.

The description of these techniques as two separate movements is merely to help you learn. When you have mastered them, you should flow from *peng* to *lu*, rather than stopping at *peng*. The change of arm direction from moving forward to rolling back should be continuous and circular, as in a figure of eight, and not abrupt and angular as in a forward

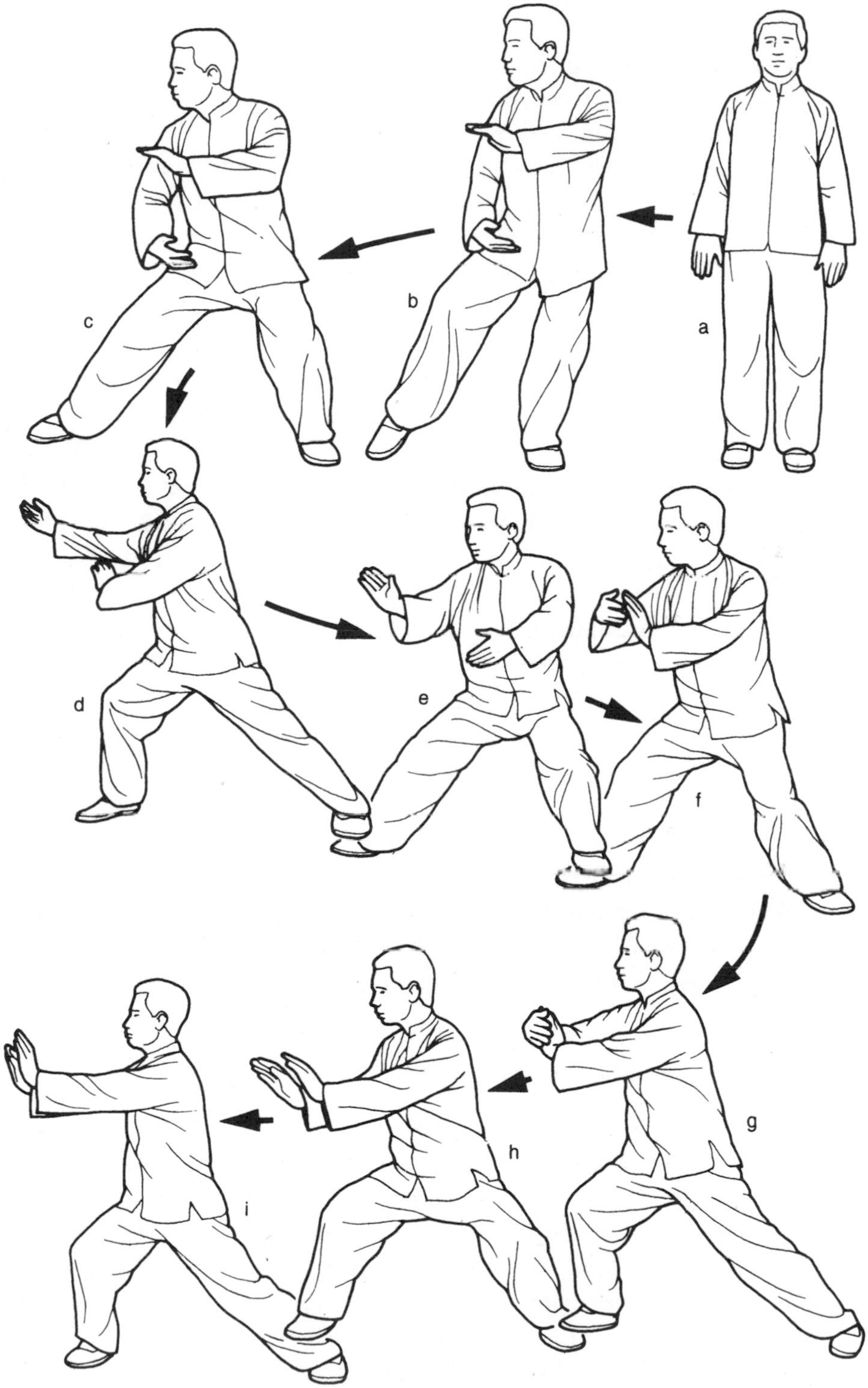

Fig 5.8 The four primary hand movements

and a backward line. This continuous, circular motion is basic in Tai Chi Chuan, and should be applied to all patterns.

Continuing from the movement of the *lu* technique, reverse the rotation of your waist from right–left to left–right, and press your right forearm forward, with your left palm pressing at your right wrist to add power *(figures 5.8f and g)*. This technique is called *qi*, or pressing. The reversing of your waist rotation must not be abrupt or angular; it should be continuous and circular, again like a figure of eight, and there must not be any break in the flow from the *lu* to the *qi* techniques. Similarly the change of direction by your hands, from rolling back to pressing forward, should not be abrupt but continuous, also in a figure of eight.

After pressing with the *qi* technique, lower your body by bending your left leg but without moving your feet, and simultaneously lower both wrists *(figure 5.8h)*. Then, with your force coming from your left heel, turn to a right Bow-arrow Stance and strike out both palms, in a technique called *an*, or pushing *(figure 5.8i)*. You may recall Li Yi Yu's advice, as quoted in the previous chapter, that 'Force starts from the heel, is controlled by the waist, materialized at the hand, and executed from the spine, with full mindfulness.'

These four techniques – *peng, lu, qi* and *an* – are the four primary Tai Chi Chuan hand movements. After the *an* technique, transfer your weight to your left leg and rotate your waist and your right foot towards the left so that you do a left about turn. Bring your left leg towards your right leg for a momentary False-leg Stance, then move your left leg forward to repeat the four techniques on the other side. Complete the routine by returning to your initial Infinite Ultimate Stance, raising your hands, palms up, above your head, then lowering them, palms down, to your side.

The Four Secondary Hand Techniques

The four secondary hand techniques – *lie, cai, zhou* and *kao* – are performed as follows. From the Infinite Ultimate Stance momentarily transfer your weight to your right leg, move your left leg a little step to your left, then transfer your weight to it and stand in a False-leg Stance. Rotate your body to your right and hold an imaginary ball of *chi* with your left palm above and your right below in a preparatory pattern called Holding the Cosmos *(figure 5.9a)*. Move your right leg forward to a right Bow-arrow Stance, and spread your right arm diagonally forward and up, and your left arm slightly down and back as shown in *figure 5.9b*. This is *lie* (pronounced 'liat'), or spreading.

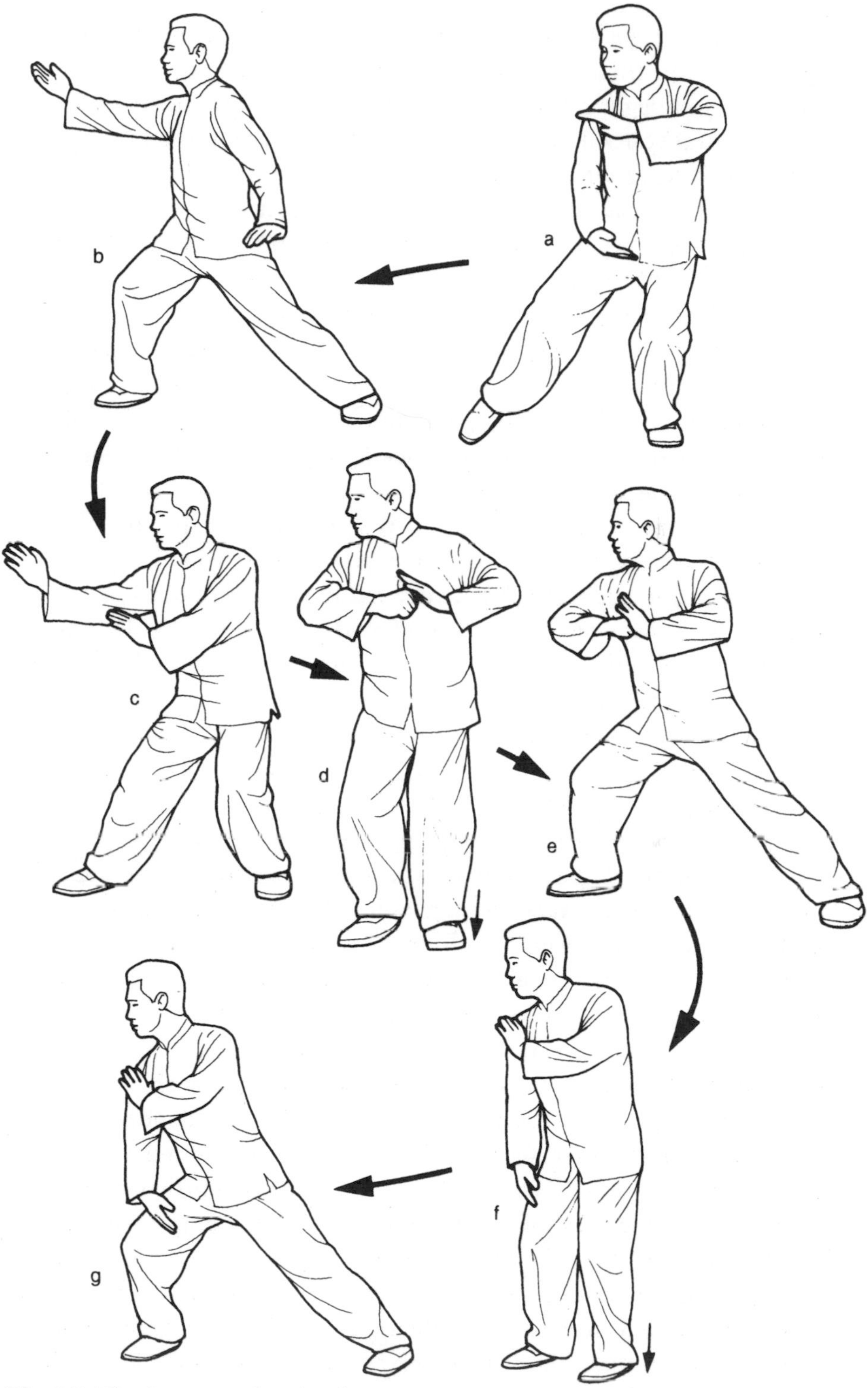

Fig 5.9 The four secondary hand movements

Bring your right leg back to stand in a Four-six Stance, with your right leg still in front, and hold your right palm in front and your left palm near your right elbow as shown in *figure 5.9c*. This technique is *cai*, or taking, and you will recognize the pattern as Playing the Lute.

For the next pattern, momentarily transfer your weight to your right leg, then bring your left leg forward and stamp it on the ground close behind your right leg, thus transferring your weight to your left leg. Your left knee should be bent. At the same time hold your right forearm horizontal, with your right elbow ready for striking and your left palm behind your right fist, as in *figure 5.9d*. Continuing from this stamping, and using your back foot for anchorage, 'throw' your body forward with your right elbow as the striking point *(figure 5.9e)*. This is *zhou*, or elbowing. The force originates from your back foot, is controlled by your waist, and manifested at your right elbow.

The next pattern, *kao* or leaning, is similar except that the striking point is the shoulder instead of the elbow. Stamp your left leg close behind your front right leg, bend your left knee, lower your body *(figure 5.9f)*, and 'throw' your body forward with your right shoulder as the striking point *(figure 5.9g)*. Pay particular attention to the following two points. Although you throw your body forward, you must not overdo it; your centre of gravity, which is now raised from the abdomen to the chest, should still be between your legs. Secondly, the striking force comes from your back leg, not from your shoulder.

After performing these four techniques on the right side, turn around and repeat the whole procedure on the left. Complete the training with the Infinite Ultimate Stance, closing your eyes gently, clearing your mind of all thoughts, and remaining still for a few minutes.

The shoulder strike is one example of *kao* or the leaning technique. Another example of *kao* is as follows, if your opponent has trapped both your hands, and attempts to push you backwards *(figure 5.10a)*, follow the momentum of the push by 'swallowing', ie pulling your abdomen back without moving your feet *(figure 5.10b)*. Then when the opponent's body is close to your shoulder *(figure 5.10c)*, rotate your waist and swing your left leg backward anti-clockwise, felling him or her with your shoulder *(figure 5.10d)*. Notice again that the force comes not from the shoulder, but from the feet, controlled by the waist.

Here is a further example of *kao* in use in combat. Suppose your opponent attacks you with a straight right punch – the most common form of attack in many martial arts *(figure 5.11a)*. 'Swallow' the punch by sitting back in the Four-six Stance, and simultaneously push at the

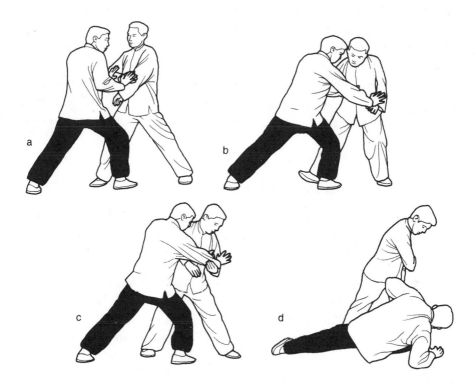

Fig 5.10 Felling an opponent with *kao*

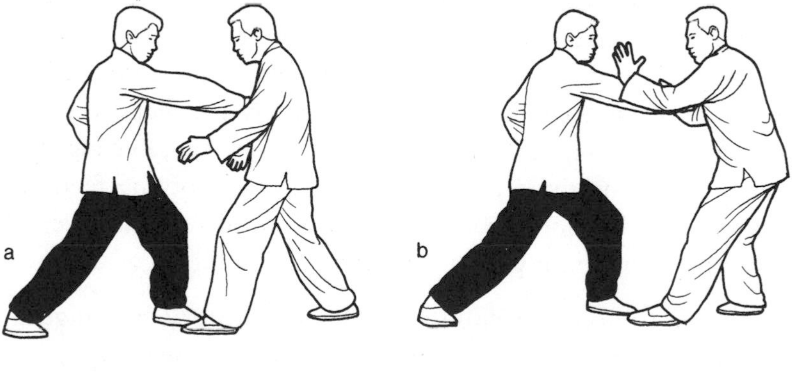

Fig 5.11 Dislocating an opponent's elbow with *kao*

opponent's wrist with your right hand, and at the elbow with your left forearm, in the pattern Playing the Lute *(figure 5.11b)*. In a real combat, this will dislocate the person's elbow, so you must be careful when practising this technique with a partner.

You will remember that in the *cai* technique we also used Playing the Lute. This shows that the same pattern may be used for different techniques; conversely, the same technique can also be implemented in different patterns.

Does Tai Chi Chuan Cause Knee Injury?

In her doctoral thesis completed in December 1991, Dr Jay Dunbar pinpoints a serious problem concerning contemporary Tai Chi practitioners in the United States. She says:

> Over 60% of the 216 Taijiquan teachers surveyed reported injuries to the knees in themselves or their students as a result of performing Taijiquan (T'ai Chi Ch'uan).
>
> This finding, the most shocking of the study in my opinion, highlights the need for all Taijiquan teachers to review their teaching methods and take steps to counteract this problem.
>
> The incidence of knee injuries in the national population might make this data seem less surprising. In 1989, The New York times reported that, according to the American Academy of Orthopedic Surgeons, knee injuries constitute 26% of all injuries — the largest category.
>
> In 'Save Your Knees,' (1988) Fox and McGuire state, 'the knee is the most venerable joint in the body ... an estimated 50 million Americans (one in every 4 or 5) have suffered or are suffering knee pain or injuries.' Knee problems are especially prevalent in sports, such as aerobics, skiing, tennis, volleyball, basketball, cycling ...
>
> Taijiquan's measured pace, careful placement of the feet, and postural considerations should make it an ideal rehabilitative and preventive exercise for present or potential conditions of the knee.

It is significant to note that throughout the long history of Taijiquan and other forms of martial arts in China, knee injury has never been a problem at all. It appears to me that this problem is peculiar to America, as none of the Tai Chi practitioners I have met in Europe and Australia has complained to me of knee injury as a result of practising Tai Chi Chuan.

I certainly agree with Dr Jay Dunbar that 'Taijiquan teachers should acquire a working knowledge of the etiology, treatment and rehabilitation of injuries such as sprains and strains', but I disagree with her suggestion that 'Taijiquan teachers would do well at least to study texts such as Arnheim's "Modern Principles of Athletic Training" and specific guidelines to the knee such as Fox and McGuire's "Save Your Knees".' This does not imply that such conventional western texts are not useful, despite the fact that of the 50 million Americans suffering from knee problem, many of them would have read the texts. The crucial point is that if we wish to avoid suffering from knee injury as a result of practising Tai Chi Chuan, we should go to Tai Chi Chuan masters whose students do not have knee problems, and not to 'instructors who simply teach choreography', nor to people who know little about Tai Chi Chuan even though they may be experts in knee anatomy and physiology.

Traditionally, every Tai Chi Chuan master or master of any other style of kungfu is familiar with traumatology, a unique branch of Chinese medicine dealing with injuries, and which is often referred to as kungfu medicine. Tai Chi Chuan and other kungfu masters employ traumatology not to heal knee injuries due to the practice of their arts, simply because such a problem is absent, but to heal injuries like sprains, strains, dislocations, fractures, blockage of blood or energy flow, and damage to internal organs, which are not uncommon in sparring or actual fighting.

But what have the masters said about knee injury due to Tai Chi Chuan or other kungfu practice? They have said virtually nothing – simply because such a problem has never happened. If Tai Chi Chuan is practised properly (not 'played!' as this term is often used in American Tai Chi literature), the least a practitioner can have is good health, including healthy knees, of course. A moment of reflection will show how incongruous it is for an effective martial art to produce exponents with injured knees.

With hindsight it can be seen that three factors are particularly relevant for the absence of the knee problem in the type of Tai Chi Chuan taught by the masters. These three factors are balance and gracefulness in the Tai Chi movements, stable stances and agile footwork, and harmonious chi flow. All these three factors have been explained in some detail in this chapter, and chi flow will be further explained in the next chapter as well as Chapter 12.

Incidentally, this American knee problem reveals the superiority of Tai Chi Chuan, if it is practised properly, over conventional anatomical and physiological knowledge in knee function and safety. Conventional experts advise that 'attention must be paid to knee mechanics during form work, and that auxiliary exercises detrimental to the knees – such as knee rotation, hurdler's stretches, and deep knee bends – must be replaced with others that will improve knee strength and stability' Interestingly, these auxiliary exercises regarded as detrimental to the knee by western experts are regularly taught by Tai Chi Chuan and other kungfu masters to make the legs (including the knees) strong and flexible, which represents an important factor in combat efficiency. What is the result of the western and the Tai Chi Chuan approach? Not only the movement of the knee is limited, an estimated 50 million Americans have actual knee problems! On the other hand, rotating the knee is a basic principle taught by Tai Chi Chuan masters to their students as part of the process in graceful movement and in transmitting internal force from the heel to the hands. Yet not only is knee injury virtually absent among students taught by the masters; practising Tai Chi Chuan properly has been recommended to relieve existing knee problems – good news for the 50 million knee suffering Americans. But of course you have to learn from the masters, or at least from competent instructors; if you learn from those who teach Tai Chi choreography or from knee anatomists who themselves suffer from knee injury, you are likely to aggravate the American knee problem.

How do you train to have knees that are both strong and flexible? As it has been explained in this chapter, you must differentiate between 'apparent' and 'solid' movement – lead with your waist and rotate your knees! If you do otherwise, such as limiting your knee to linear movement (instead of rotating your knees) and stepping forward with your body weight (instead of transferring your weight from your 'solid' to your 'apparent' foot), you would limit and hurt your knees every time you move.

Having knees that are both 'stable' and 'mobile' or strong and flexible reflects the yin-yang principle of Tai Chi Chuan. If your knees are strong but limited to only an angular bent, or if you can rotate your knees but only in pain, your Tai Chi Chuan training is incomplete. One effective method to develop knee stability is stance training, especially the Tai Chi stance. Stability and strength are developed not just from the mechanics of the external form of the various stances, but more importantly from both internal energy building and harmonious energy flow, which conventional knee experts, understandably, may not adequately comprehend.

If injurious factors to the knee or any part of the body occur during Tai Chi Chuan practice, which may happen even among students of Tai Chi Chuan masters, these factors will be eliminated by the harmonious energy flow to the knee or any affected parts, such as during the Wuji Stance or during routine form training with mind and energy control (to be explained in Chapter 7), thus giving no chance for these factors to develop into clinical knee injuries or other disorders. If we can understand this, we can appreciate why body mechanics alone, implicit in the numerous preventive measures suggested by conventional experts, is inadequate to deal with this American knee problem.

6

The Importance of Chi Kung in Tai Chi Chuan

The Development of Internal Force

Tai Chi Chuan without Chi Kung is no longer Tai Chi Chuan; it becomes a form of gentle exercise which may provide some benefits in terms of blood circulation and recreation, but is unlikely to give the type of vitality and mental freshness commonly ascribed to Tai Chi Chuan training.

Health, Combat and Spirituality

Tai Chi students cannot defend themselves if they practise only Tai Chi sets. If you want to be effective in self-defence you must develop internal force and practise combat applications. Without internal force you cannot even develop good health – the other main reason, apart from self-defence, why people practise Tai Chi Chuan. Without both internal force and combat application, Tai Chi Chuan degenerates into no more than a dance – graceful and elegant, and admittedly, but no more than that. The application of Tai Chi Chuan in combat will be explained in later chapters; here we will be looking at internal force, which is developed mainly through Chi Kung. Indeed, Tai Chi Chi Kung and Tai Chi internal force are often used synonymously, although technically speaking Chi Kung is the method and internal force is the effect.

Chi Kung, which literally means 'the art of energy', is an umbrella term referring to hundreds of training systems that develop cosmic energy for various purposes, especially for health, combat efficiency, mind expansion and spiritual cultivation.[1] It is worth noting that both the pronunciation and the Chinese word for *chi* in Chi Kung are different from the pronunciation and the Chinese word used in Tai Chi Chuan. Chi Kung is pronounced 'Ch'i Kung' and is written *qigong* in Romanized Chinese, whereas Tai Chi Chuan is pronounced 'T'ai Ji Chuan' and is written as *Taijiquan*. For the convenience of Western readers, however the English spellings for both these terms are used here.

Chi Kung training as an integral part of Tai Chi Chuan is not only essential for effective self-defence, it is also necessary for good health. Tai Chi Chuan without Chi Kung is no longer Tai Chi Chuan; it becomes a form of gentle exercise which may provide some benefits in terms of blood circulation and recreation, but is unlikely to give the type of vitality and mental freshness commonly ascribed to Tai Chi Chuan training.

The highest attainment of Tai Chi Chuan is spiritual development, which elevates the art, like Shaolin Kungfu,[2] far beyond the level of ordinary fighting arts. Spiritual development in Tai Chi Chuan is closely related to, or even synonymous with Taoist cultivation, which is non-religious as it does not involve any dogmas or worship, and people of any religion can practise it. Taoist cultivation, which will be explained in Chapter 21, involves three stages, namely cultivating *jing* (essence) to become *chi* (energy), cultivating *chi* to become *shen* (spirit), and cultivating *shen* to return to the cosmos. Chi Kung is therefore the bridge leading from the physical (*jing*) to the spiritual (*shen*).

Tai Chi Chuan masters have divided its attainments into three levels: health, combat and spiritual development. If someone claims to have practised Tai Chi Chuan for years and is still weak and sickly, then something is seriously wrong, and often it is because his or her practice lacks Chi Kung. Practising merely the physical form of Tai Chi Chuan without Chi Kung is inadequate to equip an exponent with the stamina, power and endurance necessary for efficient fighting. Aspirants aiming for spiritual attainment in Tai Chi Chuan will lack the link between the physical and the spiritual if they do not practise Chi Kung.

The Internal Force of Tai Chi Chuan Training

For convenience, we may divide the training of Tai Chi Chi Kung into intrinsic and extrinsic, or yin and the yang aspects. Extrinsic training is performed outside a Tai Chi set, whereas intrinsic training is incorporated into the set itself. We should note that 'extrinsic' here does not mean 'external'; both extrinsic and intrinsic training involve much that is internal, although the external form is, of course, necessary.

Two excellent forms of extrinsic Tai Chi Chi Kung training were described in the previous chapter – the Infinite Ultimate and Tai Chi Stances. Another form you should practise conscientiously if you wish to obtain the full benefits of Tai Chi Chuan is known by the rather prosaic name of Tai Chi Starting Pattern. In Shaolin Kungfu, this same exercise, which is the initial stage of an advanced art known as Golden Bell, is called Lifting Water. Although prosaic, the term Tai Chi Starting Pattern is meaningful, because it not only indicates that this pattern is the starting pattern of most Tai Chi sets, but it also suggests that one should practise it for some time before learning any Tai Chi sets.

Stand still for a few seconds (or a few minutes if you intend to have a longer training session) in the Infinite Ultimate Stance *(figure 6.1a)*. Then move one of your legs to the side to form the Goat-riding or Tai Chi Stance. Simultaneously raise both arms, with your elbows fairly straight, in front of you to chest-level *(figure 6.1b)*, breathing in gently through your nose. Then lower your arms gently in front as if you were pressing on water with your palms, breathing out gently through your mouth *(figure 6.1c)*.

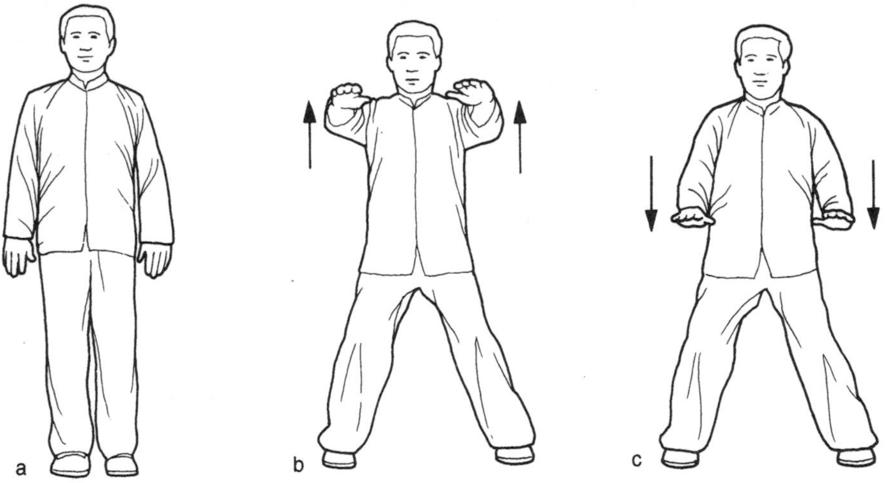

Fig 6.1 Lifting Water

After raising and lowering your arms with the correct breathing between five and ten times, you should have entered a Chi Kung state of mind, a subconscious level. Gently visualize good cosmic energy flowing into you as you breathe in, and your vital energy flowing down your arms into your palms as you breathe out. (Cosmic energy and vital energy are terms generally used to refer to energy outside and inside your body respectively.) It is very important that your visualization be done gently; if you have difficulty visualizing, just a gentle thought of cosmic energy flowing into you, and vital energy flowing to your palms, will do.

After raising and lowering your arms 30 times, with the appropriate visualization and energy flow, gently bring your feet together and remain still in the Infinite Ultimate Stance for a few minutes. You will feel internal force flowing down your arms and legs, and surging inside you. As you progress, increase the number of times you lift and lower your arms to 50 times, then gradually to 100 or more.

You may start with *zhan zhuang* (standing in a stance) and Lifting Water, then follow on without a break to a Tai Chi set, as explained in the next chapter. On the other hand, if your training session is short, you may practise them separately. Notice that both the Infinite Ultimate Stance and Lifting Water are an integral part of any Tai Chi set, which usually begins with them. When performing a Tai Chi set, however, one normally stands in the Infinite Ultimate Stance for just a few seconds, and raises and lowers one's arms only twice. If you practise them as the initial patterns of a Tai Chi set rather than as separate exercises, even though you may spend a long time over them, then they constitute intrinsic Chi Kung training.

Another example of Tai Chi Chi Kung training which may be classified as intrinsic or extrinsic depending on how we choose to practise it, is the four primary hand movements of *peng, lu, qi* and *an*, as described in the previous chapter. From the Infinite Ultimate Stance, move to the right with the *peng* or warding off technique. Breathe in gently through your nose as you carry a ball of *chi* in the False-leg Stance, and breathe out gently through your mouth as you move to a right Bow-arrow Stance with the *peng* technique. As you breathe in focus on the *chi* at your *dan tian*, and as you breathe out visualize your *chi* flowing from your *dan tian* through your forward-moving right arm to your right palm.

Then roll back with the *lu* technique, breathing in gently through your nose, visualizing cosmic energy flowing into you. As you press forward with the *qi* technique, breathe out gently through your mouth and visualize your vital energy flowing to your right arm. Then lower your palms, breathing in gently and focusing on your abdominal *dan tian*. As you push forward with the *an* technique, breathe out and visualize *chi* flowing from your abdomen, through your body and arms, and out of your palms.

Repeat the four techniques with the appropriate breathing and visualization about ten times, then repeat the whole process on the left side the same number of times. Increase the number of times as you progress. At the end of the training session, use the pattern Energy Accumulating at Energy Field described on pages 52 and 53 to focus vital energy at your abdominal *dan tian*, and remain still in the Infinite Ultimate Stance for some time.

Developing a Pearl of Intrinsic Energy

Energy training in Chi Kung falls into two main categories: increasing the amount of vital energy in the body and promoting harmonious energy flow. They may be represented as the yin and yang of Chi Kung training. An important method of increasing energy is abdominal breathing, which is best learnt in stages.

Stand in the Infinite Ultimate Stance. Place one palm gently over your *dan tian* and the other over the first palm *(figure 6.2a)*. Press gently on your abdomen for about six counts to deflate it. This does not mean that you should press it six times – it must be a smooth and continuous process, not a staccato. Hold it in about two counts, then release the pressure for about six counts so that your abdomen extends to its original level. This releasing must also be smooth and continuous. Hold this position for about two

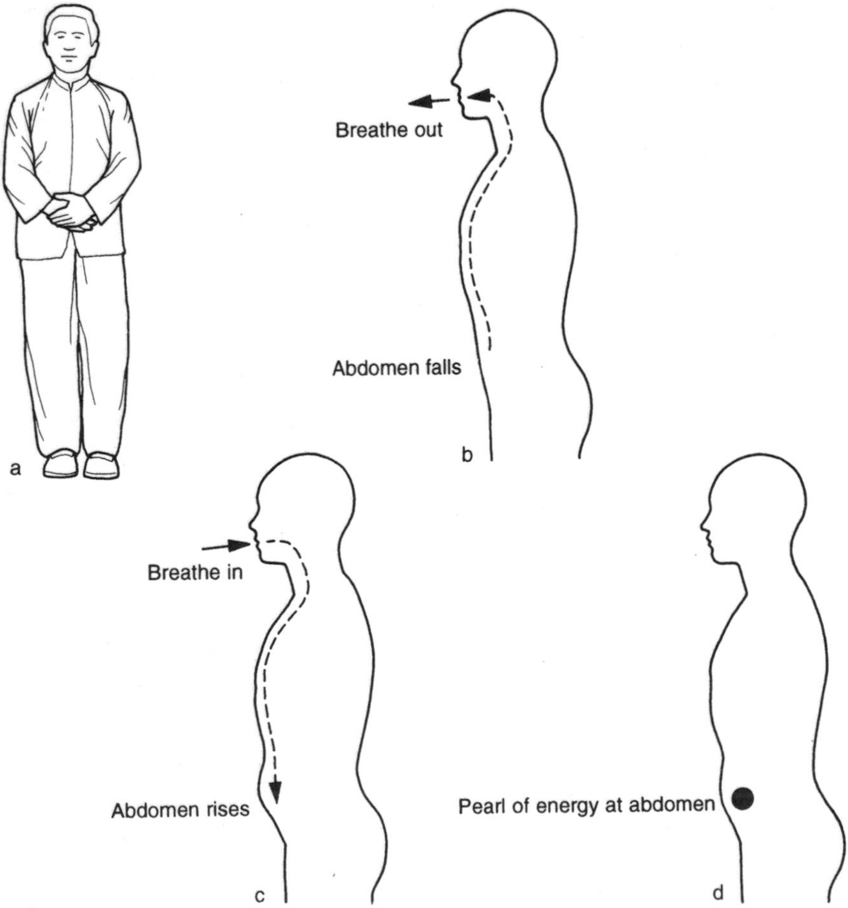

Fig 6.2 Abdominal breathing

counts, then repeat the procedure about ten times. This is the first stage of the training. Your breathing should be spontaneous, but make sure that you do not breathe in as you deflate your abdomen. Gradually increase the number of times you press and release from 10 to 36.

You should practise for at least two weeks so that the falling and rising of your abdomen becomes spontaneous, before proceeding to the second stage. Follow the same procedure as in the first stage, but as you deflate your abdomen, visualize stale energy flowing from your body out of your mouth. As you release the pressure of your palms and your abdomen rises, visualize good cosmic energy flowing through your nose into your abdomen. Practise this for at least two weeks before proceeding to the next stage.

The third stage is the abdominal breathing proper. Follow the same procedure as in the second stage, but as you deflate your abdomen and visualize stale energy flowing out, gently breathe out through your mouth. As you release the pressure and visualize good cosmic energy flowing into your abdomen, breathe in gently through your nose. After breathing in and out about 36 times, close your eyes and remain still in the Infinite Ultimate Stance. First clear your mind of all thoughts, then gently visualize a pearl of *chi* at your abdominal *dan tian*, which is about 3 inches below your navel. At first this pearl will be only imaginary, but as you progress it will become real, and it represents the primary source of your internal force.

I must reiterate that Chi Kung practice is important if you do not want your Tai Chi Chuan to degenerate into a mere dance. Without Chi Kung, Tai Chi Chuan would be unable to provide the wonderful health benefits that have traditionally been associated with it, for at best it would merely be a gentle form of physical exercise. Without Chi Kung, Tai Chi Chuan could not be an effective martial art, for it would lack the internal force that it is famous for. Without Chi Kung, Tai Chi Chuan could not be a way of spiritual cultivation, for it is *chi* that bridges the gap between its form and the development of spirit towards a unity with the cosmos. But Chi Kung should be practised under the supervision of a master or a competent instructor, and its progress must be gradual, allowing all the internal organs of your body sufficient time to become adjusted to the new power. Incorrect or hasty Chi Kung training may cause serious problems.

7

The Poetry of Energy and Mind

Tai Chi Chuan with Breath Control and Visualization

To get the best results from any Tai Chi set, you must understand its energy and mind aspects so that your poetry in motion is imbued with internal force and consciousness.

The Purposes of Set Practice

When people say they practise Tai Chi Chuan, what they usually mean is that they know how to perform one or more Tai Chi sets. But, performing a Tai Chi set is only a part, not the whole, of Tai Chi Chuan. From the point of view of our health and general daily life, developing elegant movements, energy flow and mental awareness is more important than merely performing Tai Chi sets.

Nevertheless, although set practice is not the most important part of Tai Chi Chuan training, it is still important, because it provides us with the means to learn Tai Chi patterns as well as to develop elegant movements, energy flow and mental awareness. It is also a way to learn and then to be able to execute spontaneously basic Tai Chi patterns in combat, which will be explained in subsequent chapters.

In addition to the extrinsic methods of developing internal force explained in the previous chapter, internal force can be trained as part of set practice itself. This is done mainly through co-ordinating the breathing and visualization with the physical movements of the patterns in the Tai Chi set outlined below. However, until you become familiar with the set, you will learn faster if you forget about the breath control and visualization for the time being and concentrate on performing the physical forms correctly. You can come back to the breath control and visualization when your movements are smooth and spontaneous.

The set is illustrated in a series of pictures with accompanying descriptions. In learning the set from the pictures you will probably appreciate the saying that a picture is worth a thousand words. The descriptions are there to indicate broad actions and highlight crucial points, not to explain detailed movements. Detailed instructions for the fundamental movements were provided in Chapter 5, and you should read them and *practise* if you want to get the best results from your set training in the shortest time.

The set which follows is known as the 24-Pattern Simplified Tai Chi Set, and was constructed by a council of Tai Chi Chuan masters after much thought and deliberation. This council was set up by the Chinese government to meet two pressing needs: to use Tai Chi Chuan as a convenient and inexpensive means of overcoming the country's health problems; and to find a common set with which exponents of different styles of Tai Chi Chuan could compete in newly popularized martial arts tournaments.

The 24-Pattern Simplified Tai Chi Set is predominantly of the Yang Style. For this reason, another set, known as the 48-Pattern Tai Chi Set, was devised, but although the 24-pattern set is now no longer used for Tai Chi Chuan competitions, it continues to be very popular because it is comparatively easy to learn and is effective for both health and defence.

Unless you are already familiar with Tai Chi or kungfu movements, it is not easy to learn a set from a book, no matter how well illustrated and explained. So, if you are a complete novice, it is advisable to learn from a competent instructor.

Simplified Tai Chi Set – Section 1

Perform the set described below slowly and gracefully, like poetry in motion. Pay particular attention to balance and poise in performing the various patterns; this can be attained only if you understand the finer movements of leading with the waist and differentiating between apparent and solid, as explained in Chapter 5. Remember too, that Tai Chi Chuan is an internal art, which means that if you merely perform the external patterns of the set, you will at best only perform a form of physical exercise; to get the best results from any Tai Chi set, you must understand its energy and mind aspects so that your 'poetry in motion' is imbued with internal force and consciousness.

Start from the Infinite Ultimate Stance *(figure 7.1.1a)*. It is of the utmost importance that you should be calm and relaxed, and smile from your heart. If you cannot attain this condition, it might be better for you not to proceed with the set. Feel that your whole body is charged with energy. Gently focus on your *dan tian.*

Move your right leg about 1 foot to your right to adopt a Tai Chi Stance, and slowly raise both arms to chest-level in front of you, with your fingers pointing forward and your elbows fairly straight *(figure 7.1.1b).* Simultaneously breathe in gently through your nose, and visualize cosmic energy flowing into you. Your visualization throughout this set must be done gently; forced visualization often brings harmful effects. If you find it difficult to visualize, you may instead gently think of what is to be visualized. Then lower your arms to your sides *(figure 7.1.1c),* breathe out gently through your mouth, and visualize that vital energy is flowing to your palms. This pattern is called Lifting Water or the Tai Chi Starting Pattern. Perform this pattern twice.

Next move to a transitional pattern called Carrying the Cosmos in a left False-leg Stance as shown in *figure 7.1.2a.* Breathe in gently and visualize that you are carrying a ball of *chi.* Then move to a left Bow-arrow Stance, spreading out both arms in the spreading technique, in a pattern called Flying Diagonally, also known as Wild Horse Spreads Mane *(figure 7.1.2b).* Simultaneously breathe out and visualize your vital energy flowing to your arms.

Move your right leg forward to a transitional right False-leg Stance, breathing in simultaneously *(figure 7.1.2c),* and then to a right Bow-arrow Stance, performing the right side of Wild Horse Spreads Mane *(figure 7.1.2d).* Breathe out and visualize vital energy flowing to your arms. Next, move to a transitional left False-leg Stance, breathing in simultaneously *(figure 7.1.2e),* and then to a left Bow-arrow Stance with another left side of Wild Horse Spreads Mane *(figure 7.1.2f),* breathing out and visualizing *chi* flowing to your arms.

Breathe in gently and move to a left False-leg Stance *(figure 7.1.3a);* breathe out gently and spread out both arms in a pattern called White Crane Spreads Wings *(figure 7.1.3b).*

Then make a small circle in a clockwise direction with your left hand in front of your body, and make a big circle in an anti-clockwise direction with your right hand to the right of your body *(figure 7.1.4a);* simultaneously move your front (left) leg forward to a left Bow-arrow Stance concluding with a right palm strike as shown in *figure 7.1.4b,* with your left palm at your left side near your thigh. This pattern is called Twist Knee Throw Step after the foot movement, but a more poetic name is Green Dragon Shoots Out Pearl. Breathe in as you start to make the circles with your hands, and breathe out as you conclude the right circle with a right palm strike. Visualize *chi* flowing to your right palm.

Repeat this Green Dragon pattern with a left palm strike *(figures 7.1.4c* and *d)*. Then repeat it again with a right palm strike *(figures 7.1.4e* and *f)*. The breathing co-ordination and visualization are the same as in the previous Green Dragon pattern.

Next, bring your left leg back to a left Four-six Stance *(figure 7.1.5a)*, and rotating your waist slightly to your right, place your hands as shown in *figure 7.1.5b*, in the pattern called Playing the Lute. Breathe in at the start and out at the end of the pattern. Focus your *chi* at your *dan tian*.

Then bring your left leg back to a right Four-six Stance, making a big anti-clockwise circle with your right hand ending with a right palm strike at shoulder level *(figure 7.1.6a, b* and *c)*. Breathe in at the start and out at the end of the pattern. Visualize *chi* flowing to your right palm. This pattern is called Reversed Rolling of Biceps or, more fancifully, Repulse Monkey.

Repeat Repulse Monkey with a left palm strike at a left Four-six Stance *(figures 7.1.6d* and *e)*. Repeat both the right and the left Repulse Monkey *(figures 7.1.6f–i)*, thus performing the Monkey pattern four times. Breathe in as you begin each pattern and out as you complete it. Visualize *chi* flowing to your palm.

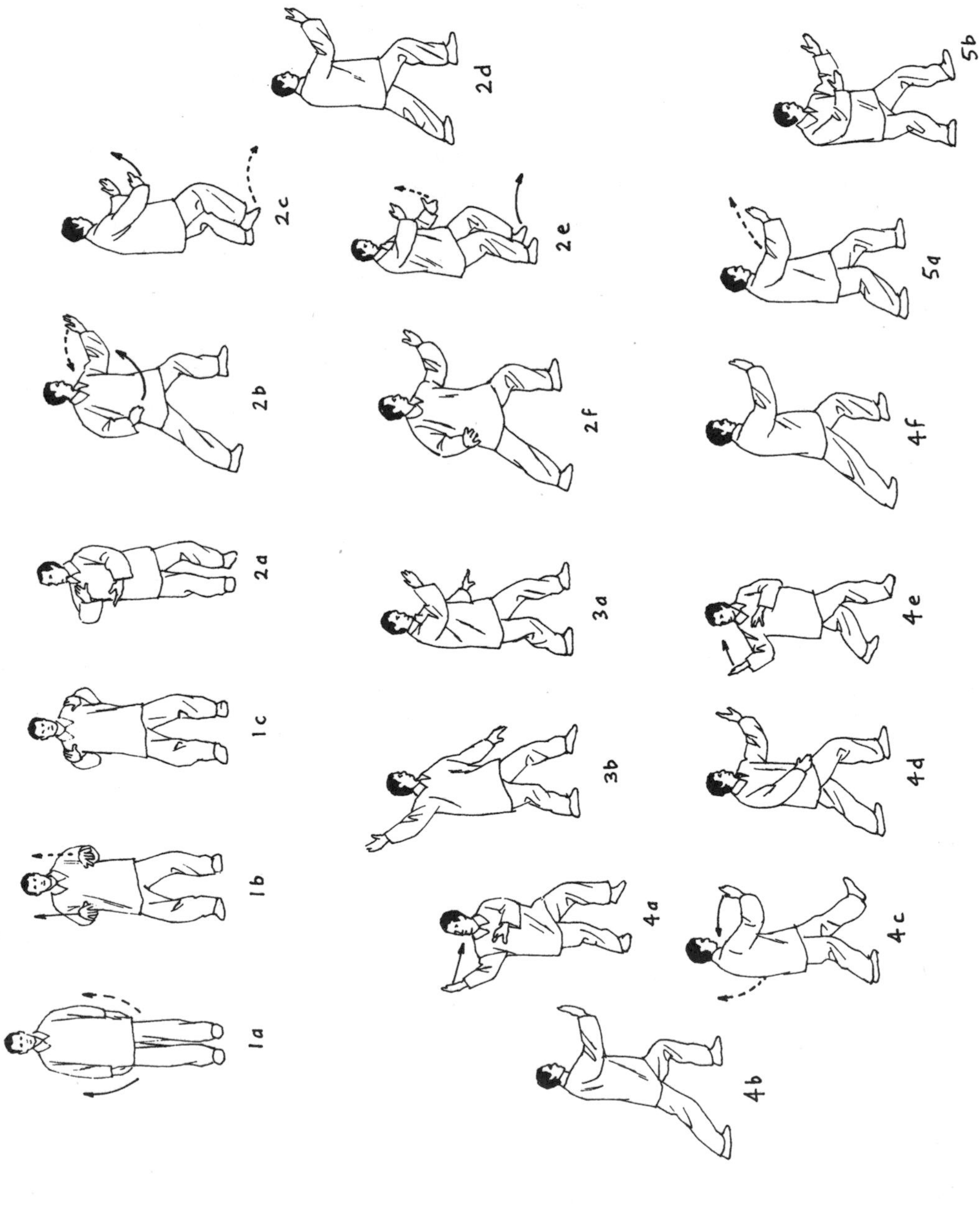
1a
1b
1c
2a
2b
2c
2d
2e
2f
3a
3b
4a
4b
4c
4d
4e
4f
5a
5b

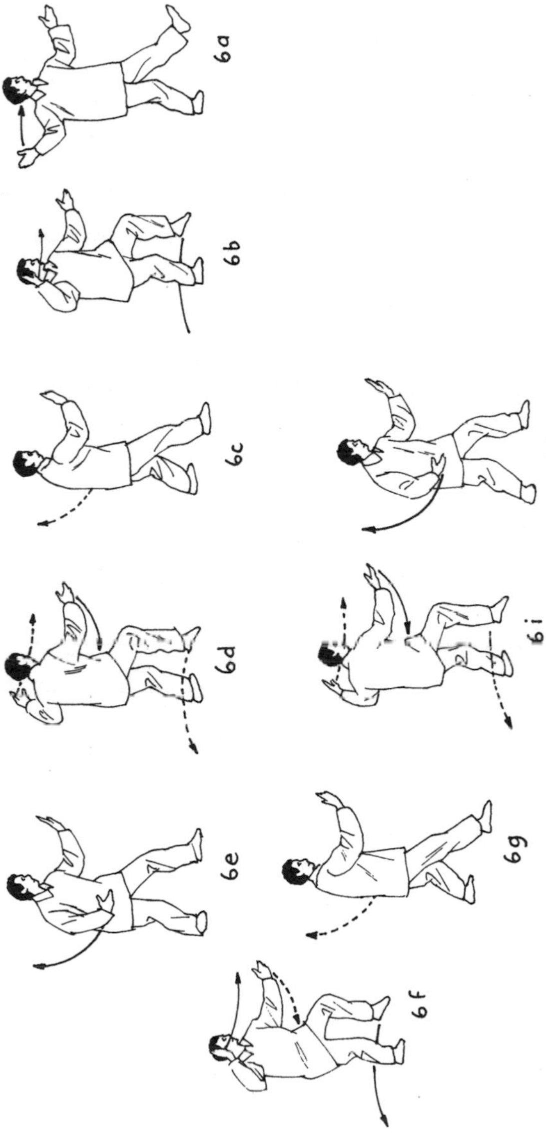

Fig 7.1 Simplified Tai Chi Set – Section 1

Simplified Tai Chi Set – Section 2

From the left Repulse Monkey turn right about to a transitional right False-leg Stance *(figure 7.2.7a)*, then to a right Bow-arrow Stance with the *peng* or warding off technique *(figure 7.2.7b* and *c)*. Breathe in as you carry the ball of *chi*, and out as you execute the *peng* technique, visualizing *chi* flowing to your outstretched hand.

From the *peng* technique, roll-back with the *lu* technique *(figure 7.2.7d)*, breathing in simultaneously and focusing on your *dan tian*. Next, move to the *qi* or pressing technique *(figures 7.2.7e* and *f)*, breathing out and visualizing *chi* in your right forearm. Breathe in and lower your stance *(figure 7.2.7g)*, then push out with the *an* technique, breathing out and visualizing *chi* striking out at the same time *(figure 7.2.7h)*.These four techniques – *peng, lu, qi* and *an* – constitute a pattern known as Grasping Sparrow's Tail.

Repeat this pattern on your left side*(figures 7.2.7i–o)*. The breathing and visualization are the same as for the right side.

Turn right into a Tai Chi Stance, and continuously move your right hand in a large clockwise circle and your left hand in a large anti-clockwise circle in front of you. As you continue to rotate your hands, move sideways to your left *(figures 7.2.8a–f)*. Breathe in as you move your left leg, and breathe out as you move your right leg to the left. Visualize vital energy flowing to your arms and hands. These patterns are called Cloud Hands.

Breathe in and bring your left foot close to your right to stand momentarily in a left False-leg Stance, and hold your hands as shown in *figure 7.2.9a*. Then move your left leg forward into a left Bow-arrow Stance, and strike out your left palm *(figures 7.2.9b* and *c)*, in a pattern known as Single Whip, simultaneously breathing out and visualizing your *chi* flowing to your left palm.

Simplified Tai Chi Set – Section 3

From Single Whip turn to a pattern called High Patting Horse as shown in *figures 7.3.10a* and *b*. Breathe in at the start of the pattern, and breathe out as you move your right hand out.

Stand on your left leg and cross your hands in front of your face, breathing in as you do so. Then separate your hands and kick out your right heel, breathing out *(figures 7.3.11a, b* and *c)*. This pattern is called Cross-Hands Thrust Kick. Lower your right leg diagonally forward and execute a pattern called Double Bees Buzzing at Ears, focusing your *chi* at your two fists *(figures 7.3.12a* and *b)*, and breathe out quite forcefully through your mouth.

Bring your right foot close to your left foot, and make a left about turn. Stand on your right leg and cross your hands in front of your face, breathing in. Then kick out your left leg in a Cross-hands Thrust Kick, breathing out *(figures 7.3.11d, e* and *f)*.

Lower your left leg forward to a pattern called Single Whip Low Stance, as shown in *figures 7.3.13a* and *b*, and breathe in gently. Without moving your feet move your body forward to a low left Bow-arrow Stance *(figure 7.3.13c)*. Continue moving your body forward to stand on your left leg in a pattern called Golden Cockerel Stands Alone *(figures 7.3.14a* and *b)*, breathing out gently in the process. Focus on maintaining good balance.

Lower your right foot to perform the Single Whip Low Stance pattern, as shown in *figures 7.3.13d* and *e*, and breathe in. Move your body and right palm forward *(figures 7.3.13f)* into a right Bow-arrow Stance, then stand on your right leg in the pattern Golden Cockerel Stands Alone *(figures 7.3.14c* and *d)*, and breathe out. Next, place your left leg forward to execute a pattern called Jade Girl Threads Shuttle *(figures 7.3.15a* and *b)*. Breathe in at the start, and breathe out at the end of this pattern; focus your *chi* at your striking palm. Next, move your left leg across your right in a transitional stance known as a Unicorn Step *(figures 7.3.15d* and *e)*, and then move your right leg forward to another Jade Girl Threads Shuttle pattern *(figure 7.3.15f)*, with the same breathing and visualization co-ordination as in the first Jade Girl pattern.

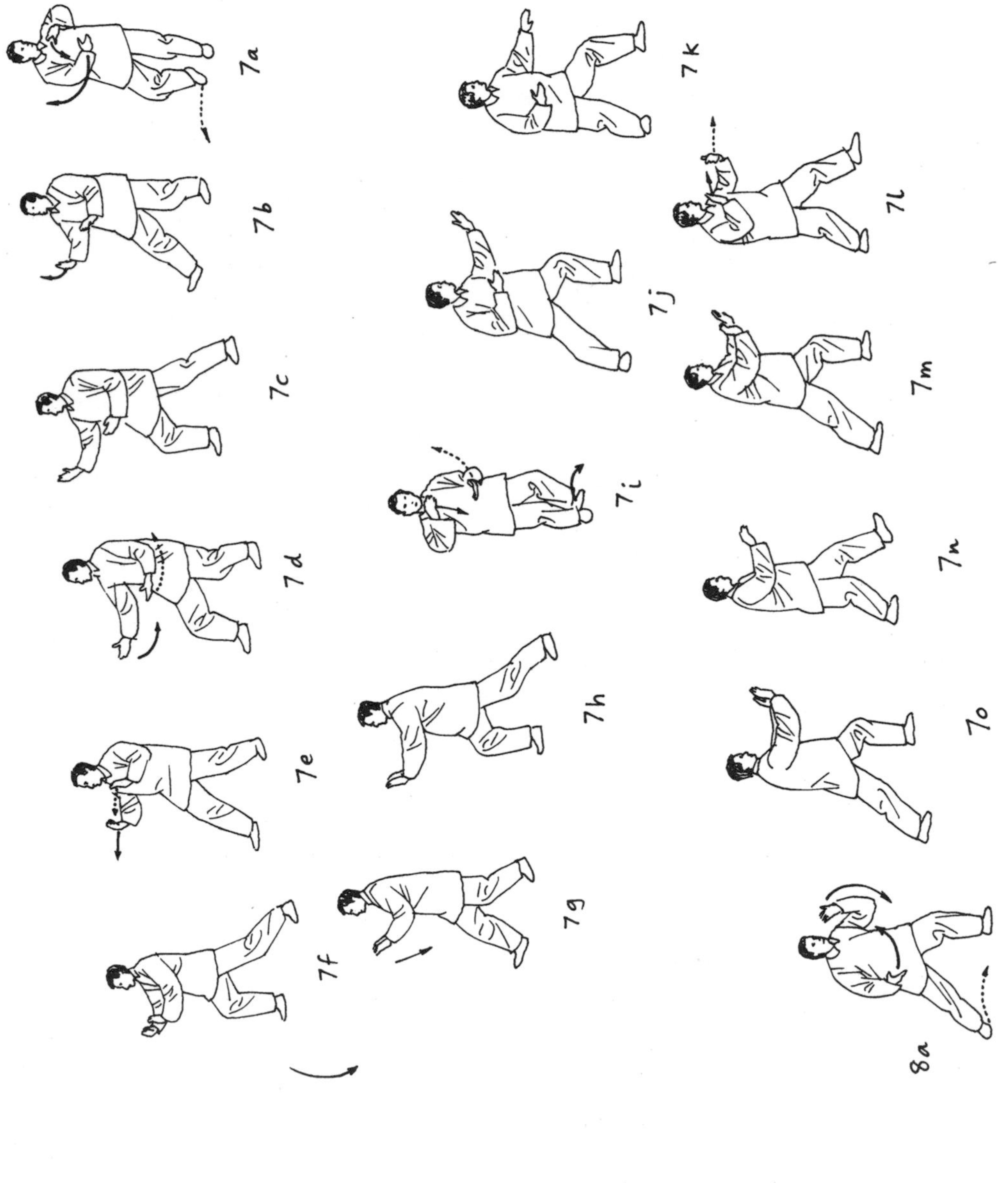
7a
7b
7c
7d
7e
7f
7g
7h
7i
7j
7k
7l
7m
7n
7o
8a

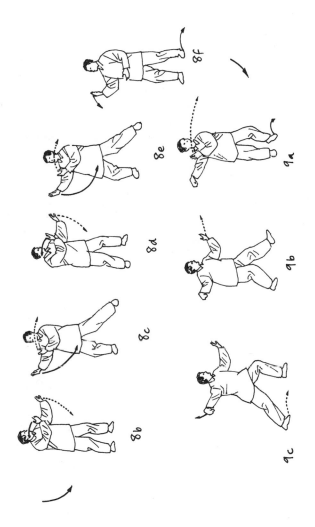

Fig 7.2 Simplified Tai Chi Set – Section 2

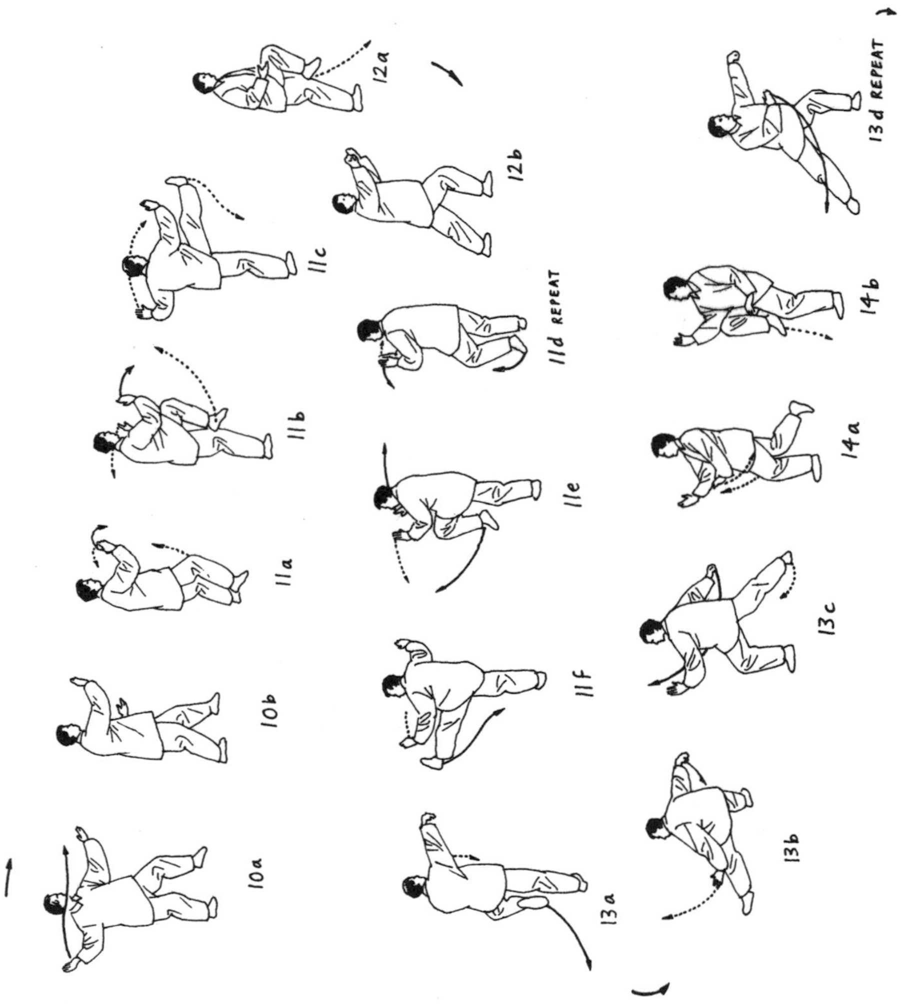
10a
10b
11a
11b
11c
12a
13a
11f
11e
11d REPEAT
12b
13b
13c
14a
14b
13d REPEAT

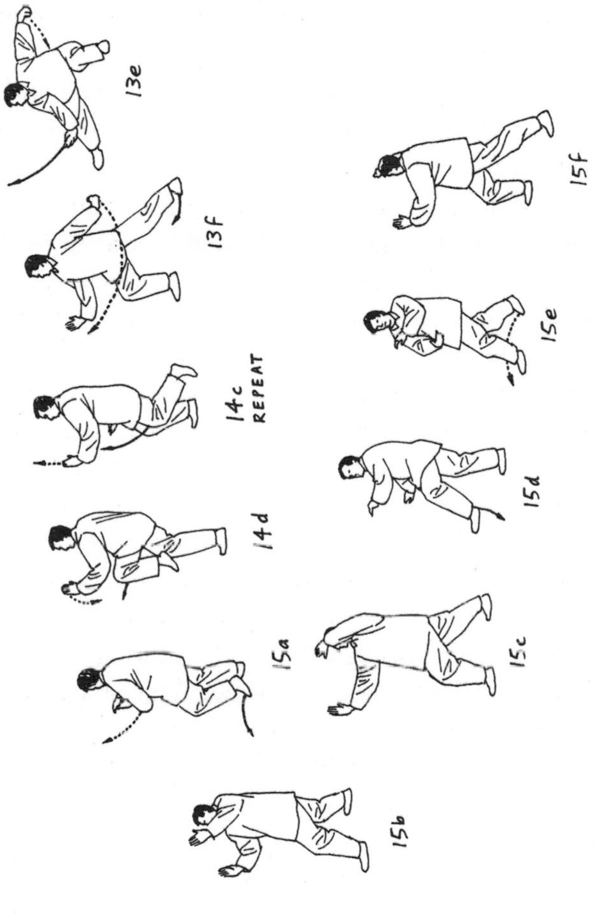

Fig 7.3 Simplified Tai Chi Set – Section 3

Simplified Tai Chi Set – Section 4

From Jade Girl Threads Shuttle move to a pattern called Needle at Sea Bottom, as illustrated in *figure 7.4.16*. Breathe in as you shift your leg, and breathe out as you chop your right palm down. Visualize your *chi* flowing to your striking hand. Then move your right leg forward for an Elbow Strike *(figure 7.4.17)*. Your breathing should be spontaneous. In this pattern, and in the next, take care that you do not lean your body so far out that your balance is upset.

Next stamp your left leg on the ground close to and behind your right leg *(figure 7.4.18a)*, and move your right leg forward with a Shoulder Strike *(figure 7.4.18b)*, breathing out fairly forcefully as you strike. Focus your *chi* at your striking shoulder. The striking technique of this pattern is known as lean, or *kao*, but do not be misled by this term. It does not mean that you lean your shoulder against your opponent. The striking force of this attack is derived from shooting your body forward from your back leg with your shoulder as the striking point, and not from bending your shoulder forward from your waist.

Form a transitional Unicorn Step *(figure 7.4.19a)*, then take a big step forward with your left leg so that it is now the front leg of a low Bow-arrow Stance, and execute a left palm strike, with your right palm above your head *(figure 7.4.19b)*. Breathe in as you move your right leg back, and breathe out as you move your left leg forward. Visualize your *chi* shooting out from your back to your striking palm. This pattern is frequently called Fan Going Through the Back, although it is more likely that the term is an adulterated form of Dodge Then Extend Arm, as the two sound alike in Chinese.

Without moving your feet but adjusting your toe positions accordingly, make a right about turn and swing your right fist, with the knuckles at the back of the fist as the striking point *(figures 7.4.20a* and *b)*. Breathe in as you move your left palm, and breathe out as you swing your right fist. Visualize *chi* flowing along your right arm to your fist. This pattern is known simply as Swinging Fist.

Turn to a transitional Unicorn Step, with your left arm held in a vertical block *(figure 7.4.21a)*. Breathe in and move your left leg forward, and then punch out your right fist, breathing out forcefully, with your left arm still held in a vertical position *(figure 7.4.21b* and *c)*. Focus your *chi* at your right fist. This pattern, which is subtle in its combat application, is known by the rather prosaic name of Move–Intercept–Punch.

Place your left palm beneath your right forearm, pull your right fist back, changing it into a right palm, and shift your body backwards without moving your feet *(figures 7.4.22a* and *b)*, breathing in at the same time. Then change back into a left Bow-arrow Stance, simultaneously move both palms forward and breathe out *(figure 7.4.22c)*. This pattern is known as Like Sealed as if Closed.

Turn right and bring your left leg towards your right so that both legs are about a shoulder width apart *(figure 7.4.23a)*. Stand in a Goat-riding Stance and bring both hands up and cross them in front of your face *(figure 7.4.23b)*, in a pattern called Cross-Hands. Breathe in gently and visualize cosmic energy flowing into you. Then lower your hands to your sides and bring your right leg close to your left, to stand in an Infinite Ultimate Stance *(figure 7.4.24)*. Breathe out gently and gently let your *chi* sink to your *dan tian*.

Close your eyes gently and remain in the Infinite Ultimate Stance for a while, ranging from a few seconds to a few minutes. If you have performed the set correctly, with the appropriate breath control and visualization, you will find your body swaying gently, moved by the vital energy flowing harmoniously inside you. You will also feel calm and pleasant, yet charged with energy. Enjoy this graceful swaying for some time, then gently still it by focussing on your *dan tian*. Remain still for some time before completing the standing meditation by rubbing your palms and warming your eyes with them to open them.

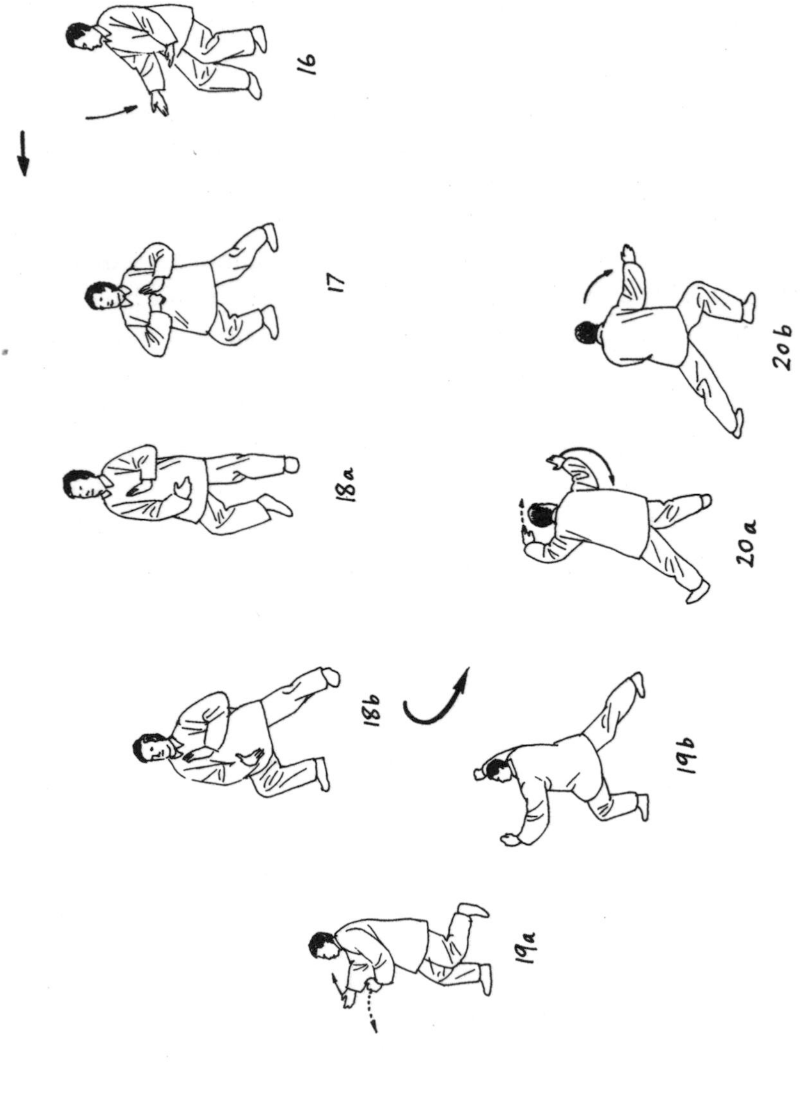
16
17
18a
18b
19a
19b
20a
20b

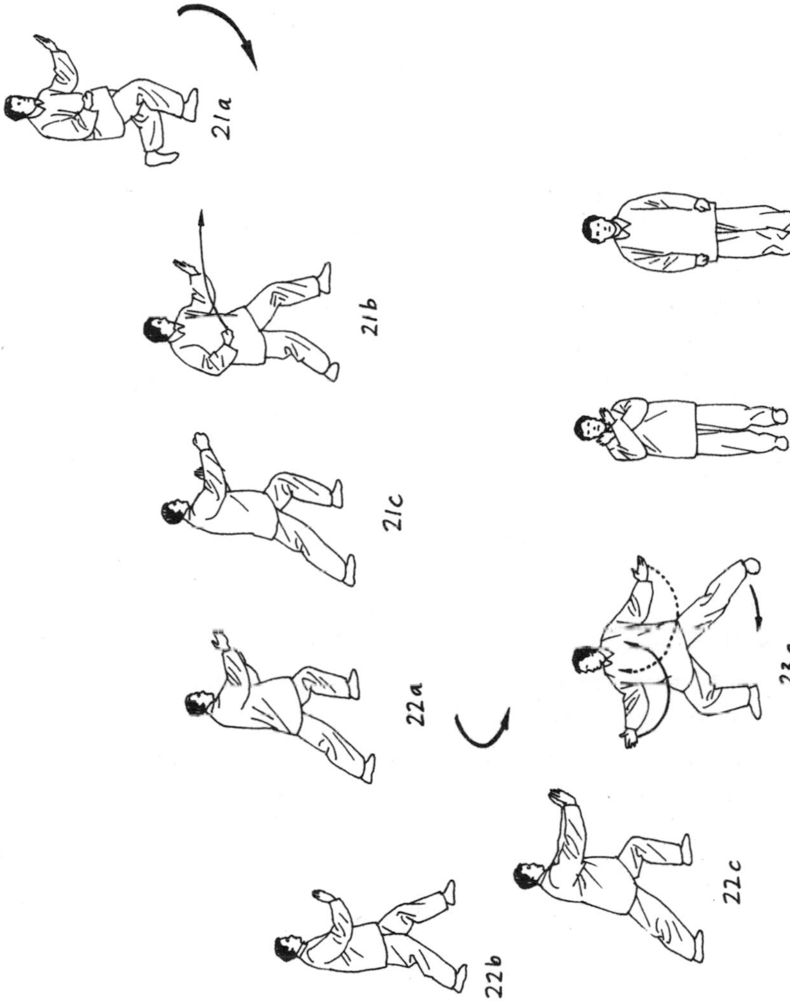

Fig 7.4 Simplified Tai Chi Set – Section 4

There are actually 36 patterns in the Simplified Tai Chi Set, but if we ignore repetitions, there are 24 different ones. Because of the cultural and linguistic differences between Chinese and English these names, which are poetic in Chinese, may appear odd when translated into English. The names of the 24 patterns of the Simplified Tai Chi Set are as follows:

1 Lifting Water
2 Flying Diagonally
3 White Crane Flaps Wings
4 Green Dragon Shoots Out Pearl
5 Playing the Lute
6 Repulse Monkey
7 Grasping Sparrow's Tail
8 Cloud Hands
9 Single Whip
10 High Patting Horse
11 Cross-Hands Thrust Kick
12 Double Bees Buzzing at Ears
13 Single Whip Low Stance
14 Golden Cockerel Stands Alone
15 Jade Girl Threads Shuttle
16 Needle at Sea Bottom
17 Elbow Strike
18 Shoulder Strike
19 Dodge Then Extend Arm
20 Swinging Fist
21 Move–Intercept–Punch
22 Like Sealed as if Closed
23 Cross Hands
24 Infinite Ultimate Stance

The 48-Pattern Tai Chi Set

The 48-Pattern Tai Chi Set, which incorporates many patterns from the Chen-style of Tai Chi Chuan and is particularly suitable for combat purposes, is divided into six sections for convenience and illustrated in the charts below. If you are not sufficiently familiar with Tai Chi Chuan, it will be difficult to learn this 48-pattern set from the illustrations, and you can use this presentation simply for your interest. If you *can* learn the set from the illustrations – which is a poor alternative to learning from a competent instructor – you should perform it with appropriate breathing co-ordination and visualization so that it flows poetically, with internal force and mental awareness.

The names of the 48 patterns are as follows:

Section 1

1 White Crane Flaps Wings
2 Green Dragon Shoots Out Pearl
3 Single Whip – left side
4 Playing the Lute
5 Roll Back and Press
6 Move–Intercept–Strike – left side
7 Grasping Sparrow's Tail – left side

Section 2
8 Leaning with Slanting Body
9 Punch Below Elbow
10 Repulse Monkey
11 About-Turn Palm Strike
12 Playing the Lute
13 Twist Knee, Plant Fist

Section 3
14 White Snake Shoots Venom
15 Kick and Tame Tiger
16 Swinging Fist – left side
17 Thread Fist Low Stance
18 Crane Standing Among Cockerels
19 Single Whip – right side

Section 4
20 Cloud Hands – right side
21 Wild Horse Spreads Mane
22 High Patting Horse
23 Right Thrust Kick
24 Double Bees Buzzing at Ears
25 Left Thrust Kick
26 Cover Hand Rising Fist
27 Needle at Sea Bottom
28 Dodge Then Extend Arm

Section 5
29 Left and Right Snap Kicks
30 Green Dragon Shoots Out Pearl
31 Advance to Get and Hit
32 Like Sealed as if Closed
33 Cloud Hands – left side
34 Swinging Fist – right side
35 Thread Shuttle – left and right
36 Retreat Step Thread Palm

Section 6
37 False-leg Press Palm
38 Single-leg Lift Palm
39 Lean on Horse Stance
40 Turn Body to Roll Back
41 Rising Palm Lower Stance
42 Advance to Cross-fists
43 Single-leg Ride Tiger
44 Turn-about Sway Lotus
45 Shooting Tiger
46 Move–Intercept–Punch – right side
47 Grasping Sparrow's Tail – right side
48 Cross-hands

Practising a Tai Chi set with the proper co-ordination of movements, breathing and visualization enables us to develop internal force as well as mental focus. It also familiarizes us with Tai Chi patterns which can be used for attack and defence.

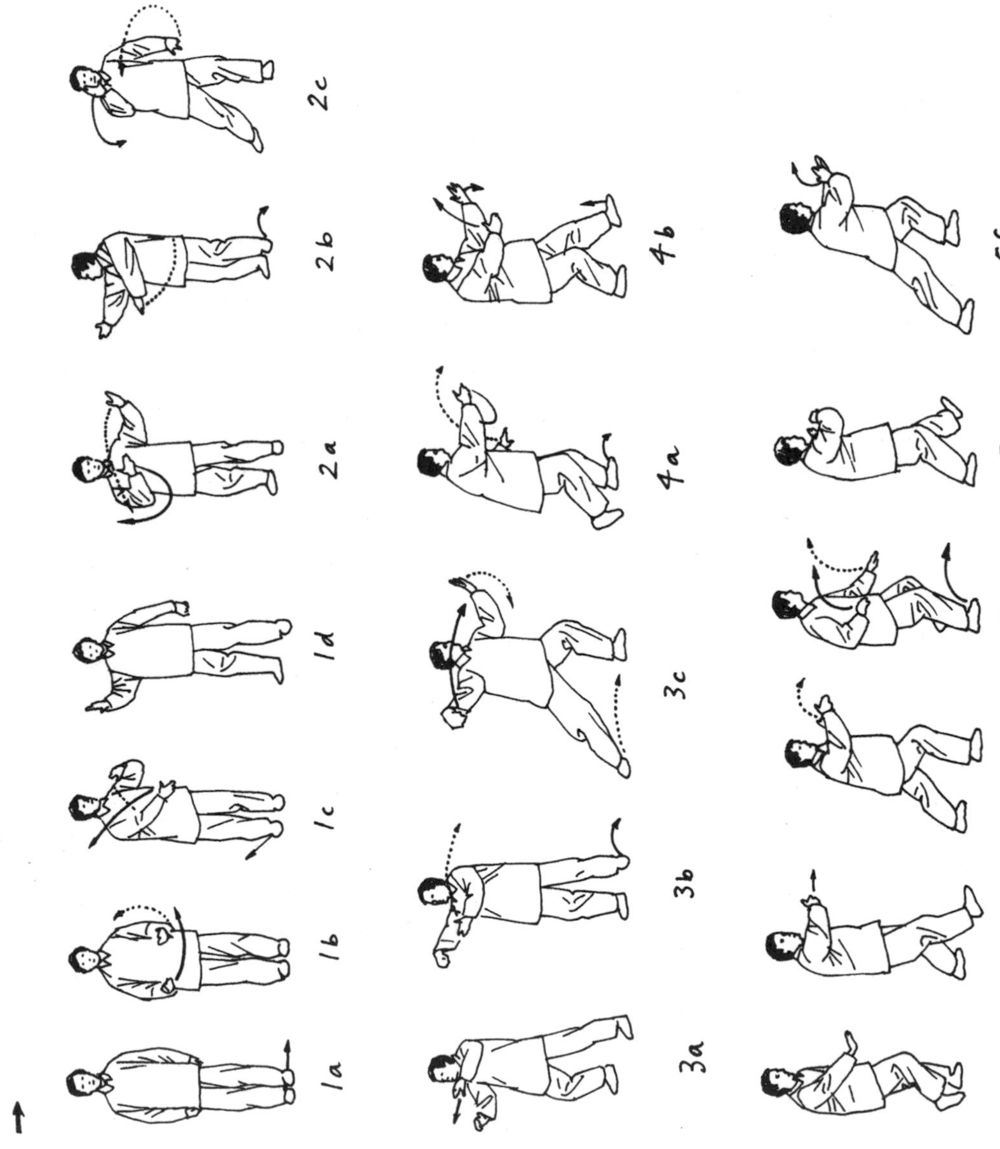
1a
1b
1c
1d
2a
2b
2c
3a
3b
3c
4a
4b
5a
5b
5c
5d
5e
5f

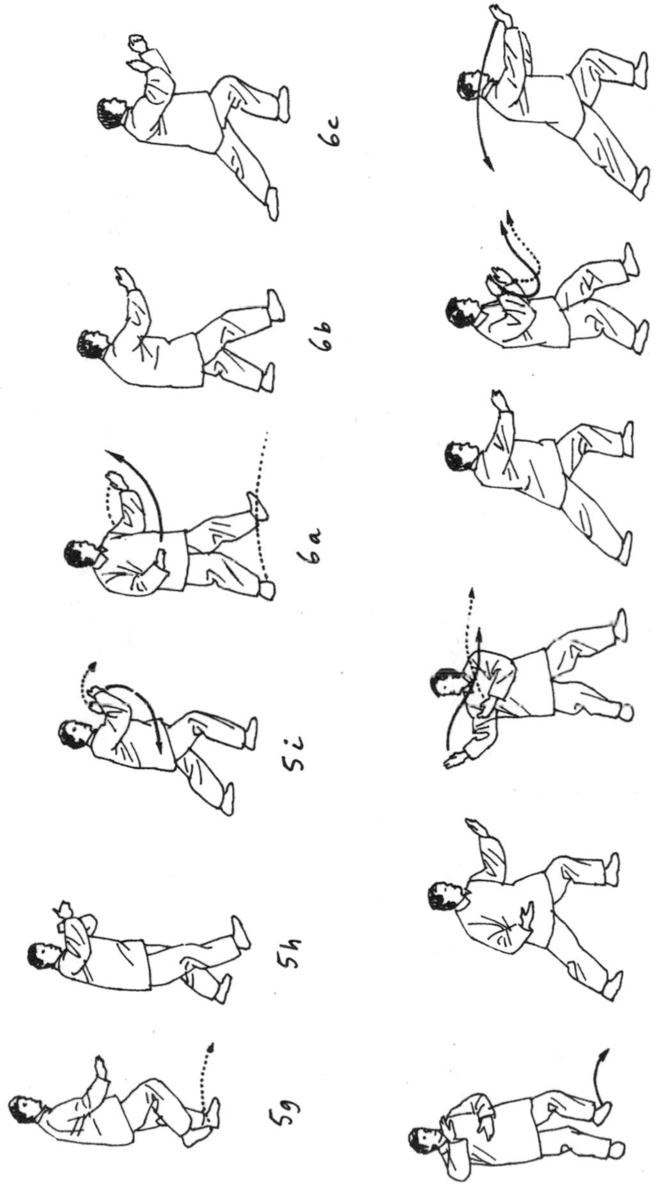

Fig 7.5 48-Pattern Tai Chi Set – Section 1

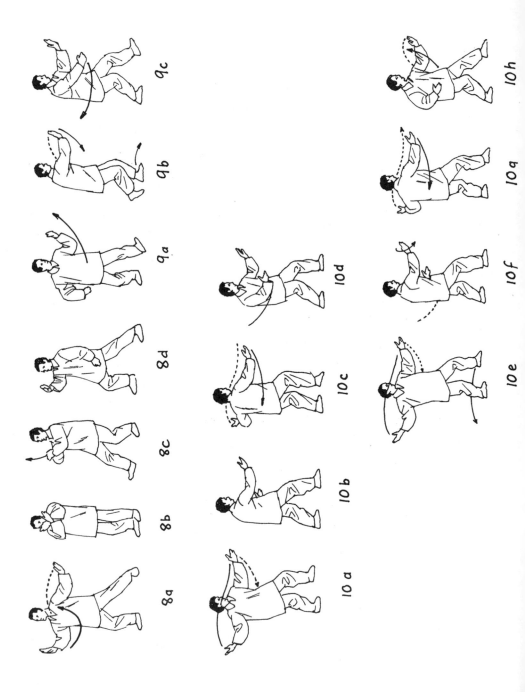

8a
8b
8c
8d
9a
9b
9c
10a
10b
10c
10d
10e
10f
10g
10h

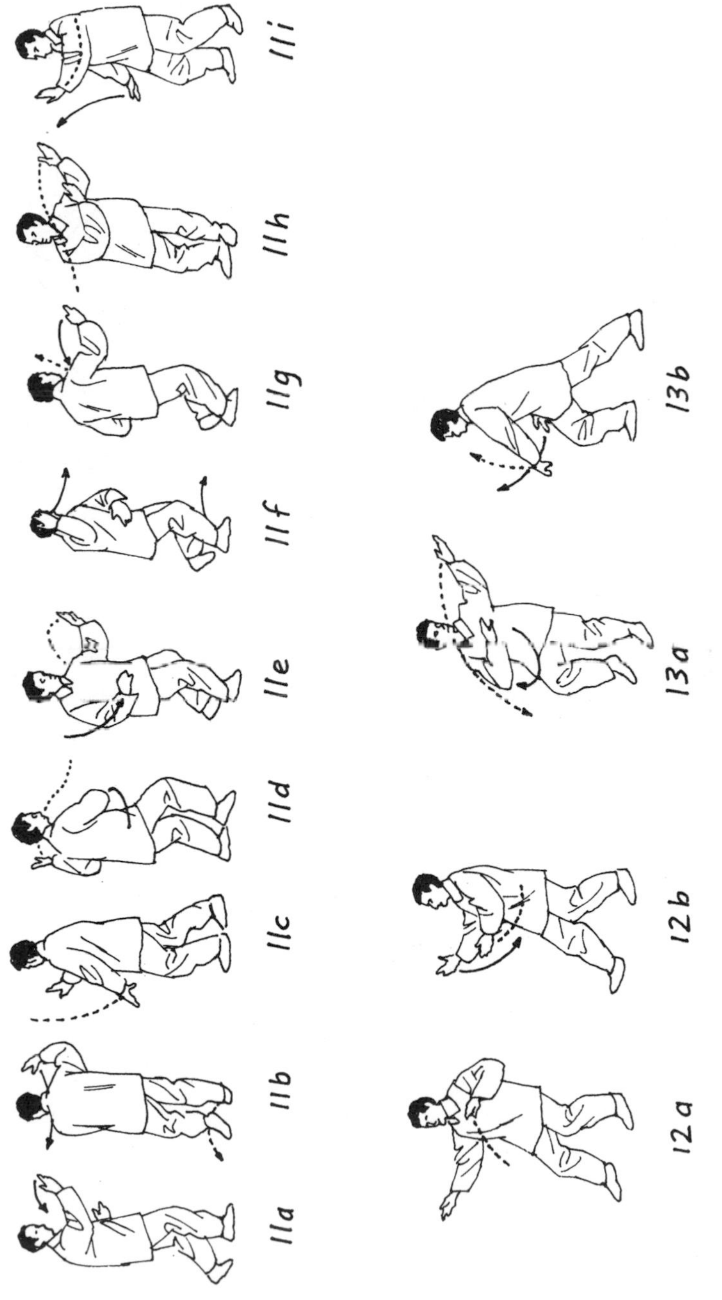

Fig 7.6 48-Pattern Tai Chi Set – Section 2

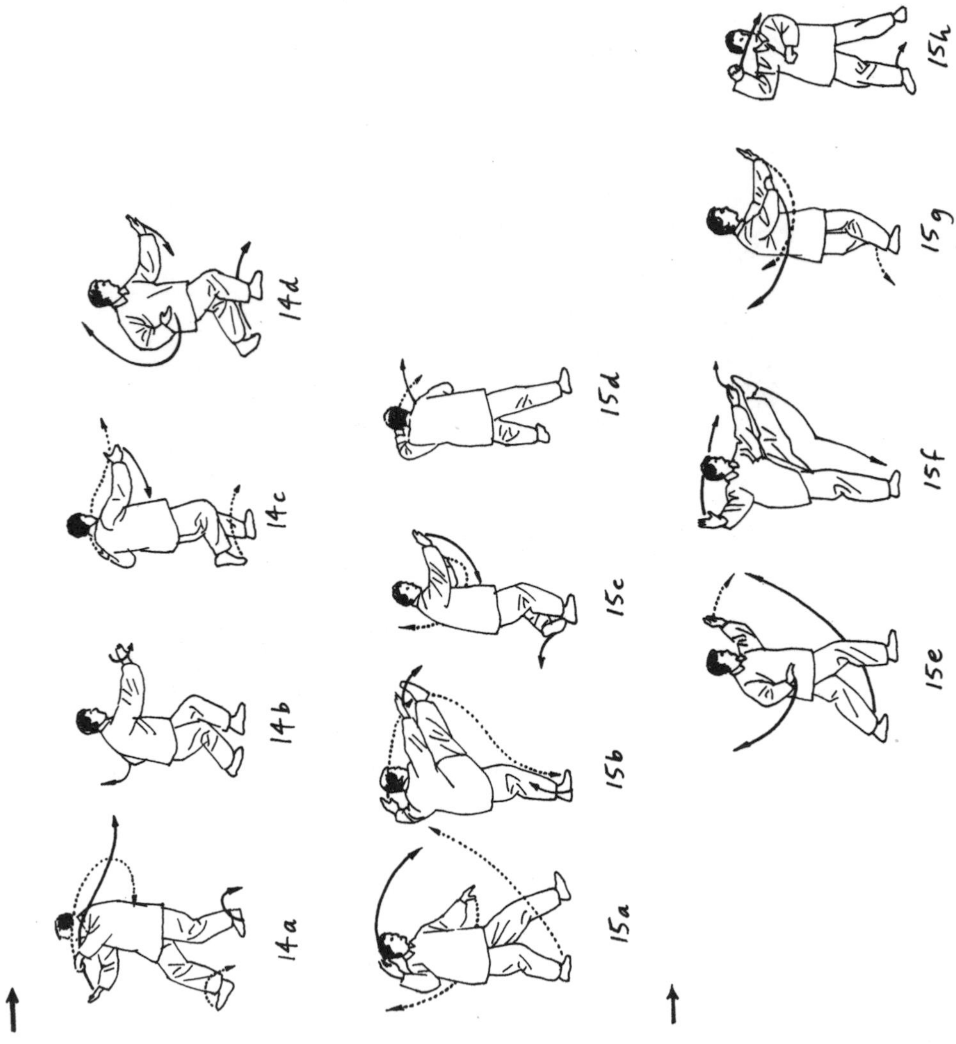

14a
14b
14c
14d
15a
15b
15c
15d
15e
15f
15g
15h

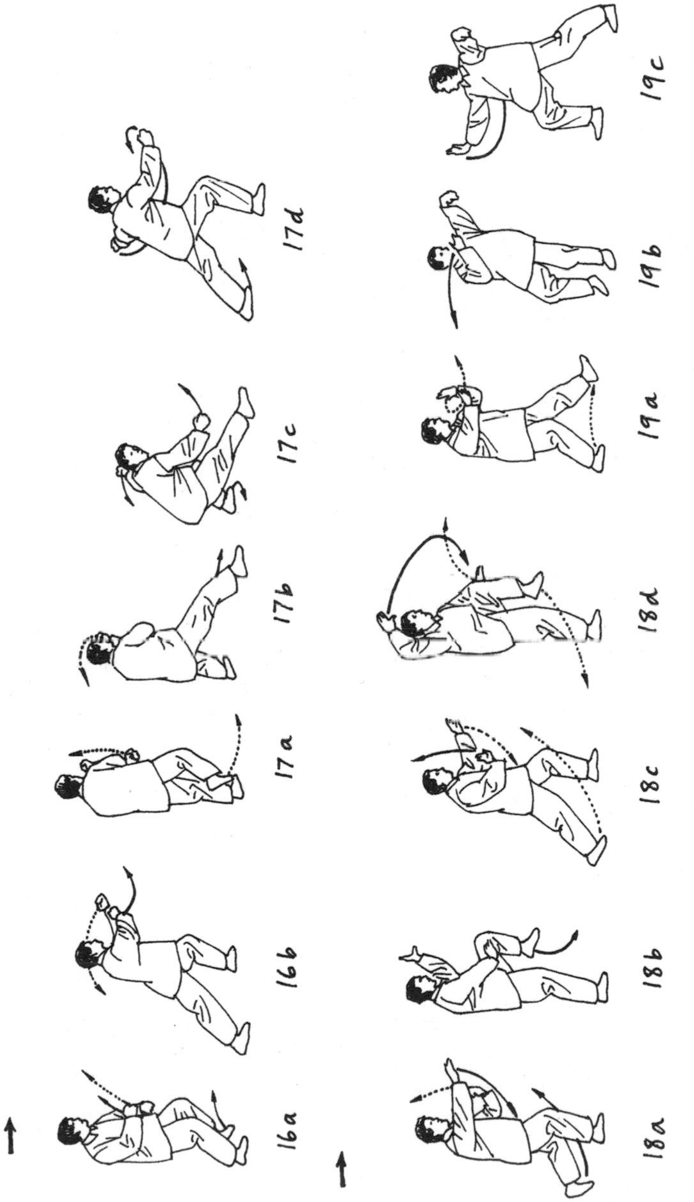

Fig 7.7 48-Pattern Tai Chi Set – Section 3

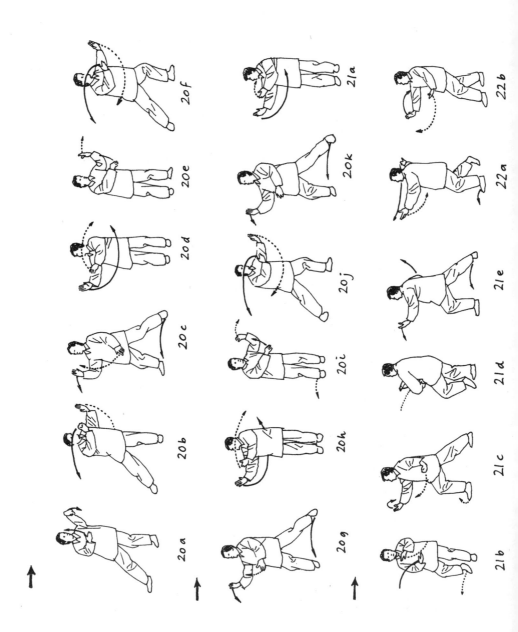
20a
20b
20c
20d
20e
20f
20g
20h
20i
20j
20k
21a
21b
21c
21d
21e
22a
22b

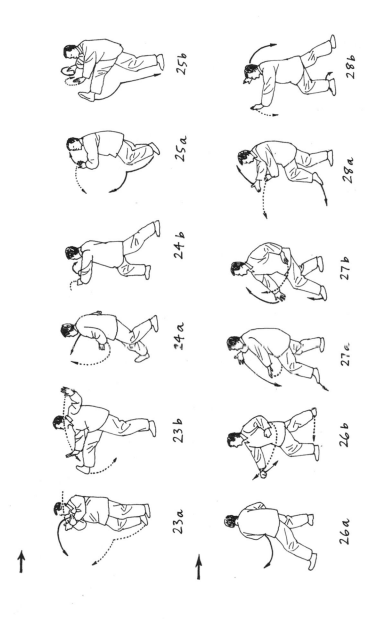

Fig 7.8 48-Pattern Tai Chi Set – Section 4

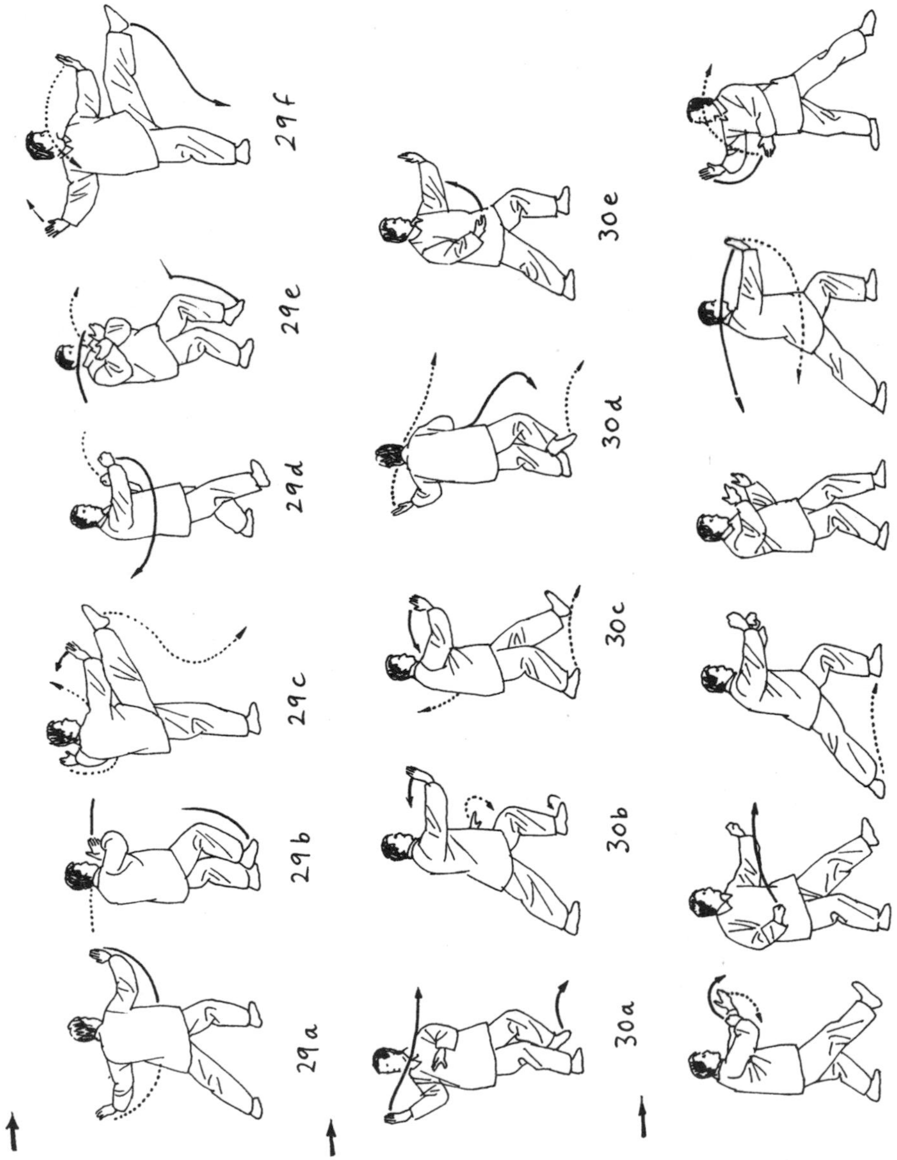
29a
29b
29c
29d
29e
29f
30a
30b
30c
30d
30e
31a
31b
31c
32a
32b
33a

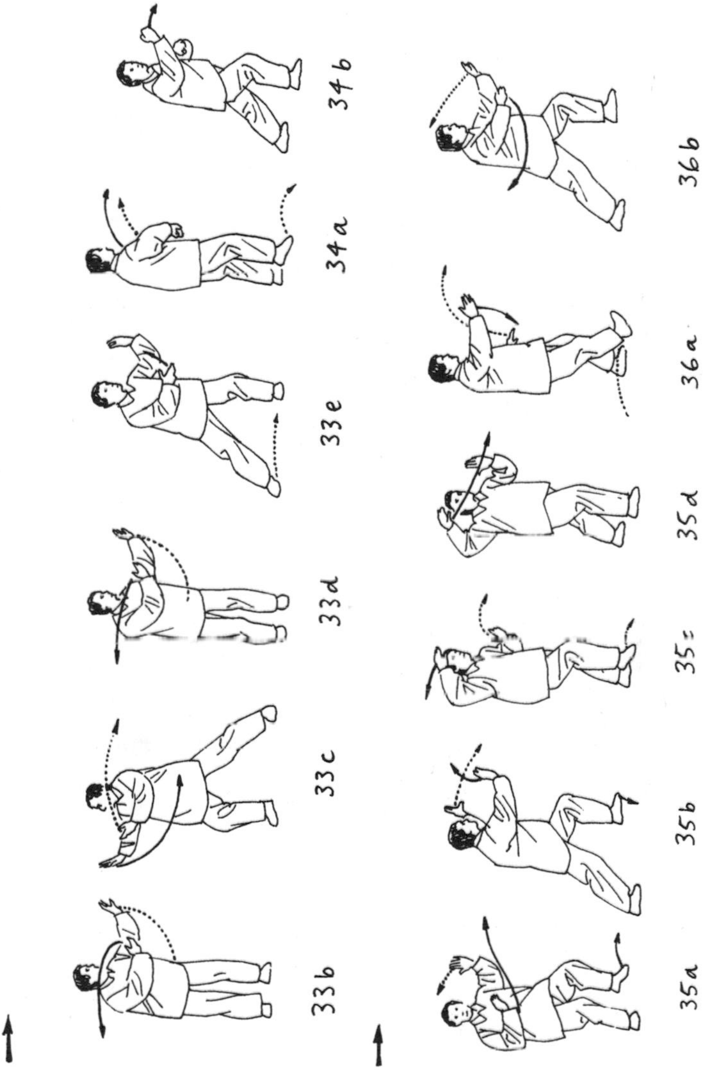

Fig 7.9 48-Pattern Tai Chi Set – Section 5

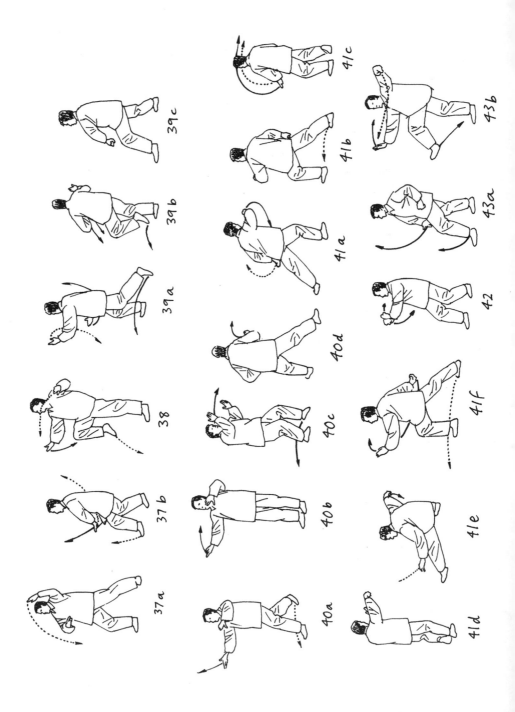
37a
37b
38
39a
39b
39c
40a
40b
40c
40d
41a
41b
41c
41d
41e
41f
42
43a
43b

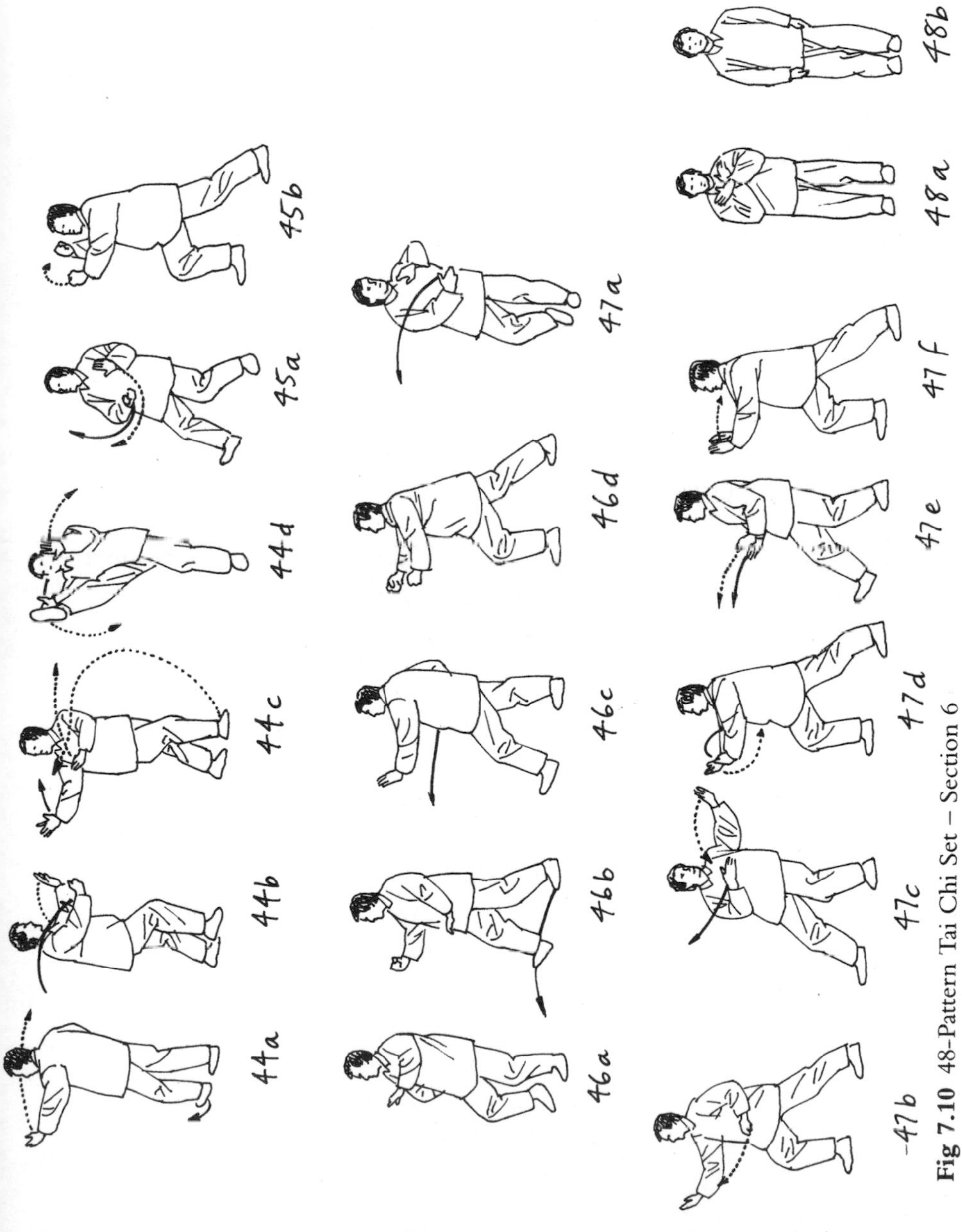

Fig 7.10 48-Pattern Tai Chi Set – Section 6

8

Techniques and Skills of Pushing Hands

How to Sense Your Opponent's Weakness

If you are hasty in your training, as most students unfortunately are, you will find that eventually you merely know the theory behind Pushing Hands but lack the necessary skills to execute the techniques.

The Principles of Pushing Hands

Would you like to develop the skill to sense not only your opponent's movements but also his or her emotions, to use your opponent's strength against him- or herself, and to react with grace and elegance? All these skills can be developed by practising an ingeniously devised system of Tai Chi Chuan training known as *tui shou* or Pushing Hands.

Unlike Tai Chi set practice, there are no fixed sequences in Pushing Hands training. Nevertheless, past masters have handed down the following principles to enhance our practice:

- '*Chi* at *dan tian*, body upright'. Focus your intrinsic energy at your *dan tian*, or the vital energy field in your abdomen, and your body should be relaxed and well balanced.
- 'Use will, but not strength'. Use your heart (or mind) to sense the opponent's movements, and to direct your *chi* flow accordingly, but do not use brute or mechanical strength in your own movements.
- 'Listen to his intention, exploit his strength'. Sense the combative intention of your opponent's movements, follow their momentum, then exploit this momentum.
- 'Move later, arrive earlier'. Your initiative should be a logical result of your opponent's initiative, and is therefore made later. But your move, although it is initated later, accomplishes its purpose earlier than your opponent's. In other words, do not attack first but let your opponent

attack you, and as you neutralize that attack, strike before he or she can recover.

- 'Neutralize locally, strike with the whole body'. Neutralize your opponent's attack at the point of attack, but marshal your whole body (see below) to strike back. For example, if your opponent pushes at your arm or your chest, you merely roll back your arm or rotate your waist to neutralize the attack; it is unnecessary, and unwise, to move your whole body.
- 'Rooted at feet, executed at legs, controlled at waist, materialized at hands'. When you attack with your hands, your power comes not from them but from your feet, executed through your legs and controlled by your waist. For example, if you push your opponent, the power of the push does not come from your palms, but is channelled all the way from your feet through your legs, body and palms into your opponent.

These six principles serve as guidelines as well as the objectives of Pushing Hands training. In other words, as you practise the exercises, bear them in mind, and your training will lead to the development, among other benefits, of the skills associated with them, such as good balance, elegance and the ability to turn your opponent's strength against him or her.

Sharpening Your Skills of Perception

Before attempting Pushing Hands, you must be familiar with the basic Tai Chi forms (see Chapter 5) and have developed some internal force in your Chi Kung training (see Chapter 6); otherwise you will not gain the benefits of this wonderful aspect of Tai Chi Chuan.

You and your training partner face each other in a right Bow-arrow Stance with your right arms in contact in the *peng* or warding off position, and your left hands near your right elbows *(figure 8.1a)*. Without moving the body or changing stance, your partner pushes his or her right arm forward using the *peng* technique. Yielding to this movement, roll back your right arm using the *lu* technique; still continuing the momentum, move your partner's arm round in an arc and then push forward using the *peng* technique. In this way each of you alternately push forward and roll back your arms.

Your arms should be in constant contact (as they should be in all Pushing Hands exercises), and should move in a continuous oval *(figure 8.1b)*. Sometimes you can move them in a figure of eight *(figure 8.1c)*. Repeat this exercise using the left arms in a left Bow-arrow Stance –

indeed, all Pushing Hands exercises should be done twice, once with each arm. This particular exercise is called *peng-lu*, or warding off and rolling back.

Sometimes, one of you may succeed in pushing your arm forward so close to the other person's body that the latter has difficulty diverting it away to continue the exercise *(figure 8.1d)*. This difficulty can easily be overcome if the defender sinks back by bending the back leg and shifting the body back *(figure 8.1e)*. As soon as the attacking arm has been pushed away in a curve, and without breaking the momentum, shift the body forward, without moving your feet, to re-establish the Bow-arrow Stance, and push your arm forward to continue the exercise.

The simplicity of this *peng-lu* exercise is deceptive. The purpose of the training is not just to develop the techniques of *peng* and *lu*, which can be learnt in five minutes, but to develop sensitivity and internal force in the arm, which will take many months of *daily* practice. If you perform this *peng-lu* movement continuously (and correctly) at least 100 times per session, focusing your mind on your arm to sense your partner's movement and flowing with that movement without the slightest resistance, you may get some idea of what is meant by developing sensitivity. And if you practise for a few sessions daily for at least 100 days, you should find that your arm is moved not by your muscular action but by flowing *chi* in your arm. You will also discover that this *chi* not only generates internal power but also follows the direction of your mind.

You may have heard or read that practising Tai Chi Chuan, or any style of kungfu, successfully demands a great deal of patience and self-discipline. Practising this seemingly simple exercise at least 100 times per session, for a few sessions per day, for at least 100 days, will give you some idea of how much patience and self-discipline is needed. But you will certainly be rewarded. Apart from patience and self-discipline, which are in themselves highly desirable qualities, you will develop sensitivity and internal force, as well as experiencing directly the saying that there is much profundity in simplicity.

Throwing Your Partner Off the Ground

As your flowing meditation and perception become enhanced through your *peng-lu* exercise, you can sense not only the intention and direction of your partner's arm movement, but also that person's balance and emotion. When you sense that your partner's balance or emotional state falters, for example through a momentary break in momentum or an

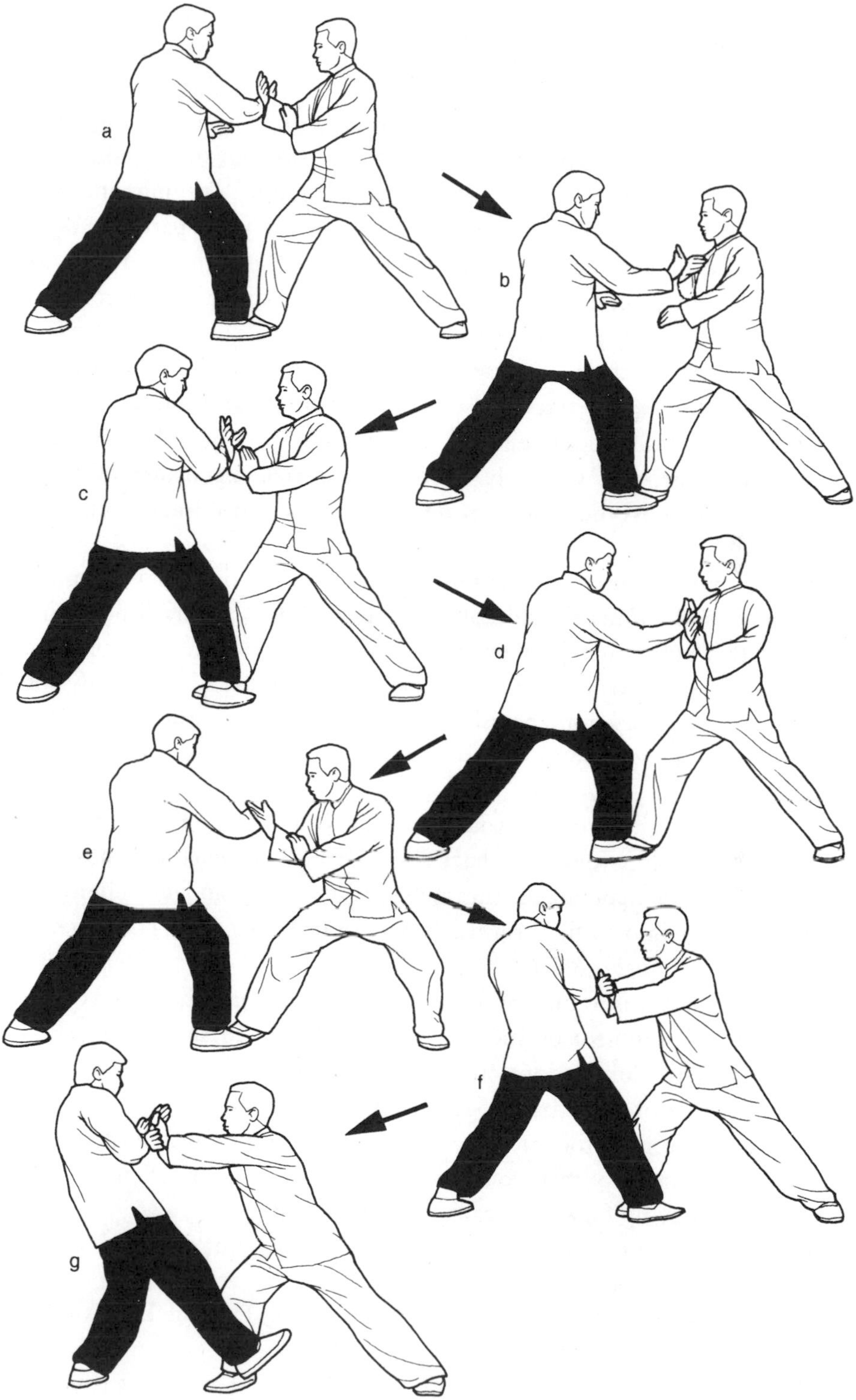

Fig 8.1 The *Peng-Lu* exercise

indication of uncertainty, you can exploit this opportunity and push him or her over. One basic way of accomplishing this is the *qi* or pressing technique *(figure 8.1f)*. As you push forward using the usual *peng* technique with your right arm, place your left palm on your inner right wrist, and change the *peng* technique to the *qi* technique, pushing simultaneously with your right forearm and left hand at your partner's body, making him or her fall backwards *(figure 8.1g)*. But remember that the power of your push comes not from your right forearm nor your left palm, but from your back leg.

Do not attempt this technique unless you have spent at least two weeks on the simple *peng-lu* exercise to develop sensitivity and internal force – in fact two months would be better. If you are impatient or lack the necessary discipline, you will only learn the external mechanics of the *qi* technique and miss the chance of developing the more important internal skills.

At first when one of you has sensed a weakness in the other and presses or pushes, the other should not resist but let him- or herself be pushed away so that both can experience what it is like to push and to be pushed. Then you should resume the *peng-lu* exercise, with the objective of sensing an opening for another push. If the push is unsuccessful in sending the partner off the ground, then continue the *peng-lu* exercise without a break.

At a later stage, as soon as you sense that you are being pushed, lower your stance, ie shift your body backwards, bend your back leg and lower your body, thus neutralizing the attack *(figures 8.2a* and *b)*. Then shift your body forward to the original Bow-arrow Stance, and continue the *peng-lu* exercise *(figure 8.2c)*.

If your partner is too far away for you to use the *qi* technique, you can overcome this problem by moving your legs forward simultaneously as you press. This can be done in one of the following two ways. Root yourself firmly on your back leg and take a big step forward with your front leg as you press forward *(figures 8.3a* and *b)*. Immediately drag your back leg forward so that you resume your Bow-arrow Stance. This method of moving forward is called the drag step.

Alternatively, bring your back leg a bit forward, but still behind your front leg *(figure 8.3c)*, and using this back leg as an anchor, propel your body forward with the *qi* technique *(figure 8.3d)*. This method is called the push step.

Notice that in both methods, the pressing force comes not from the pressing arm but from the back leg. You should also notice that while

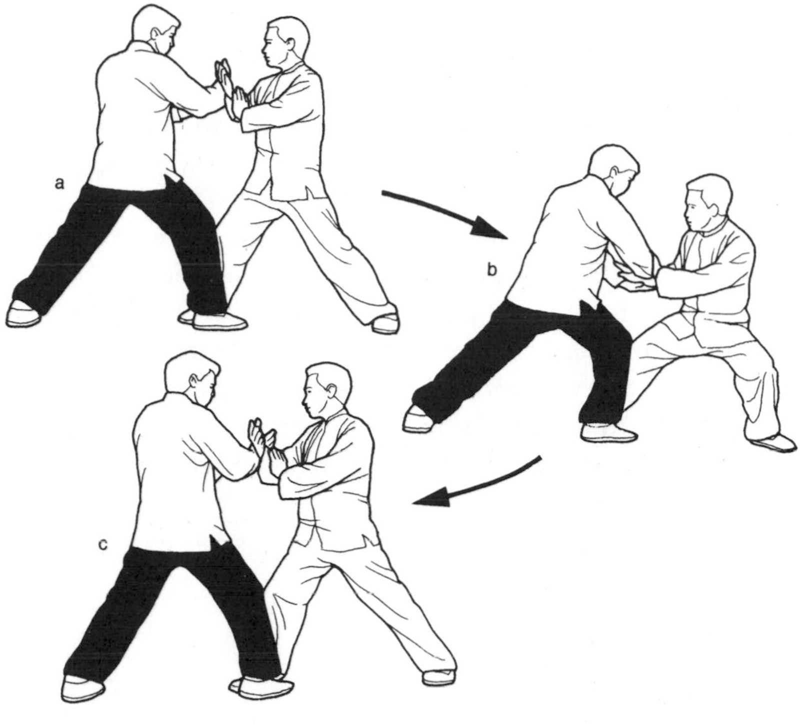

Fig 8.2 Neutralizing an opponent's push

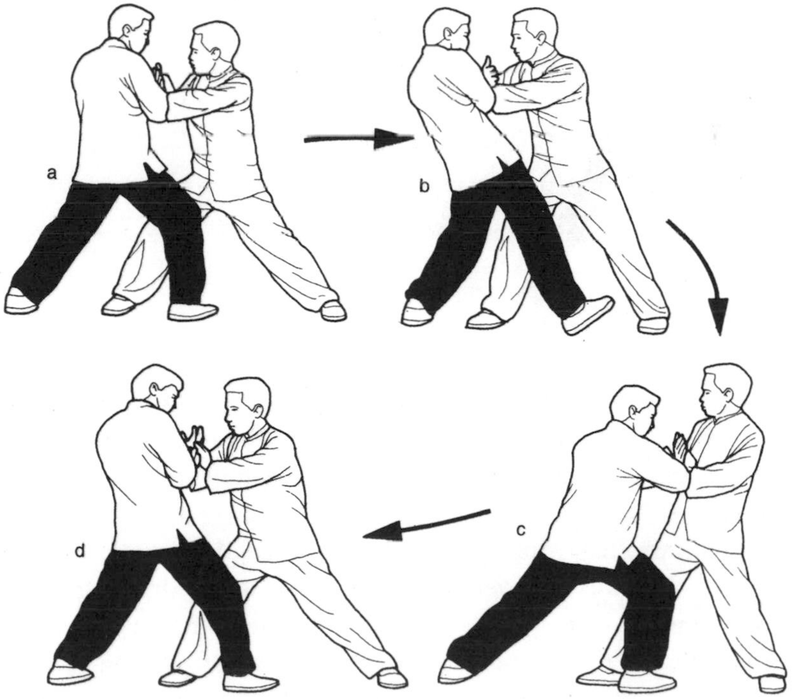

Fig 8.3 Drag step and push step

both methods are forceful, there is an innate weakness: if your opponent can sense and exploit the moment when you have just begun but not completed your step, he or she can easily fell you. This moment of weakness, alternatively known as the golden moment of attack, is described as 'when old strength is spent, but new strength has not started'.

One effective way of neutralizing the *qi* technique is the *an* or pushing technique. If your partner presses forward without moving the feet *(figure 8.4a)*, follow the momentum but simultaneously shift your body backwards without moving your feet, and lower your partner's right hand with your left hand, and your partner's left hand with your right hand, as shown in *figure 8.4b*. At the golden moment when the other person's old strength is spent but new strength has not started, push forward with the *an* technique *(figure 8.4c)*.

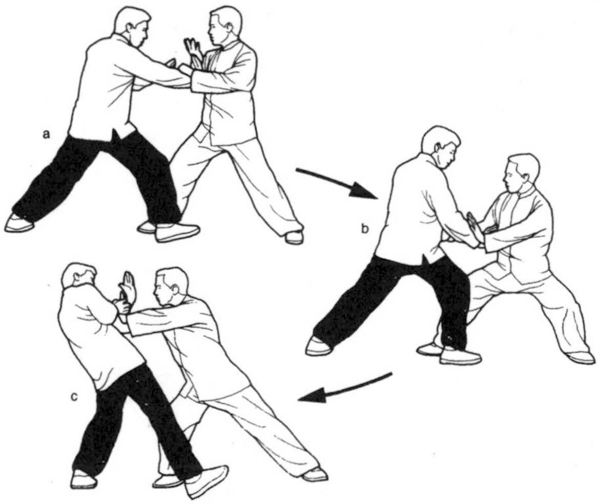

Fig 8.4 The *Qi-An* exercise

If your partner does move the feet forward, using the drag or the push step, you should move your feet backward to deny the other person any advantage he seeks. This can be done by using the pull step or the roll step as follows.

Figure 8.5a shows that your partner, having moved forward, has an advantage over you. You can overcome this advantage by moving your back leg back, pulling your front leg along and, following the momentum, lower your partner's hands *(figure 8.5b)*. This way of moving back is called the pull step. At the golden moment, push forward with the *an* technique *(figure 8.5c)*.

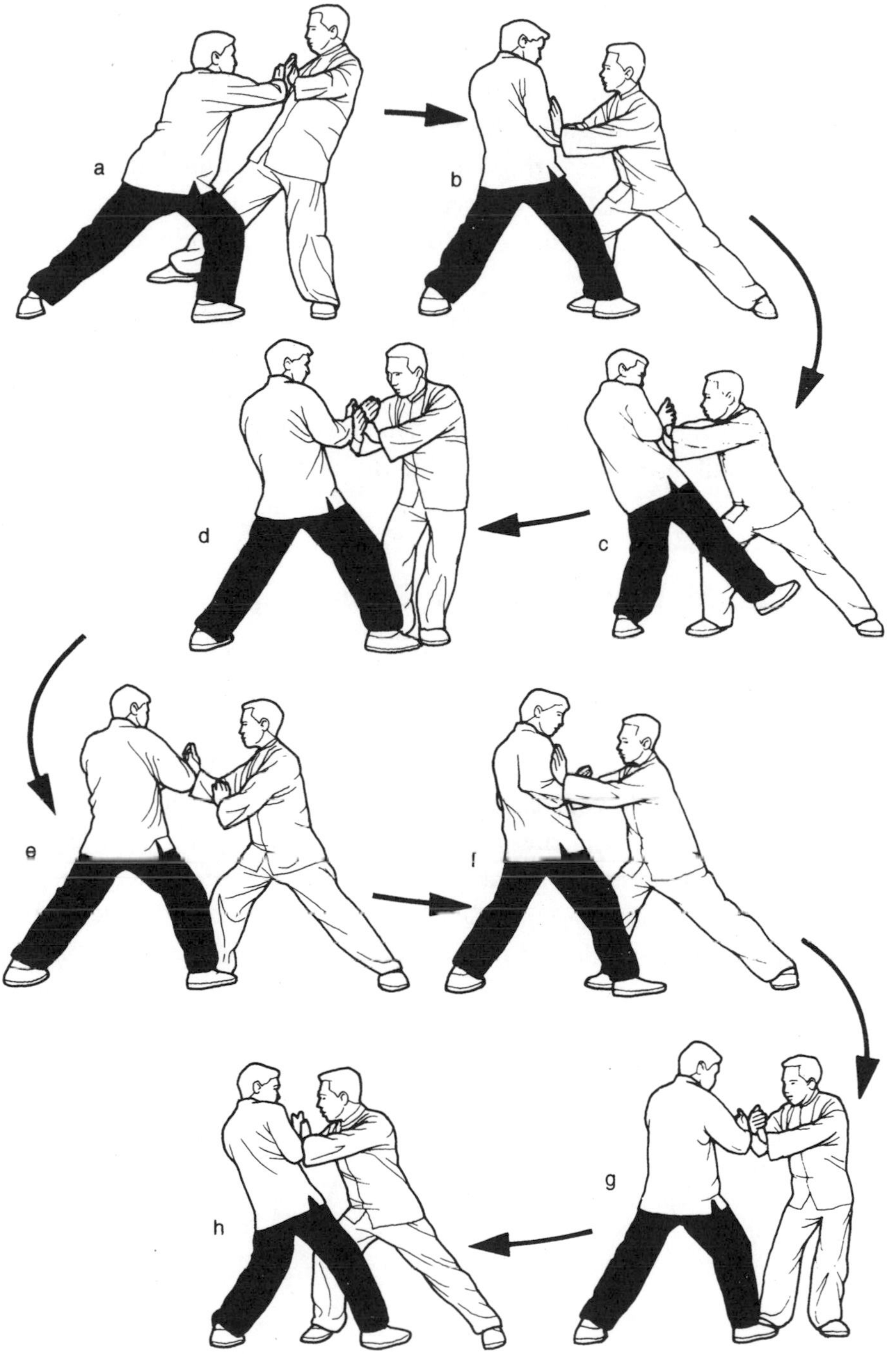

Fig 8.5 Pull step and roll step

Alternatively, as your partner moves forward, move your front leg a short distance back, but still in front of your other leg *(figure 8.5d)*; as your partner presses forward, move your back leg back, thus neutralizing the press *(figure 8.5e)*. This method is called the roll step. Then using the *an* technique, push your partner back *(figure 8.5f)*.

When either person is thrown off the ground, come back to resume the exercise. If an attack is unsuccessful because it is poorly executed, or if a successful attack is also successfully neutralized, continue the exercise without break.

When there is a lot of space between you and your partner, you will have to move forward while pushing. You can use the drag or the push step to do so or, if you are fairly advanced, you can use a half-roll step while lowering your partner's hands. Move your front leg a short distance back, but still in front of the other leg *(figure 8.5g)*. Then move the same leg forward as you push *(figure 8.5h)*.

Seeking the Best Angle and Closing Up

It may not be easy to push someone with a solid stance off the ground, even if he or she fails to neutralize your attack. One way to overcome this problem is to seek the best angle from which to push; this is usually from one side instead of from the front. Let us assume that you are facing north. As you guide your partner's arm towards him or her in an oval or a figure of eight, using the *peng* technique, move your front leg (your right leg if you are standing in a right Bow-arrow Stance), diagonally forward to north-east, move your left leg forward and turn left so that you are standing in your left Bow-arrow Stance facing west *(figure 8.6a)*. Push from your partner's left side with both palms, using the *an* technique.

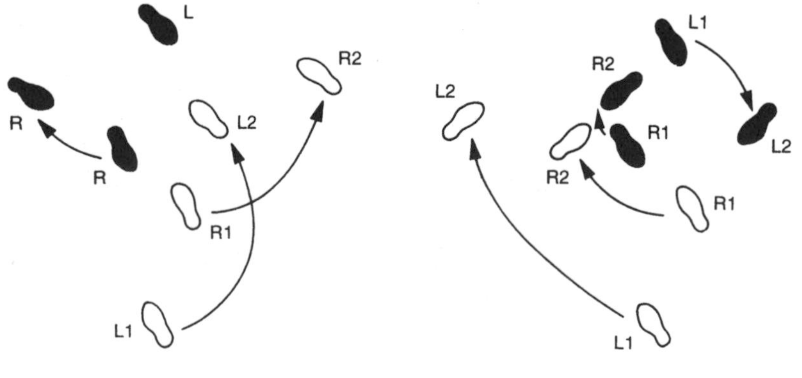

Fig 8.6 Attacking from the side

To neutralize this attack, if you are the defender, move your right leg, if you are standing in a right Bow-arrow Stance, back in the direction of north-west, and turn left so as to stand in a left Bow-arrow Stance facing east *(figure 8.6a)*.

Instead of moving to your partner's left (your right side), you can of course move to the right. When your partner is pushing towards you (not when you are pushing towards your partner as above), guide his or her arm towards your right, move your back (left) leg diagonally forward to the north-west *(figure 8.6b)*, followed by your front (right) leg. Turn right to stand in a right Bow-arrow Stance facing east, and push with both palms at your partner's right side. To neutralize your advantage, your partner could move the back (left) leg diagonally forward in the direction of south-east and turn right into a right Bow-arrow Stance to face you.

Another way of gaining an advantage is to close up an opponent, especially one who is pushing you with both hands. *Figure 8.7a* shows one partner pushing the other's right arm with both hands. To neutralize such a push, lower your body backwards and simultaneously place your left hand under your right arm. Move your left hand forward as you pull back your right arm in what is known as the threading technique *(figure 8.7b)*. Then shift your body forward (or move a step forward if necessary) and push your partner's left arm so that it is bent at the elbow with the forearm pressing against the right arm so that it is difficult for him or her to use both hands *(figure 8.7c)*. Later when you are doing combat application, you may close up your opponent with one hand and strike with the other.

But it is easy to neutralize a closing up if you know how. All you need to do is to sink back *(figure 8.7d)*, and ward off your opponent's arm *(figure 8.7e)*. Then you can continue with the exercise.

A good opportunity to use this technique is when your partner attempts to gain the advantage of a better angle. Suppose you are both in the right *peng* or warding off position in the right Bow-arrow Stance and your partner attempts to move to your left to push you, using the foot movements illustrated in *figure 8.6a*. Move your front right leg back and to your right, turn left to face your partner, sink back to neutralize the push, thread with your left hand and close up. Your partner can neutralize this move by sinking back and warding off with the left arm. Now, as both of you are in the left *peng* position in the left Bow-arrow Stance, you can continue the whole sequence of exercises on your left side.

You will have noticed that the exercises described so far all use the *peng, lu, qi* and *an* techniques, the four primary hand movements which collectively constitute the pattern known as Grasping Sparrow's Tail,

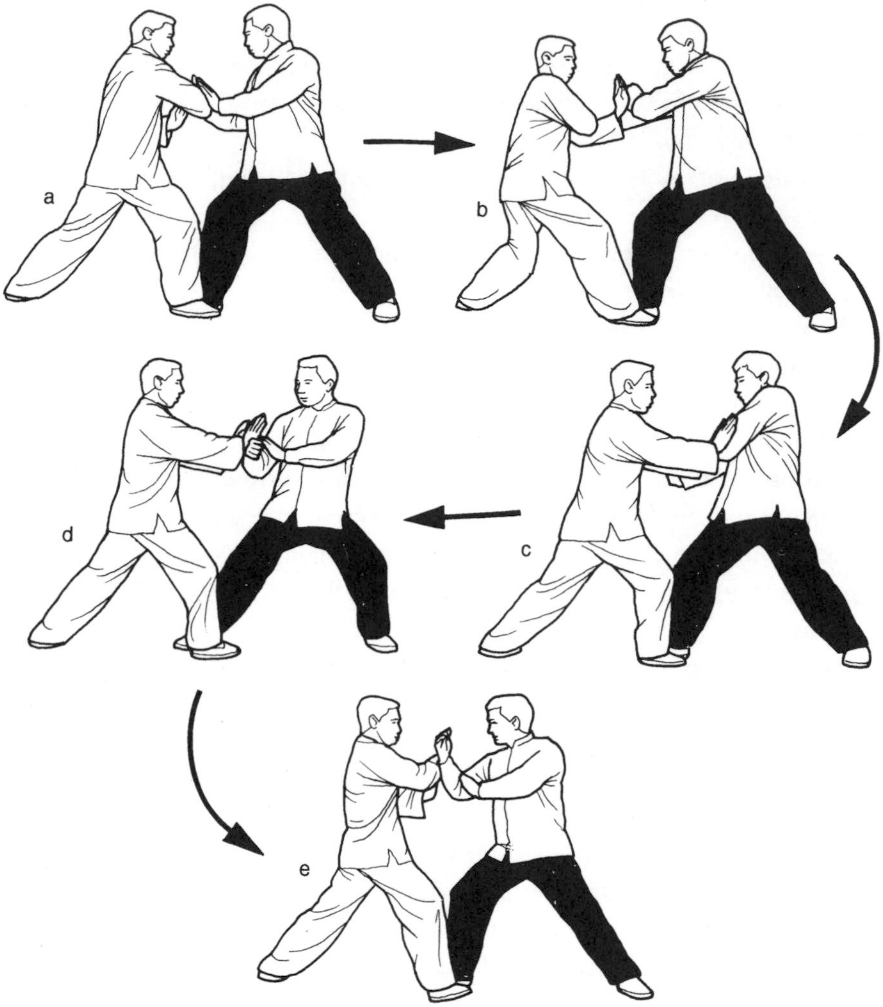

Fig 8.7 The closing up technique

considered by many masters as the most important pattern in Tai Chi Chuan. Moreover all five of the basic leg movements – moving forward, moving back, moving to the left, moving to the right and remaining in the centre – are also used.

You will probably get more enjoyment from your Pushing Hands training if you treat it as a game. Draw a circle, about 3 feet in radius, around you and your partner, leaving you no room to move back. Play Pushing Hands inside the circle, scoring a point each time you push your partner out, with the first to get three points as the winner. At first, do not allow the feet to be moved from the standing position. Next, say that only the attacker's feet may be moved (so that the defender can sense it and exploit the opening). Finally, allow both of you to move your feet. Later you can draw an outer circle with a radius of about 4 or 5 feet, so that the defender can retreat out of the inner circle into the outer circle. Give one point every time one of you is forced out of the inner circle, and three points every time you are pushed out of the outer circle, with the first to gain ten points as the winner. *Figure 8.8* shows just such a playing area.

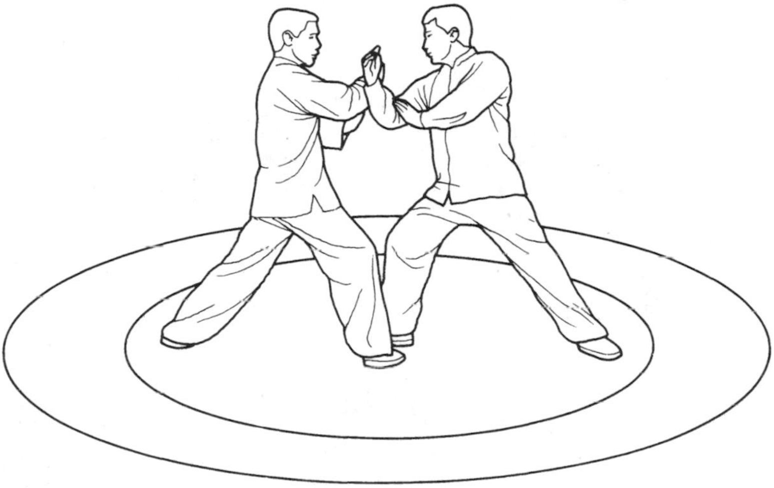

Fig 8.8 Inner and outer circles for Pushing Hands

Advanced Techniques of Pushing Hands

When you have practised Pushing Hands sufficiently using the four primary hand movements, you can move on to use the four secondary movements. You can start with the standard *peng-lu* oval, or continue from the pushing or closing up attack described earlier. Remember that Pushing Hands does not follow a prearranged routine; as in free sparring, all the hand and leg movements in Pushing Hands are made spontaneously for each situation as it arises.

When your partner pushes at you from the standard *peng-lu* oval, you can respond with any of the four primary hand movements or with any of the four secondary hand movements, as we are about to see. You can also use any of the five basic leg movements to complement the hand movements.

Let us start the more advanced part of our training with the *peng-lu* oval, with the right arms in contact and at the right Bow-arrow Stance *(figure 8.9a)*. As your partner pushes with the right arm, follow the momentum. Guide the arm to your right, shift your body back into a

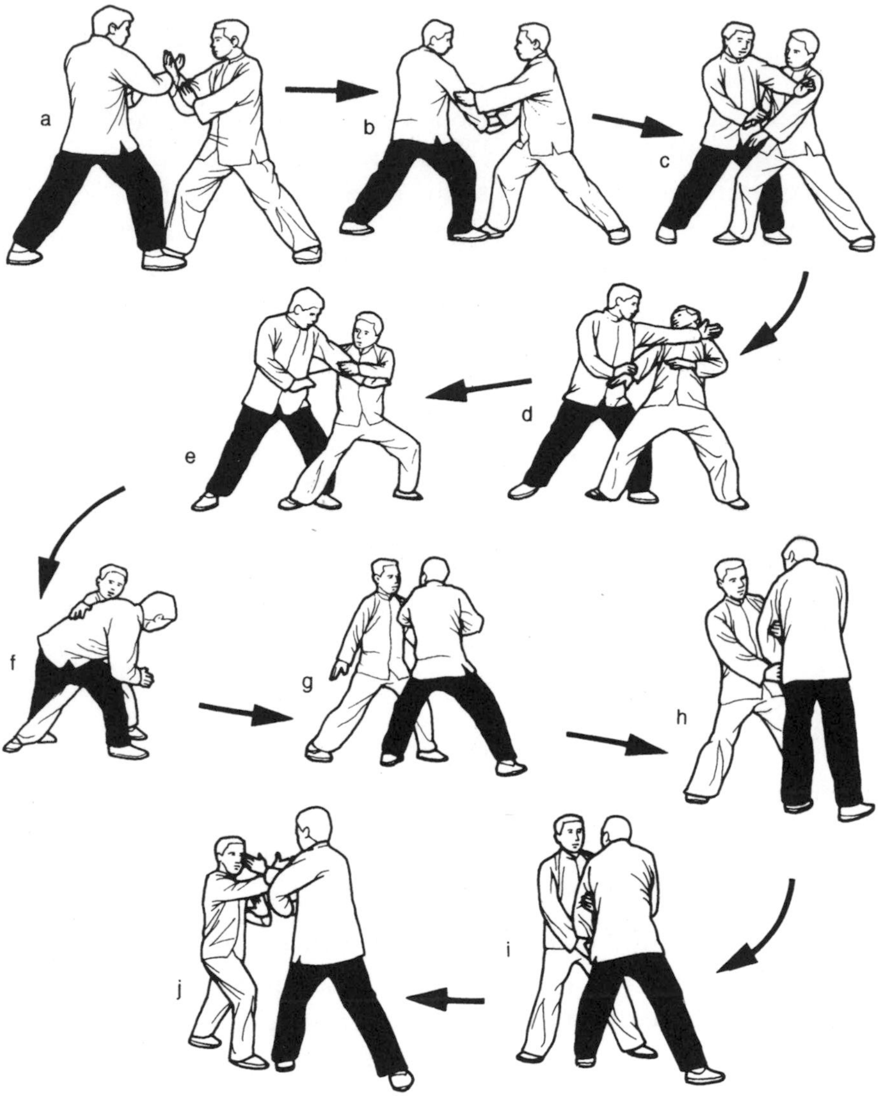

Fig 8.9 Advanced Pushing Hands

right Four-six Stance and grip the wrist with your right hand and the elbow with your left hand *(figure 8.9b)*, using the *cai* or taking technique in the pattern called Playing the Lute.

To counter this attack, your partner can move the back left leg forward and place it behind you to act as an anchor *(figure 8.9c)*, at the same time spreading the left arm across your chest, pushing you backwards, while the right hand prevents your hands from striking back, using the *lie* technique with the pattern Flying Diagonally *(figure 8.9d)*.

However, you can easily overcome this attack with a seemingly simple technique. As you sense this spreading attack, move your back leg just a little further back *(figure 8.9e)*, turn left, pull your partner's left wrist with your left hand, and his or her waist with your right hand so that he or she falls over your right leg *(figure 8.9f)*. This is the *lu* or rolling back technique. Do not be alarmed to find that this *lu* technique is different from the one described earlier in the basic Pushing Hands exercises. One technique may be implemented in many ways with different functions. You will learn yet another application of this technique later in the chapter.

Your partner can overcome your attack by moving the back leg forward, thus avoiding falling, turning left into a left Bow-arrow Stance and jabbing you with the left elbow *(figure 8.9g)*. This is the *zhou* or elbowing technique.

You in turn should take one step back, maintaining your grip on your partner's left arm and twist it back *(figure 8.9h)*. This is the *cai* or taking technique.

Your partner can then move the back leg forward, and using it like a propeller, thrust the front leg deep in between your legs, ramming the left shoulder onto your solar plexus *(figure 8.9i)*.

You should take back either leg and lift up your arm into the *peng* or warding off position *(figure 8.9j)*. Your partner then also adopts the *peng* position as protection in case you strike the upper body. From this position you can both continue with Pushing Hands.

Pushing Hands and Combat Efficiency

The basic and advanced exercises described in this chapter will give you some idea of how you can practise the art of Pushing Hands. Allow your movements to develop spontaneously from each situation, and pay careful attention to the six principles explained at the start of this chapter. For instance, in the *lu* technique above, you should be able to pull your partner almost effortlessly if you correctly sense the *lie* or spreading attack, and execute your pull at the right time. If your perception, timing, spacing or other factors are wrong, your pull will not work, even if you use brute strength – and that of course, would defeat the whole purpose of Pushing Hands training.

Your main objective, therefore, is first to listen to your partner's or opponent's weakness, which includes any faulty moves as well as any emotional distractions, and then to exploit that weakness. You should not, as many novices do, try to push or pull your partner if no favourable opening arises, as that will result in a clumsy contest of brute strength.

It needs to be emphasized again that the essence of training is developing skills, not merely learning techniques. Different people progress at different rates but as a rough guide you should, having spent some time on internal force training and familiarized yourself with a Tai Chi set, spend at least six months practising these Pushing Hands exercises.

While Pushing Hands provides an excellent preparation for combat, as well as providing many other benefits, it is insufficient by itself for fighting. How would you defend yourself if an opponent in actual

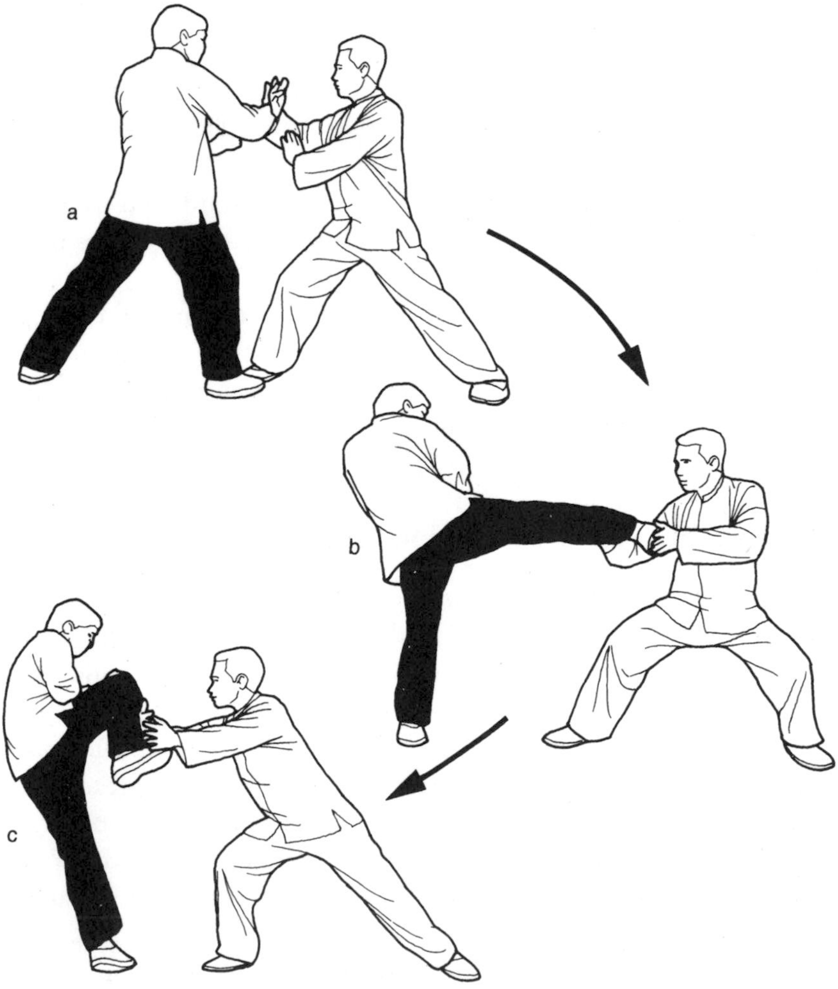

Fig 8.10 Overcoming a side kick with the *lu* Technique

combat suddenly gave you a side kick or a round-house kick while you were engaged in Pushing Hands?

Figure 8.10a shows two exponents in the *peng-lu* position. In *figure 8.10b* one launches a side kick; following the momentum, the other holds the kicking leg with the *lu* technique. And in *figure 8.10c* the defender throws the opponent away with the *qi* technique.

In *figure 8.11a* one exponent closes up the other's arm. In *figure 8.11b* the opponent moves the front leg a short distance back and threads the left hand, thus neutralizing the close-up, following with a round-house kick with the other leg *(figure 8.11c)*. The defender lowers his or her stance backwards to avoid the kick. Then just as the kick passes, the defender moves forward with a drag step and fells the opponent with a *lie* or spreading technique before the latter has recovered from the attack *(figure 8.11d)*. The Tai Chi Chuan exponent can overcome the assailant because besides having the combative skills derived from Pushing Hands training:, he or she knows and effectively applies combat techniques, which will be explained in detail in the next chapter.

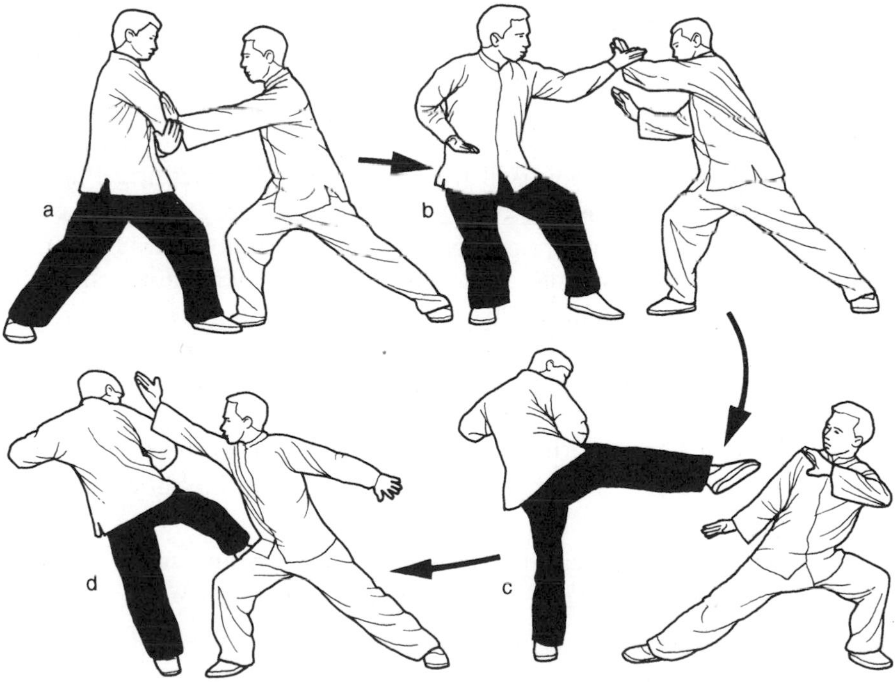

Fig 8.11 Overcoming a round-house kick with *lie*

9

Specific Techniques for Combat Situations

Applying Tai Chi Chuan Patterns for Self-defence

Requirements for Combat Proficiency

It is worth remembering that Tai Chi Chuan is not a gentle dance, not even a set of health exercises; it is basically a martial art. And it is not an ordinary martial art. Unlike most others, it is graceful and elegant even when it is used in fighting, and it abhors aggression which is a prominent feature of many fighting systems. Interestingly, because of the nature of Tai Chi Chuan itself, aggression actually detracts from the exponent's ability to fight well – as you will have discovered in practising Pushing Hands, where mental calmness and physical elegance are essential to good performance. But even more significant is that at its highest levels Tai Chi Chuan expands the mind and cultivates spirituality, two features that will be discussed in some detail in Chapters 12, 13 and 21.

To enjoy the rewards of Tai Chi Chuan as an effective martial art, you need to be proficient in the following:

- basic Tai Chi Chuan forms and movements, which can be developed by practising a Tai Chi set, such as the 24-pattern Simplified Tai Chi Set
- internal force, which can be developed by practising static and dynamic Chi Kung, as in the Tai Chi Stance and Lifting Water
- combat skills like sensing the opponent's movements, sound judgement, good timing, reflexive action and fluidity of movements, which can be developed in Pushing Hands
- combat techniques, such as the appropriate actions to take against aggressive moves in order to obtain the best technical advantage, which

can be learnt by practising specific individual techniques and short series of combat sequences
- combat principles, which summarize tactical and strategic considerations in given situations, and which can be culled from the writings of past masters

This list shows that if you learn only the Tai Chi forms and nothing else, you will at best only derive 20 per cent of the potential benefits of Tai Chi Chuan for self defence, since form is only one of the requirements. And since self-defence is only one of the many benefits of practising Tai Chi Chuan – the others being health and fitness, emotional stability, mind expansion and spiritual joy – even if you spend your whole life practising the art, you will only gain 20 per cent of 20 per cent of the potential benefits – ie only 4 per cent.

Of course, this analysis is not accurate, but it does show how much you will be missing if you concentrate on form alone. This book aims to supply the knowledge you need to increase the benefits you derive from your practice, but the actual work must be done by you.

From Lifting Water to Repulse Monkey

Although many people are impressed with the beauty of a Tai Chi Chuan performance, all its forms and movements are based on martial considerations, not on pleasing spectators. Here I will explain the martial functions of the 24 patterns of the Simplified Tai Chi Set we learnt in Chapter 7. A basic approach is to practise their specific techniques, or *san shou* in Chinese, ie to learn and practise applying a particular pattern or technique in a specific combat situation.

To apply the techniques efficiently, it is necessary to have a stable stance, good balance and internal force. The application of some Tai Chi Chuan techniques may be difficult if it is not backed by sufficient internal force.

Lifting Water, also called Tai Chi Starting Pattern, is a technique for developing internal force, but it also has a combat function. If someone is holding your wrists *(figure 9.1a)*, you can release them by using this pattern *(figure 9.1b)*.

In the hands of a master, Flying Diagonally can be a very versatile pattern. In addition to being used to knock an opponent down, it can be used as follows. If your wrists are being held, as in *figure 9.1c* you can release the hold by a typical Tai Chi circular turn *(figure 9.1d)*,and strike your opponent's face with the side of your palm *(figure 9.1e)*.

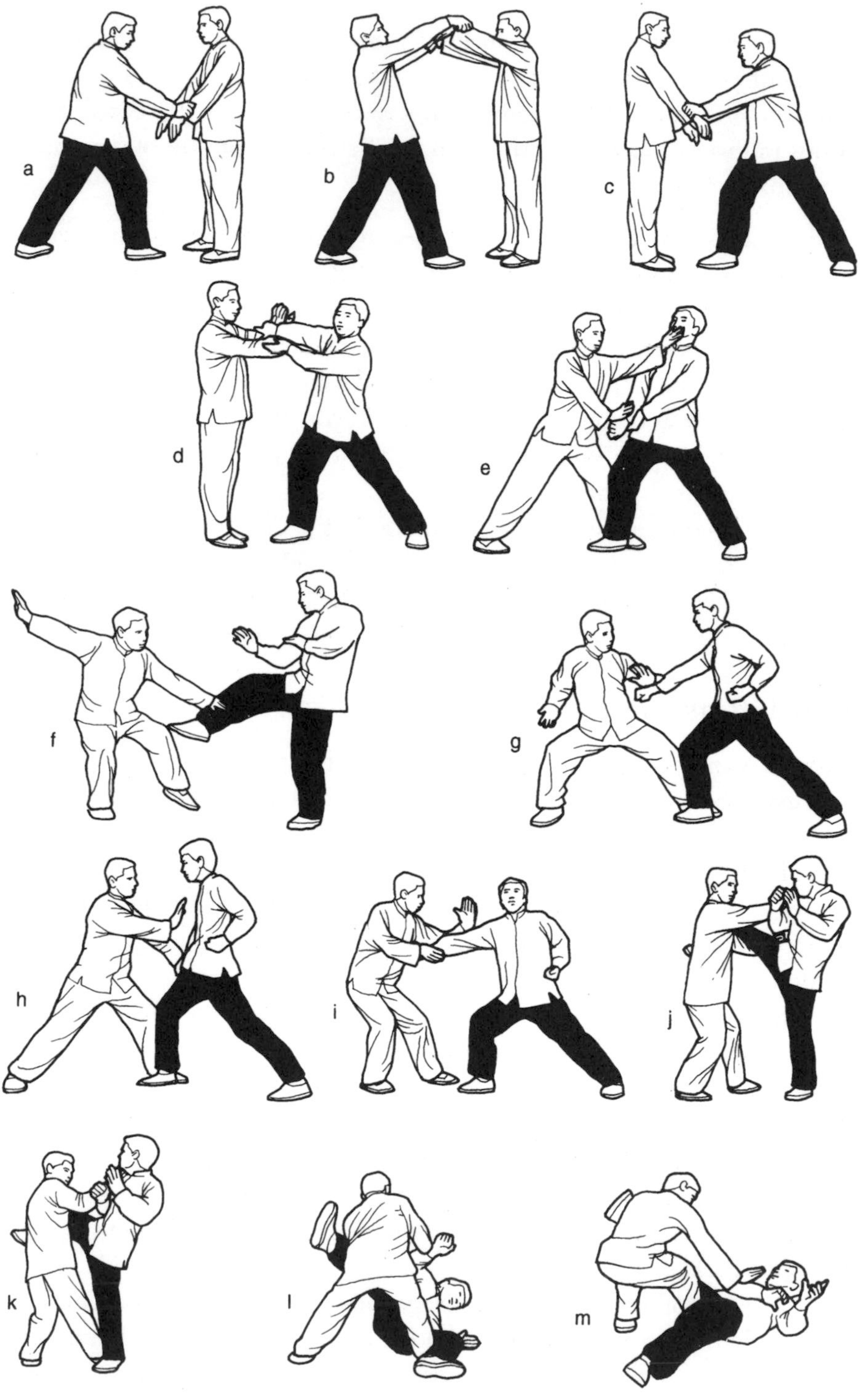

Fig 9.1 Applications of Tai Chi Chuan patterns (1)

If your opponent executes a snap kick, you can respond with White Crane Flaps Wings *(figure 9.1f)*. If you are attacked with a thrust punch, you can swallow the attack by shifting your body back without moving your legs, sweep aside the punch *(figure 9.1g)*, then strike back with your other palm *(figure 9.1h)*. This is Green Dragon Shoots Out Pearl.

Another effective counter against a thrust punch, which is a very common form of attack in most styles of martial art, is Playing the Lute. Following the momentum of the punch, shift your body backwards and grip your opponent's elbow and wrist with your hands, as in one of the Pushing Hands techniques described in the previous chapter. If, instead of gripping the elbow, you strike it with the base of your forearm while you grip the wrist with your other hand and straighten the arm for your strike *(figure 9.1i)*, you can dislocate the elbow; so be very careful when you try this technique in sparring.

Repulse Monkey is a very effective counter against the ferocious Siamese Boxing whirlwind kick, and one which comes as a total surprise to most people. If someone attacks you with a right whirlwind or roundhouse kick, instead of moving away as many defenders would do when faced with a fast, powerful kick, move your left leg diagonally towards the opponent, and place your left forearm underneath his or her thigh so that you not only foil the kick but also hold the leg up *(figure 9.1j)*. Guard your opponent's hands with your right hand. The kick cannot hurt you because the striking point, the shin, is behind you, and you have intercepted the kick at the weakest point, the thigh. Move your right leg forward to hook the other leg and push the opponent back with your right hand *(figure 9.1l)*. Squat on your opponent's abdomen or thigh (if he is a man, be careful not to squat on his genitals) and control him or her with your right hand while your left hand still holds the attacking leg *(figure 9.1m)*. Position yourself so that you are safe from any possible counter.

The Profundity of Grasping Sparrow's Tail

If you are impressed with the application of Repulse Monkey against the ferocious whirlwind kick, you will be even more impressed by what you can do with the innocent-looking Grasping Sparrow's Tail. It can be used to counter almost any attack, if you know how. Using only this pattern as his principal move, Yang Lu Chan, the first patriarch of Yang-style Tai Chi Chuan, defeated all the martial arts masters he met and earned the title 'Yang the Ever Victorious.' It is not easy to describe in writing the versatility and profundity of this seemingly simple Tai Chi pattern, but

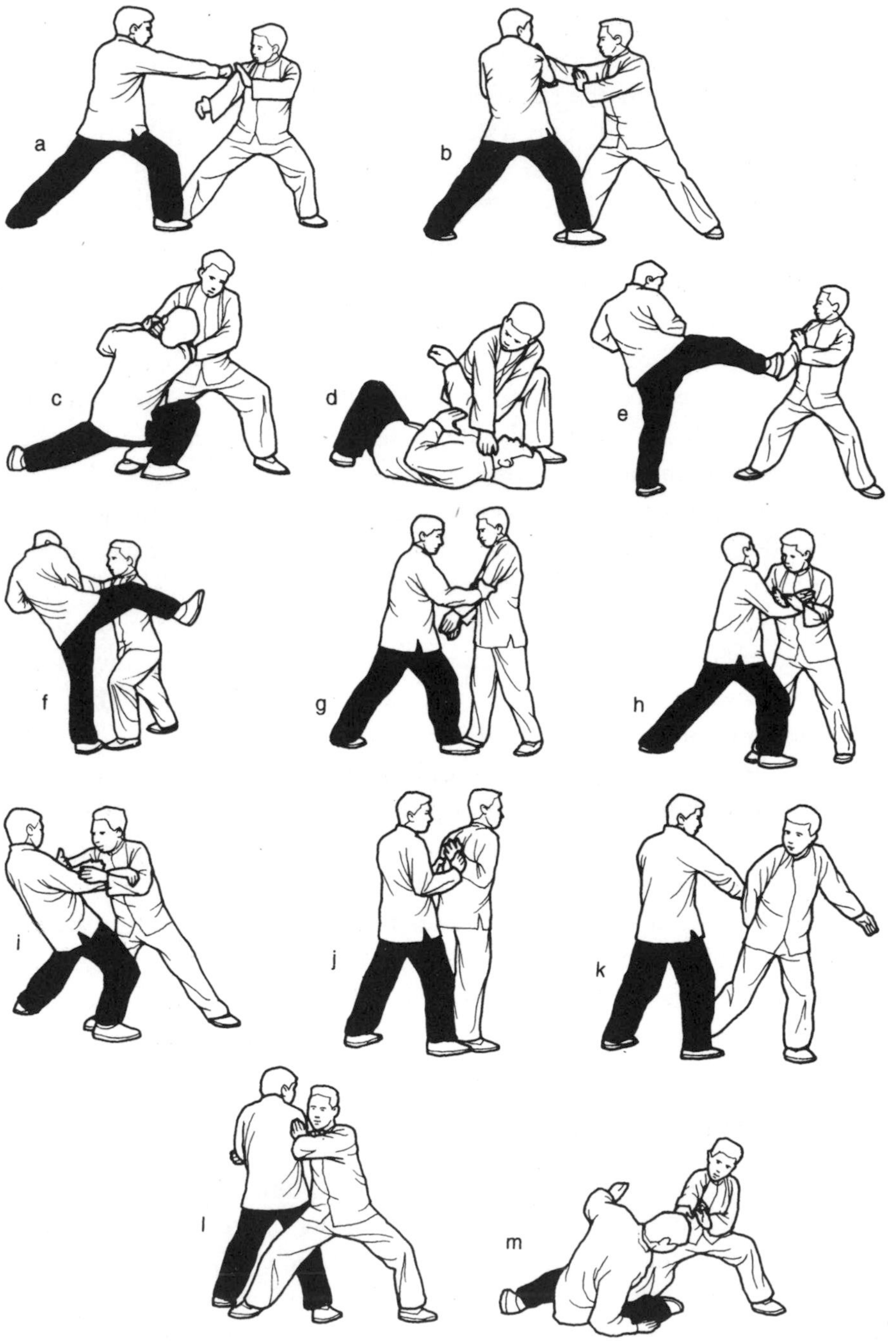

Fig 9.2 Some applications of Grasping Sparrow's Tail

the following are some examples of the ways it can be used against all the four different categories of attack.

If an opponent launches forward with a straight punch *(figure 9.2a)*, sink back to avoid it and ward off with the *peng* technique *(figure 9.2b)* when it is at its fullest extent. Before the opponent can pull it back, roll back with the *lu* technique to the neck, causing him or her to fall backwards, *(figure 9.2c)*. Control the opponent on the ground, with your knee on the ribs and your hand still at the throat *(figure 9.2d)*.

If an opponent executes a powerful side kick *(figure 9.2e)*, move to one side to avoid it, then move forward with the *an* or pushing technique, felling the opponent before the leg can be withdrawn *(figure 9.2f)*.

In *figure 9.2g* an opponent is shown holding your arms and trying to push you over with a hip throw in *figure 9.2h*. Move your left leg backward to stand in a right Bow-arrow Stance, thus foiling the throw, and simultaneously bring your right forearm round and above your opponent's arms so that they are locked between your body and your right arm. Use your left hand to help to hold them together *(figure 9.2i)*. If you press forward with your body, your opponent will have to release you and fall back to avoid suffering great pain in the wrist and fingers. Press further with a *qi* technique. Hold your opponent so that the fall does not break the backbone!

What would you do if someone twisted or bent your right arm behind your back, as in *figure 9.2j*? You can get out of this situation with a simple *lu* technique. Move your body slightly forward and, following the momentum of the twisting or bending, straighten your arm *(figure 9.2k)*. Place your right leg behind your opponent's leg or legs, sit in a Horseriding Stance *(figure 9.2l)* and smoothly follow through with a *lu* or rolling back technique. Your assailant will fall backwards *(figure 9.2m)*.

Whenever you knock a partner or opponent to the ground, you must be very careful not to break the backbone, which can result in paralysis. One effective way to minimize the impact of a fall is to hold the opponent's arm tight as he or she drops. Your stance must of course be firm, or else you might fall on top of the other person.

From Cloud Hands to Needle at Sea Bottom

Using Cloud Hands as a blocking technique, as in *figure 9.3a*, illustrates the principle of 'using minimum force against maximum strength'. *Figure 9.3b* shows how a huge attacking force has to be met by an equally huge defending force when met head-on, a situation that never occurs in Tai

Chi Chuan but is encouraged in some martial arts and is common in wrestling. *Figure 9.3c* shows that less force is needed to *deflect* the oncoming force.

The effectiveness of a deflecting block is enhanced when its direction is not straight but circular, and further enhanced when the circular

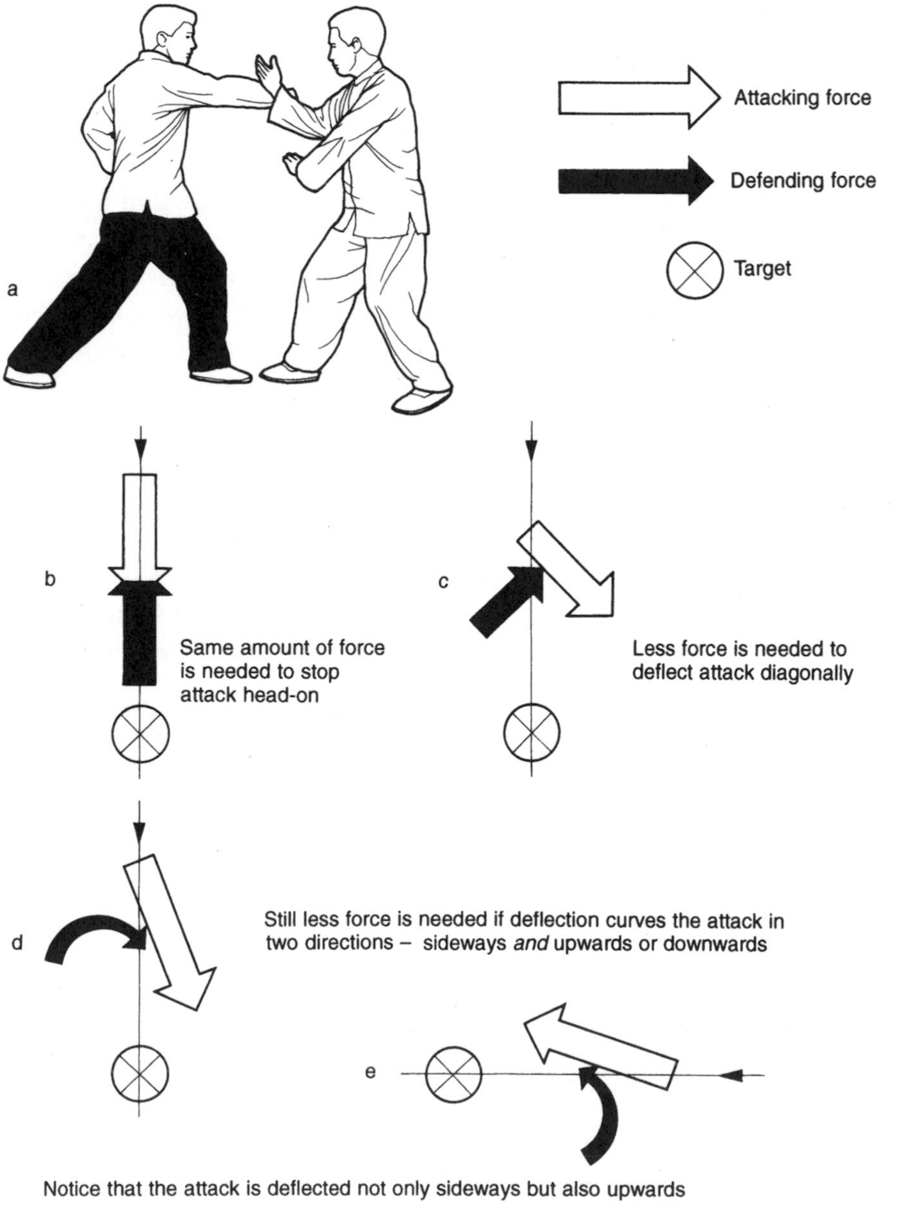

Fig 9.3 Using minimum force against maximum force

deflection follows the direction of the attacking momentum, as in *figure 9.3d*. In Tai Chi Chuan, moreover, the deflection is at more than one plane; in addition to moving the attacking force sideways in a curve following its forward momentum, as in *figure 9.3d*, it also moves it diagonally upwards, as in *figure 9.3e*, which shows the deflection as viewed from one side.

Cloud Hands, with appropriate breathing and visualization, is also a very useful method for developing internal force.

If your right wrist is gripped by your opponent's right hand, you can make a small anti-clockwise circle with your right hand and grip your opponent's wrist in return, at the same time striking the right ribs with your left palm, using Single Whip *(figure 9.4a)*. In this pattern, you must be careful that the opponent's right hand does not slip your grip to strike your face.

In High Patting Horse, you grip your opponent's right elbow, lock the opponent's right forearm between your body and your left upper arm, and jab your fingers at the throat *(figure 9.4b)*. If your opponent gives you a round-house kick, a side kick or a thrust kick, move a step diagonally in front and kick at the attacking thigh or abdomen with Cross-hands Thrust-kick *(figure 9.4c)*.

If someone grabs you from the front, before he or she can get a tight hold, strike the attacker's temples or ears with Double Bees Buzzing at Ears *(figure 9.4d)*.

The Single Whip Low Stance is a very useful pattern to counter almost any type of kick. When someone attacks you with a kick, irrespective of whether it is a high, middle, low or round-house kick, lower yourself into the Single-whip Low Stance *(figure 9.4e)*. Golden Cockerel Stands Alone is a knee attack on your opponent in close-body combat *(figure 9.4f)*. If your opponent chops at your head, you can lower your stance and apply Jade Girl Threads Shuttle, intercepting the attack above the elbow and striking with your other palm *(figure 9.4g)*.

Needle at Sea Bottom is an adroit counter against a snap kick *(figure 9.4h)*. It is also effective for releasing your arm from a grip. Before your opponent can tighten the grip, you can release it by jerking your arm down sharply; if the grip is already tight, you have to make a circular twist of your hand before you jerk your arm down. In either case, you must watch out for an attack on your face, which will be exposed. If it comes, you can respond with the Jade Girl pattern described earlier.

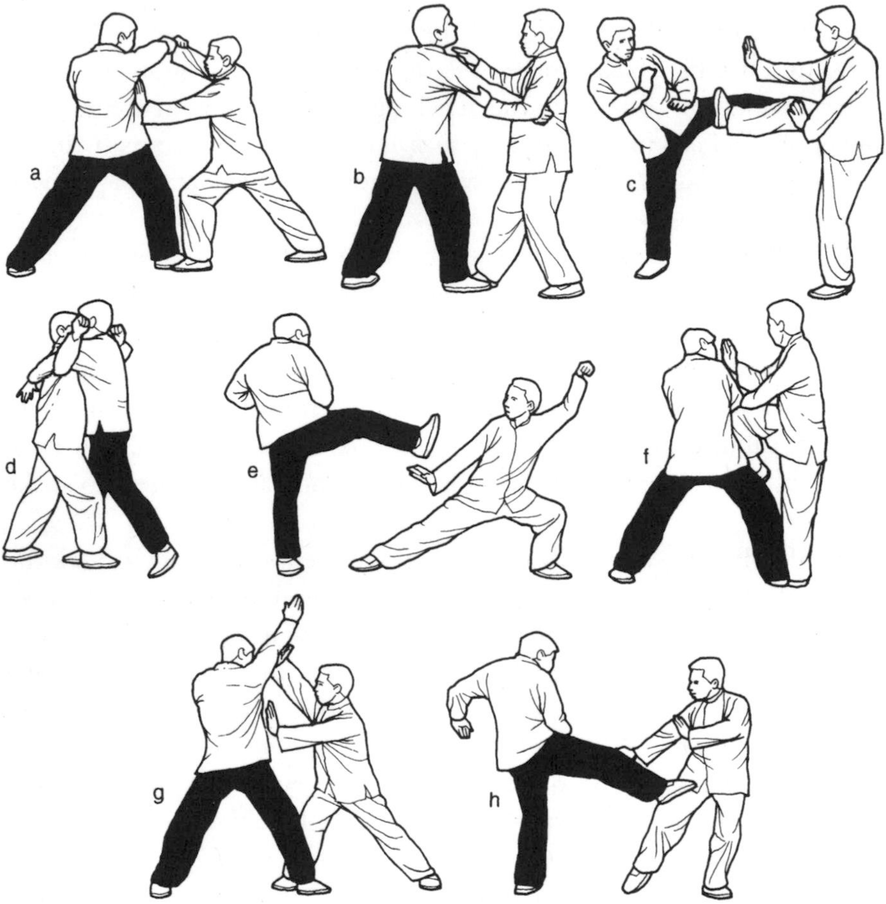

Fig 9.4 Application of Tai Chi Chuan patterns (2)

The Final Eight Patterns

Another way to counter a wrist grip, especially if you are being pulled, is an elbow strike. Use your free hand to hold the hand gripping your wrist, so preventing your opponent from suddenly releasing it to strike your face. Move forward along with the momentum of the pull, and bend your elbow to strike the opponent's face or chest *(figure 9.5a)*. If your arm is gripped with both hands, one at your wrist and the other at your elbow, move forward to strike with a Shoulder Strike *(figure 9.5b)*.

Dodge, Then Extend Arm is a useful counter against high kicks. As your opponent attacks you, lower your body, 'float' the kick with one

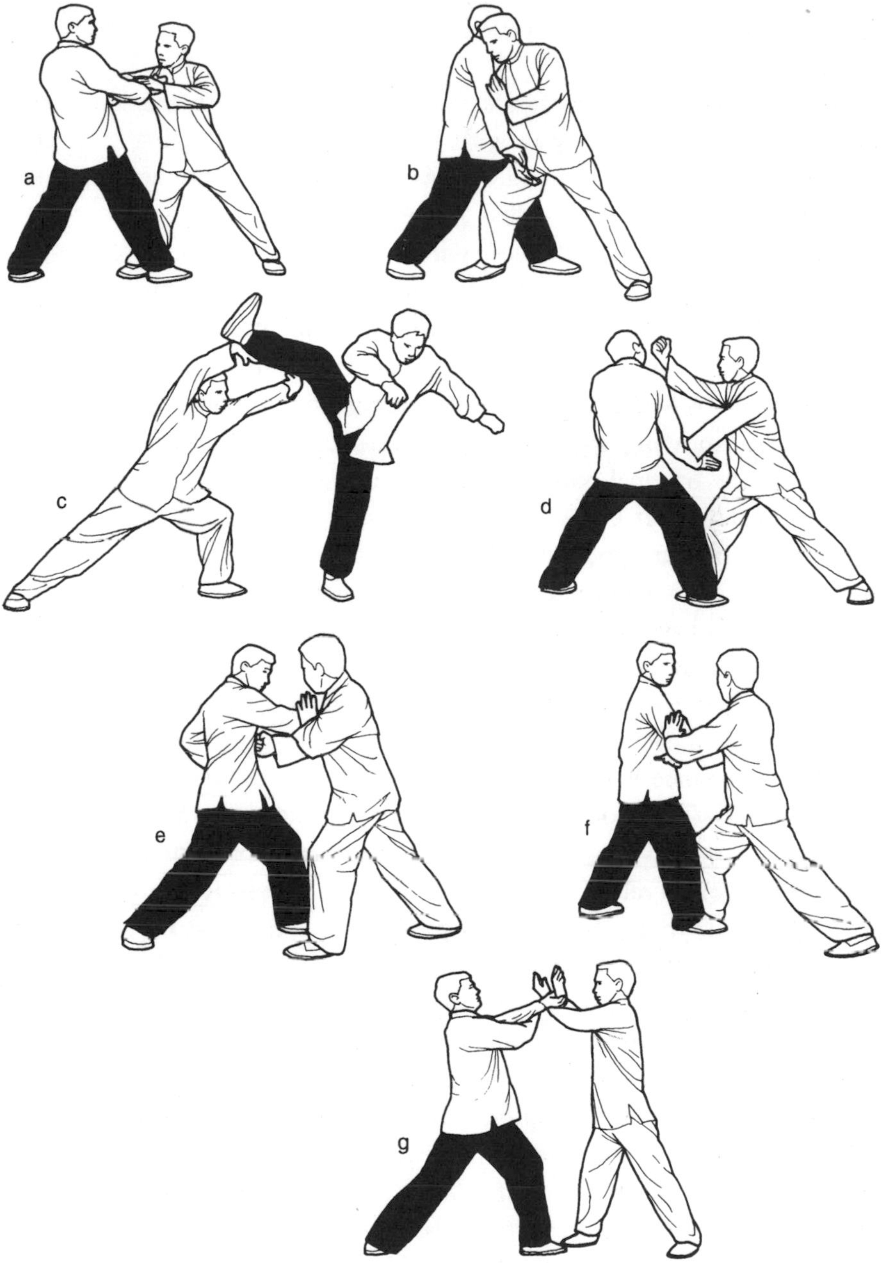

Fig 9.5 Application of Tai Chi Chuan patterns (3)

hand and strike the exposed thigh with the other *(figure 9.5c)*. This is just one example of how exposed and dangerous high kicks are for the attacker.

If someone is about to attack you from behind with the hand, turn around, sweep the hand away with your left hand and swing your right fist, with your reversed knuckles as striking points, at the attacker's face *(figure 9.5d)*, in the pattern called Swinging Fist.

If your opponent attacks you with a powerful, straight right punch, move yourself slightly to your left, intercept and gently push aside the attacking arm with your left palm or arm, and move in to strike the opponent's ribs with your right vertical fist below the arm *(figure 9.5e)*. If you execute this Move–Intercept–Punch correctly, your opponent will be hit without knowing where the strike has come from, just when he or she thinks the original punch has been successful!

Like Sealed As If Closed is a useful pattern to close up an opponent *(figure 9.5f)*. If your opponent is holding your wrists, you can release them by swinging your arms up into the Cross-hands position *(figure 9.5g)*. The opponent will have to release the hold because this technique will cause the holding arms to knock each other.

The last pattern in the Simplified Tai Chi Set, the Infinite Ultimate Stance, is not meant for direct fighting, but for you to relax your mind and body, enhance harmonious *chi* flow and attain a heightened state of consciousness. This non-fighting pattern does not contradict my earlier assertion that all the patterns in the Tai Chi set have combat functions. By training you to relax, to experience energy flow inside your body, and to have a clear mind, this pattern provides the essential ingredients for combat efficiency.

But you will probably not be able to fight efficiently yet, because in real combat, or even in friendly sparring, your opponent or partner is unlikely to use only one attacking pattern. The training in specific techniques explained in this chapter, where you learn *and practise* an appropriate technique to overcome a specific combat situation, supplies the foundation for efficient fighting, but by themselves individual techniques are inadequate to meet a continuous series of attacks. Even if you can counter attacks inflicted individually, you may be unable to do so if they are applied continuously in a series. One effective method of training for continuous fighting is known as *da shou*, or combat sequences, which will be described in the next chapter.

10

Combat Sequences and Tactics

Techniques, Tactics and Skills for Effective Fighting

We should never forget that basically Tai Chi Chuan movements are devised for fighting.

Martial Arts as Sports

There are countless ways a fighter can attack an opponent. One common way is to throw a punch from the shoulder and swing the body to add weight – a typical technique when the attacker is not trained in martial arts. A trained person would improve on these natural movements. A boxer, for example, would lift the forearms to protect the head, and shift about from one leg to another for better agility.

Nevertheless, a boxer would also punch from the shoulder and swing the body to add momentum, because this would give the best technical advantage within the limits of the rules of boxing. A wrestler, who follows a different set of rules, would fight differently. Similarly, exponents of Judo, Karate or Taekwondo fight in the way that is best suited to the rules and regulations of their arts. Hence, a judoka would not punch an opponent, a karateka would not lock an opponent's neck, a taekwondo exponent would not grab an opponent's leg, because such actions are not allowed by their contest rules. This also explains why blocking an opponent's punch, breaking an opponent's lock or disengaging from an opponent's grab is not normally taught in a Judo, Karate or Taekwondo class. If we remember that these arts are meant for sports, where rules are applied for safety reasons, it is hardly surprising to find that they are inadequate against forms of attack that go beyond their rules.

Kungfu, including Tai Chi Chuan, was never meant to be a sport, although at the present time, because of changing needs and conditions, the Chinese government has been promoting it as such. There are many benefits in practising this art as a sport, among them the promotion of health and an artistic expression of culture. However, too much emphasis on kungfu as a sport or a demonstration form, without paying attention to its primary function as a martial art gives an unbalanced view.

One result of this situation is that many modern instructors and performers of *wushu*, the current Chinese term for martial arts, including Tai Chi Chuan, cannot fight, although their demonstrations may be magnificent. The crucial point is that *wushu* can serve its martial, health, demonstration and other functions very well if the practitioner knows how, and is prepared to spend time and effort on it.

The Depth and Scope of Tai Chi Chuan

We should never forget that basically Tai Chi Chuan movements are devised for fighting. The term itself means 'cosmos kungfu'. Unlike many other martial arts, there are no rules or restrictions for fighting in Tai Chi Chuan or in any other kungfu styles, although Tai Chi Chuan exponents, like Shaolin disciples, would generally not maim their opponents with such drastic techniques as jabbing their fingers into the opponents' eyes or damaging their genitals with a kick, not because they are restricted by rules but because the training and philosophy of the art generate a genuine care for all humanity including an opponent. Hence, despite the lack of safety rules, it is far safer to practise Tai Chi Chuan as a martial sport, and less damaging but no less effective to use Tai Chi Chuan in a real fight.

Tai Chi Chuan not only has a continuous history of its own going back more than 500 years, but at the time when it evolved from Shaolin Kungfu, the latter already had 1,000 years of development behind it. In other words, the fighting skills and techniques we learn in Tai Chi Chuan have been evolved and refined for 15 centuries, which is a very long time compared with some martial arts with a history of less than 100 years. This is one reason why both the fighting skills and the techniques in Tai Chi Chuan are so subtle.

Initially fighting techniques were crude, perhaps not very different from those an untrained person would use today. Over long periods of trial and error, experienced fighters discovered that by adapting certain stances and punching in certain ways, they gained certain technical advantages. For example, instead of standing with feet apart and punching from the shoulder as in boxing, kungfu masters discovered that they would have more stability in their stance and more power in their punch if they used the Bow-arrow Stance and punched from their waist.

Gradually, the masters discovered that tactics and skills are often more important than just techniques for effective fighting. Through long years of both study and actual fighting, they also evolved many methods of implementing the relevant tactics and developing the necessary skills. This development took a long time, with the result that not only were the techniques complex after many centuries, but the methods used to acquire the skills or force had become so subtle that they were no longer meaningful to the uninitiated. Hence, not only advanced methods like energy flow and visualization, but even basic training like stances, transferring of body weight and waist rotation, are not understood by many modern martial arts students, whose arts may not have the length and depth of development of Tai Chi Chuan.

A very significant development in the history of martial arts occurred in 527CE, when Shaolin Kungfu was institutionalized at the famous Shaolin Monastery in China. Before this time, a warrior had to invent his own fighting methods, or at best learn some useful techniques from a teacher; there was little or no continuity in passing on fighting methods through the generations. But since its establishment, fighting methods have been taught systematically at the Shaolin Monastery as an art to be passed on from generation to generation. What a student practised was not his own invention, not even his teacher's invention, but a body of skills, techniques and rich philosophical knowledge accumulated through the ages.

For the first time, martial art was taught not in an *ad hoc* manner for personal needs, but as a properly organized system, which enabled the art to develop to an extent that would not have been possible in any learning based on personal attainment. When Zhang San Feng, the first patriarch of Tai Chi Chuan, evolved the system from Shaolin Kungfu, he bequeathed to it the great benefits of an institutionalized development going back 1,000 years.

In addition to this tremendous advantage of continuous development, Tai Chi Chuan is not limited by rules like boxing, wrestling, Judo, Karate, Taekwondo and other martial sports. Tai Chi Chuan exponents do not swing the body forward like boxers when they punch, first because doing so would upset their balance, which would in turn make it easy for an opponent to throw them to the ground, and secondly because they do not need the extra weight swinging the body adds since they can inflict more damage by using internal force. Boxers, on the other hand, do not worry so much about poor balance because boxing rules do not allow opponents to exploit their poor balance to throw them to the ground, and the wearing of boxing gloves minimizes the effect of internal force, so that it is an advantage to add power by swinging the body forward.

Similarly, because no rules are followed in real fighting, Tai Chi Chuan exponents are trained to take extra precautions when attacking an opponent, which exponents of wrestling, Judo, Karate, Taekwondo and some other martial sports may not bother about because of the protection provided by the rules on safety. The methods used in these other sports would, moreover, give away technical advantages which the opponent could exploit.

For example, if you were to go low to tackle an opponent's legs, as a wrestler might do, you would offer your head as a target to be hit in a pattern like Green Dragon Shoots out Pearl *(figure 10.1a)*, which could result in serious injury. If you were to grab an opponent's clothing in preparation for a throw as in Judo, the opponent could easily raise one knee to strike hard at your genitals, possibly maiming you for life, in the pattern Golden Cockerel Stands Alone *(figure 10.1b)*.

If you were to charge in widely with typical Karate punches and without providing adequate cover while attacking, you would expose yourself

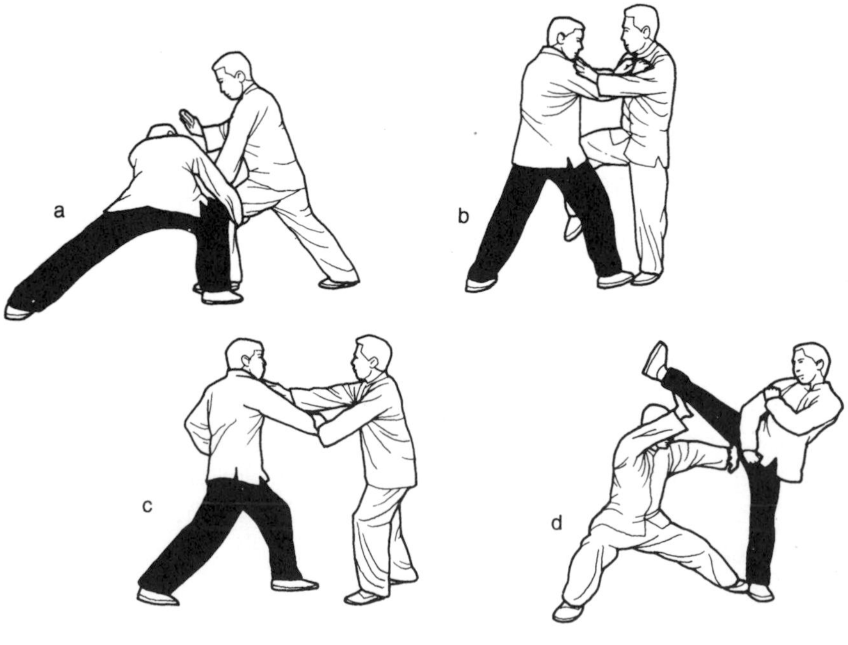

Fig 10.1 Postures to be avoided in Tai Chi Chuan

to dangerous counter attacks, such as a thrust to the throat with the pattern High Patting Horse *(figure 10.1c)*. If you were to kick high, as in Taekwondo, there would be a good chance of your genitals being damaged by the pattern Dodge, Then Extend Arm *(figure 10.1d)*. The crucial point to bear in mind whenever you initiate an attack is not whether your opponent knows how to counter attack, but the fact that you must not give such technical advantages to an opponent in the first place.

Because there are no rules in real fighting, Tai Chi Chuan exponents are trained to defend themselves from any form of attack. This is obviously a clear advantage over martial sports where practitioners are mainly trained to defend against attacks that are allowed under their particular rules. Many Judo students, for example, do not know how to counter kicks, and Taekwondo students do not know how to counter throws, because such attacks are not allowed in their sports.

The Why and How of Combat Sequences

Learning and practising the application of appropriate patterns to overcome specific combat situations is an essential step to combat efficiency, but by themselves specific techniques are insufficient. In a fight, an opponent does not normally inflict one attack, and then wait for you to counter with the appropriate specific technique. You will usually be subjected to a series of attacks, often before you can recover from the first one if you are untrained.

From their practical experiences as well as their analysis of combat, the masters have discovered that because of the technical advantages to be gained from given combat situations, certain arrangements of the sequences of attack and defence are preferable. For example, if an opponent directs a punch at you and, as soon as you ward it off, follows it with another punch, linking the two smoothly together as if they were one continuous pattern, the chances of hitting you are higher than with two punches executed separately. On the other hand, if you are aware of this tactic of continuous instead of staccato attack, and are prepared for it, you can not only defend against it more effectively, but are also more likely to be successful with a counter attack.

In theory, when you initiate an attack there are countless ways in which your opponent can defend against it, but in practice any defence generally falls within a range of a few patterns. This is because these patterns provide certain technical advantages in that particular combat situation. The opponent *can* respond with patterns outside this range, but to do so would be unwise. Hence, the masters have worked out sequences of attack and defence that are commonly used, and such training is known as *da shou*, or combat sequences.

Besides enabling students to become familiar with series of attack and defence patterns arranged logically to derive tactical advantages in given combat situations, combat sequence training also develops essential combat skills like spacing, timing, quick decision making, and adjusting to changing situations. Initially, combat sequences are prearranged, but as students progress in their training, the control of prearranged patterns is gradually loosened until eventually they are sparring freely.

Nine combat sequences are given in this chapter and the next. The initiator or attacker in each sequence is called X for convenience, and the responder is called Y. The techniques used by the initiator in all nine sequences are taken from Shaolin Kungfu; they are part of the standard practice in my Shaolin Wahnam Kungfu School. Shaolin patterns have been chosen deliberately for the attack because, since Shaolin Kungfu is the most comprehensive and extensive martial art in the world today,[1] if you can successfully defend against Shaolin techniques you can defend against typical techniques from any other martial arts. The nine attacking sequences incorporate all the four categories of attack: hitting, kicking, felling and gripping. All the patterns used by the responder are taken from the 24-pattern Simplified Tai Chi Set (see Chapter 7), except the poise pattern known as Lifting Up Hands (see Chapter 5) which is used at the start and end of each sequence.

Learning a Tai Chi set from a book is daunting enough; learning combat sequences, though not impossible, is considerably more difficult. You should, therefore, seek the guidance of a competent instructor if you want to achieve good results.

Practise the sequences slowly at first, paying particular attention to accuracy of form. Later, when your form is correct, pay attention to force (but not brute strength). When you can perform the sequences well with the correct form and appropriate force, you can pay attention to speed, which will have increased remarkably without your being conscious of it.

Practise one sequence well before progressing to the next one. Remember that developing combat skills like spacing, timing and appropriate adjustment is as important as performing the techniques.

Refer to the illustrations for the forms and movements of the combat sequences. The accompanying explanations will not describe them in detail, they merely highlight crucial points.

Sequence 1 Triple Punches – Warding Off

X and Y stand facing each other at their poise patterns – X in a Shaolin pattern known as Lohan Asks the Way, and Y in the Tai Chi pattern Lifting Up Hands *(figure 10.2a)*. Use these two poise patterns at the beginning and end of all the combat sequences.

X moves the front left leg forward, uses the left hand to open Y's defence, ie push aside Y's guarding left hand, and attacks Y three times with a right, a left and then a right punch, known in Shaolin Kungfu as Black Tiger Steals Heart *(figure 10.2b)*, Fierce Tiger Speeds Across Valley *(figure 10.2c)*, and again Black Tiger Steals Heart *(figure 10.2d)*. Y pulls the left leg back to stand in a right Bow-arrow Stance, and responds with a

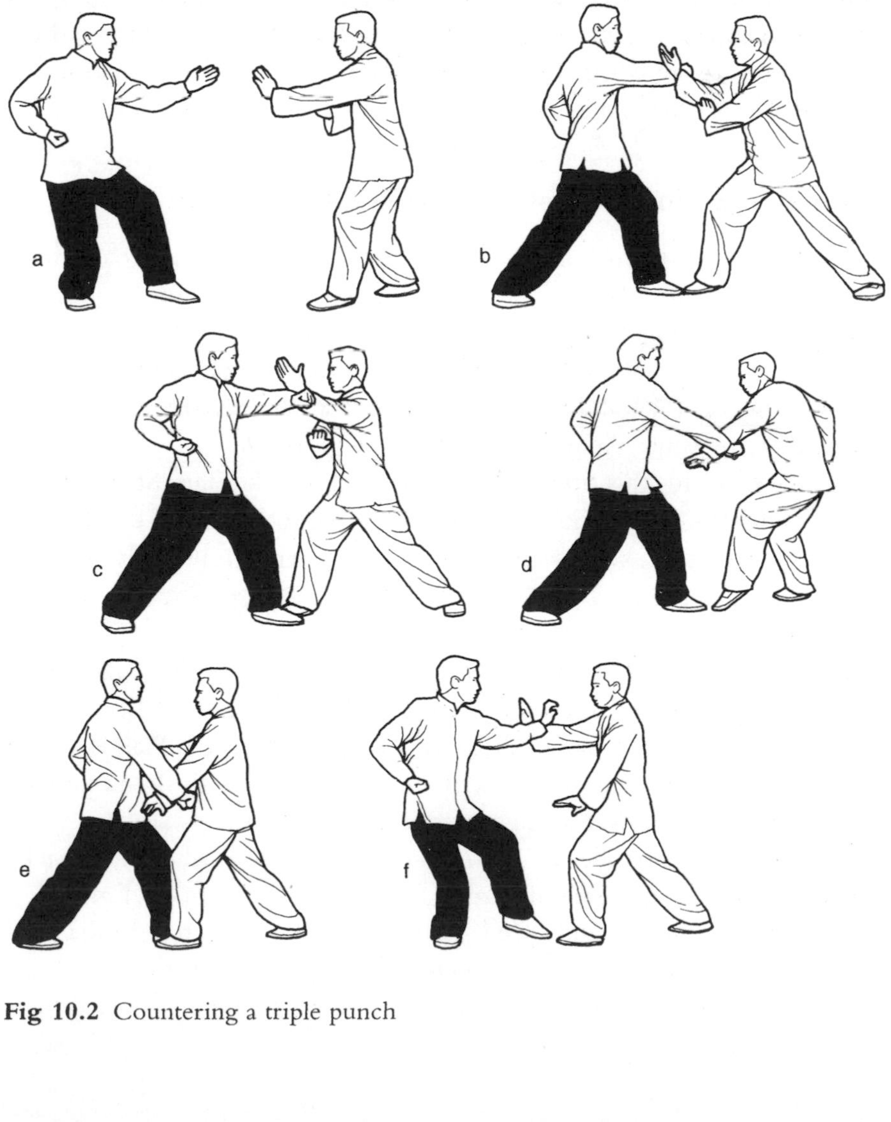

Fig 10.2 Countering a triple punch

right *peng* technique, a left *peng* technique, and then Green Dragon Shoots Out Pearl *(figures 10.2b, c* and *d)*. For the Green Dragon pattern, Y first moves the front leg back to a momentary left False-leg Stance, then moves the same leg forward to a left Bow-arrow Stance *(figure 10.2e)*.

X pulls the front leg back to a left False-leg Stance, and replies with Single Tiger Emerges from Cave *(figure 10.2f)*. Y then pulls the front leg to a left Four-six Stance, and observes X from the poise pattern Lifting Up Hands. X changes the left tiger claw, used to block Y's attack earlier, to a palm and stands at the poise pattern Lohan Asks the Way.

This is an example of a smooth continuity of three attacks; three significant factors for a successful application of this form of attack are timing, fluidity and speed. Even if you use the same attacking techniques, but lack these factors, you are unlikely to succeed. If you have these three factors you may apply other techniques and be successful, illustrating that in combat it is often skills, not techniques that are decisive.

Sequence 2 Three-level Attacks – Green Dragon

From the poise pattern Lohan Asks the Way, X attacks Y's throat with a right finger-thrust known as White Snake Shoots Out Venom. Y responds with a *peng* technique *(figure 10.3a)*. As soon as Y responds, X moves in to attack with a left low punch known as Precious Duck Swims Through Lotus at Y's abdomen. Y retreats to a left False-leg Stance, and counters with White Crane Flaps Wings *(figure 10.3b)*.

X attacks again, this time at Y's chest, with Black Tiger Steals Heart. Y moves the front leg back close to the back leg to stand in a Cat Stance, 'swallows' X's attack, sweeps aside X's punching arm, and moves the front leg forward again to strike X's chest with Green Dragon Shoots out Pearl *(figure 10.3c)*.

X moves the front leg back and defends against Y's palm strike using Single Tiger Emerges from Cave *(figure 10.3d)*. Y changes the Bow-arrow Stance to a Four-six Stance in the poise pattern Lifting Up Hands, while X changes the tiger claw into a palm and observes Y with the poise pattern Lohan Asks the Way as illustrated in *figure 10.2a*

This sequence provides an example of another combat tactic: attacking an opponent at three different levels (top, bottom and middle). Besides timing, fluidity and speed – the three decisive factors in the previous sequence – distraction plays a crucial role here. The concept of *xu-shi*, or 'apparent-solid', is important in this tactic. If, when you attack at the top level, your opponent attempts to defend, this attack becomes *xu* or 'apparent';your real intention is not to strike but to distract, so that you will have a better chance of success when you strike with the *shi* or 'solid' attack below. However, if the opponent fails to respond to your attack at the top, the attack becomes 'solid', and you actually strike.

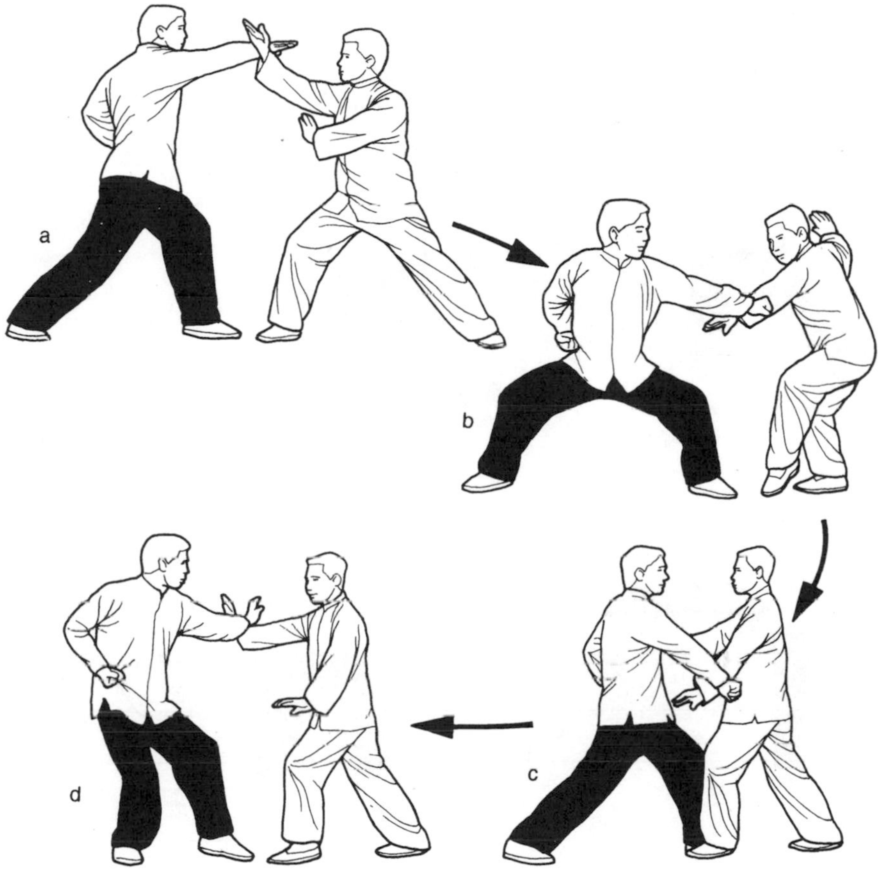

Fig 10.3 Countering a three-level attack

Sequence 3 Whirlwind Kick – Single Whip Low Stance

From the poise pattern, X moves forward and attacks with Black Tiger Steals Heart. Instead of using the *peng* technique to respond, as in the previous two sequences, Y takes a small step back with the front leg and uses Green Dragon Shoots Out Pearl to sweep aside the punch *(figure 10.4a)*, then, moving the same leg forward, strikes X with a palm strike *(figure 10.4b)*.

X moves the left leg to a left False-leg Stance to avoid the palm strike, and simultaneously 'threads' up the left hand to push Y's left arm aside *(figure 10.4c)*. X immediately kicks the right leg in an arc to strike Y's ribs with the pattern Whirlwind Sweeps Fallen Leaves *(figure 10.4d)*. Y drops into the pattern Single Whip Low Stance to avoid the sweeping kick, then as the kick passes by, rises forward and strikes X with Single Whip

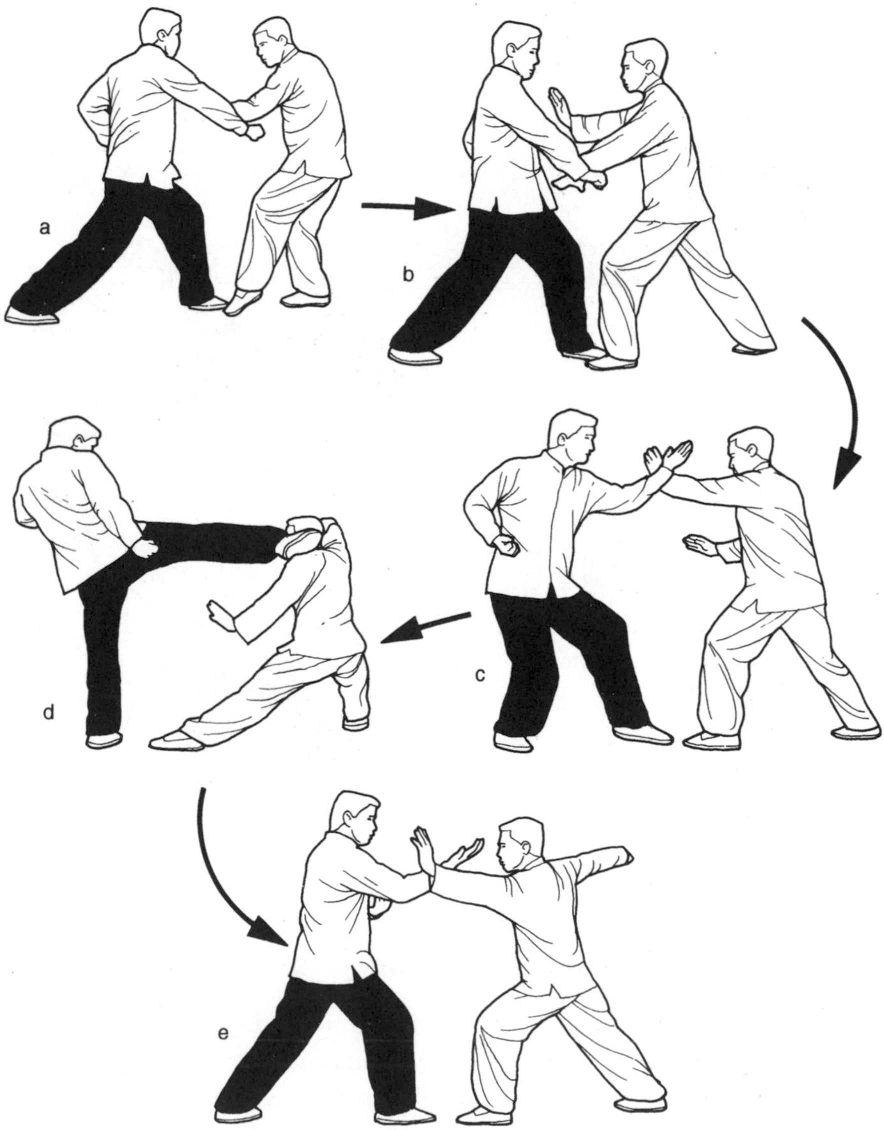

Fig 10.4 Low Stance against a whirlwind kick

(figure 10.4e). X withdraws the right leg, placing it in front, shifts the left leg back and blocks with Beauty Looks at Mirror. Then both return to their poise patterns to observe the other's next move.

This sequence gives an example of the tactic 'defence-cum-counter-attack' in the pattern Green Dragon Shoots Out Pearl. Instead of first blocking the attack and then counter-attacking in the tactic called 'first defence, then counter-attack' described in the previous two sequences, you can let your defence and attack run together in one pattern.

Sequence 4 Hiding Flowers – Playing the Lute

X again attacks with Black Tiger Steals Heart *(figure 10.5a)*. This is a very common attacking pattern, and here it represents any form of middle hand attack. If you can defend against this representative level fist attack, you can also defend against similar attacks where the opponent may use other hand forms such as a vertical fist, a leopard punch, a phoenix-eye punch, a palm strike or a spear hand.

Instead of defending, Y shifts first the right leg and then the left leg back a little while still remaining in the left Four-six Stance. Y strikes X's wrist with the right palm, and X's elbow with the base of the left fore-arm, using the pattern Playing the Lute *(figure 10.5a)*. In your practice you must be very careful not to break or dislocate your partner's elbow when you apply this technique.

To neutralize this attack, X moves the front left leg diagonally to the left, simultaneously jerks down the elbow and brings the right leg into a right False-leg Stance in a pattern called Hiding Flowers in Sleeve *(figure 10.5b)*. X immediately punches out the right fist in the pattern Precious Duck Swims Through Lotus. *Figure 10.5c* shows what the situation would be if Y failed to respond.

In fact, Y moves the right leg a little way back and simultaneously spreads out both arms, striking X's wrist with a sweeping left palm in the pattern White Crane Flaps Wings *(figure 10.5d)*. Notice that Y's sweep-ing palm is not meant to block X's attack – it is not necessary to have any defensive blocks because by shifting the right leg Y has moved away from the attack – but to strike the attacking arm. Similarly the earlier Playing the Lute was not aimed at stopping X's attack, because Y had already moved away, but to strike X's elbow.

This sequence shows an example of the tactic called 'no defence, direct counter-attack', which is more advanced than 'defence–cum–counter–attack' which was explained in the previous sequence. The

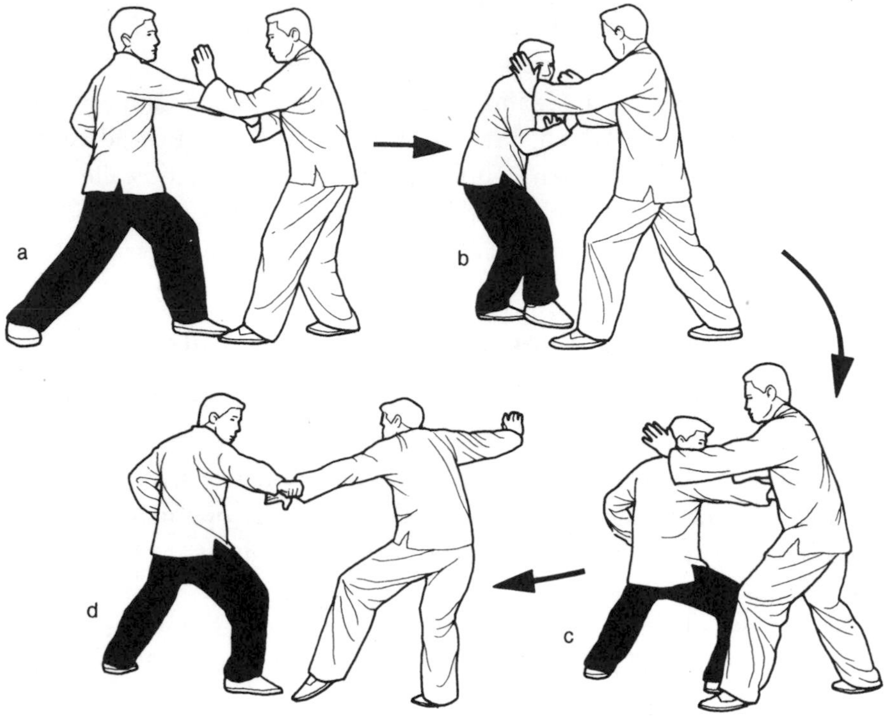

Fig 10.5 Hiding Flowers and Playing the Lute

expression 'no defence' is a misnomer, because although Y did not block or deflect X's attacks, the skilful shifting of position was in fact a form of defence. But the shifting was done at the same time as the counter-attack. Y did not shift and then attack, which would have been a case of 'first defence, then counter-attack'; instead, Y shifted and counter-attacked at the same time. If this tactic is applied properly, your opponent will be hit at the time when his or her own attacking move has just been spent.

Obviously, 'no defence, direct counter-attack' is superior to 'defence–cum–counter-attack', which in turn is superior to 'first defence, then counter-attack'. And of course you need to spend more time and effort in developing a superior tactic and the relevant techniques to implement it. But does this mean that if you are ready to spend the time and effort, 'no defence, direct counter-attack' is better than the other two tactics, or that it is a waste of time to practise 'first defence, then counter-attack' because it is inferior? The answers to both questions is an emphatic 'No!'

It is important to practise the basic tactics and techniques thoroughly before progressing to the more advanced ones. If you do not have a foundation in the more basic tactic of 'first defence, then counter-attack' it will take much longer to learn the other two. And even when you are skilful in all three tactics, there are occasions – such as assessing the opponent's power or avoiding a possible trap – when the more elementary tactic is to be preferred.

Hence, in combat sequence training we do not just learn and practise sequences of techniques, but also skills and tactics, which, especially at higher levels, are more important than techniques. You should therefore pay more attention to developing skills and appreciating tactics, and not merely learn more and more forms. The next chapter will provide further opportunity for you to develop skills and study tactics.

11

More Combat Sequences and Tactics

Some Amazing Ways to Overcome an Opponent

If you doubt whether Tai Chi Chuan tactics like using an opponent's strength against himself or herself, following the attacking momentum to lead the attacker to his or her defeat, and starting later but arriving earlier can really work in practice, you will have the opportunity to experience the effects directly if you learn to perform these combat sequences correctly.

Factors in Winning a Combat

A common misconception among many martial arts students is that fighting techniques are the sole or most important factor determining the outcome of a fight. But if you ask those who have had a lot of experience in fighting, they will tell you that of the numerous factors involved in winning a combat, techniques are probably the least important.

There is a Chinese saying which lists the decisive factors in combat in descending order of importance as follows: 'One, guts; two, strength; three, kungfu'. Here the term 'kungfu' is used loosely: it refers to techniques.

More important than techniques is what kungfu masters collectively term as *gong* (pronounced 'kung'), which includes, among other things, accuracy, power and speed. The term 'kungfu' (written as *gongfu* in Romanized Chinese) actually refers to the consistent training of this *gong*. Consistent practice in Pushing Hands for balance and quick reflexes, the Tai Chi Stance for internal force, and Grasping Sparrow's Tail for energy flow, are examples of *gong* training in Tai Chi Chuan.

Two other significant factors are the stamina needed to last the fight and a relaxed state of mind, not only to assess your opponent correctly but to allow you to apply your combat skills and techniques effectively. If you are nervous or panicky when you face an opponent, all that you have learnt and practised may be thrown to the winds. Tai Chi Chuan, if practised properly as the masters have always taught, is particularly effective in developing stamina and a relaxed state of mind.

What is meant by 'guts' is courage nurtured by the confidence derived from proper *gong* training and supported by calmness and mental clarity. Strength is the back-up force, which may be internal or mechanical, without which fighting techniques cannot be efficient. In more refined terms, 'guts', 'strength' and 'kungfu' refer to the dimensions of mind, energy and form in any martial art training.

If you bear this in mind, you will derive greater benefits from the combat sequence training that follows. In practical terms, you should do two things: one, be sufficiently trained in basic movements and internal force (explained in Chapters 6, 7 and 8) before you attempt training of combat sequences seriously; two, when practising combat sequences, apart from the visible techniques, pay attention to the invisible skills like balance and elegance, spontaneous reflexes and fluidity of movements.

If you doubt whether Tai Chi Chuan tactics like using an opponent's strength against himself or herself, following the attacking momentum to lead the attacker to his or her defeat, and starting later but arriving earlier can really work in practice, you will have the opportunity to experience the effects of these tactics directly if you learn to perform these combat sequences correctly.

The five combat sequences below continue on from the four sequences described in the previous chapter; thus the first sequence below is labelled as Sequence 5. As before the initiator, X, uses Shaolin Kungfu, and the responder, Y, uses Tai Chi Chuan.

Sequence 5 Felling a Tree – Rolling Back

From the poise pattern shown in *figure 11.1a*, X attacks Y with Black Tiger Steals Heart, and Y responds with *peng (figure 11.1b)*. X immediately places his or her right leg behind Y's right leg and sits firmly in a Horseriding Stance. X's left hand guards Y's right hand, X's right forearm presses Y's left hand against Y's body, and X's right hand presses against Y's left shoulder *(figure 11.1c)*. The description of this pattern, called Felling a Tree, may be long but it should actually be executed in a split second. In this position, if X pushes forward and Y does not counter in time, Y will fall backwards.

But Y, exemplifying the Tai Chi Chuan principle of tricking an opponent into advancing to no avail, then using minimum force against

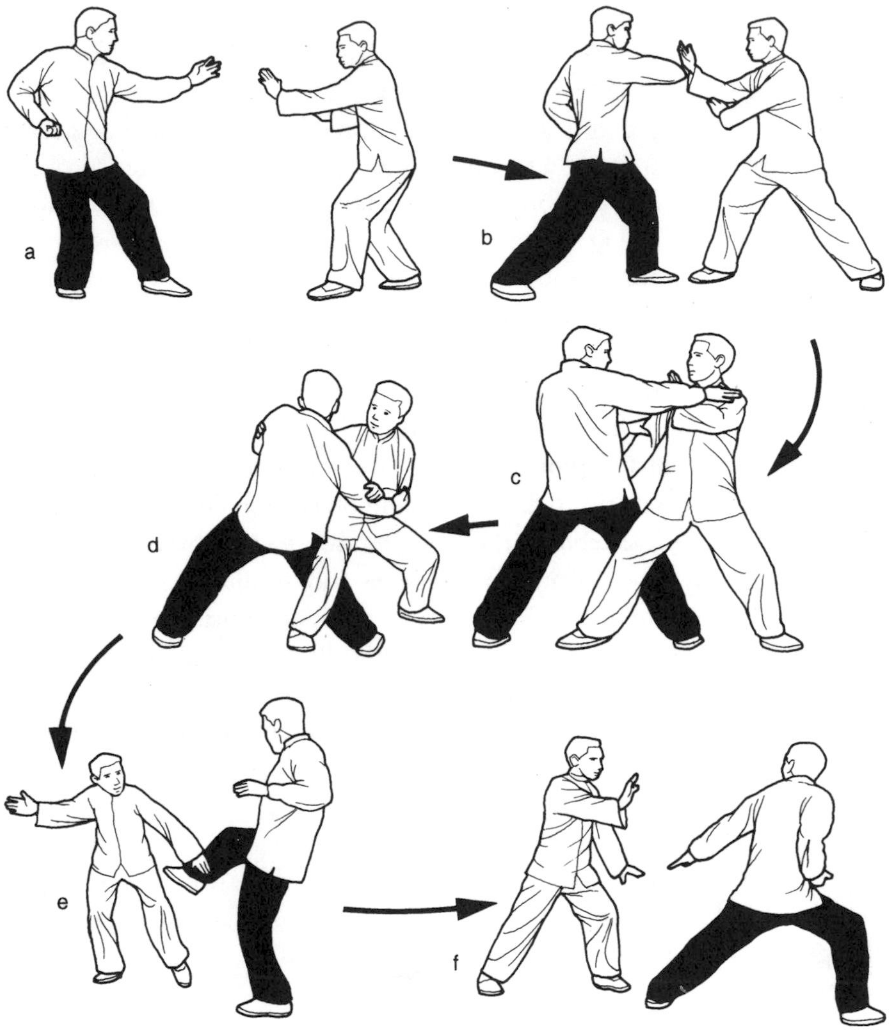

Fig 11.1 Countering a felling attack

maximum force, allows X to push forward. As X pushes, Y follows the momentum and rotates at the waist towards the left, taking a small step back with the left leg. At the same time Y grips X's right arm with the left hand and X's left elbow with the right hand, and performs the *lu* or rolling back movement. The effect is very interesting: just at the moment X expects to fell Y, Y fells X *(figure 11.1d)*!

Timing is crucial for the success of this technique. If it is executed too early, Y will be unable to exploit X's strength; if it is executed too late,

Y and not X will fall. The skill, again, is developed from Pushing Hands; in fact, such an application is common in Pushing Hands training.

Notice also that Y does not pull or push X: the force used to fell X comes from the rotation of Y's waist as well as the forward momentum of X's push. Imagine X pushing the edge of a horizontal wheel. The wheel turns and X, losing balance, falls forward.

You can avoid a fall by placing your front leg in the direction of the fall. But in this situation, X cannot move the front leg because it is being 'locked' by Y's front leg. This is another interesting effect. Initially X placed the front leg behind Y's to 'lock' it so that X could push Y backwards. But by a subtle movement of the back leg and rotation of the waist, Y turns the tables. This is another example in Tai Chi Chuan of using an opponent's strength against that opponent.

However, X overcomes this difficult situation by swinging the back left leg in a big arc behind and to the right, and then kicks up the right leg using the toes to strike at Y's ribs *(figure 11.1e)*. This pattern is known as Little Bird Shows Pointed Kick. Y takes a small step back and responds with Green Dragon Shoots Out Pearl, sweeping away X's kick with the left hand, and moving forward to strike X's chest with the right palm.

X brings the right leg back and lowers his or her stance to observe Y, letting Y's strike pass, using a pattern called Tiger Tail at Bow-arrow *(figure 11.1f)*. Then both move to their poise patterns to assess each other.

Sequence 6 Pushing Mountains – Thrust Kick

As usual, X starts with a right punch and Y responds with a right *peng* *(figure 112a)*. Of course in a real fight your opponent would not necessarily start with a punch, nor you by warding off; this is only a fairly typical opening for this combat sequence training. If your opponent, for example, started with a kick – not a wise way to initiate an attack, because that exposes a weakness right at the beginning instead of reserving the kick for the right occasion – you could sink into Single Whip Low Stance to observe the situation or, if you are competent enough, use *lu* and *li* (rolling back and pressing forward) to throw the opponent off the ground in the very first move.

One reason why our combat sequences so far have always started with the same opening is to facilitate the development of the ability to make reflexive decisions in combat. Later, when these combat sequences are being performed well, either the initiator or the responder can continue in different ways from the same opening. At first, however, it is advisable to limit the options to only two or three. In other words, from the same opening the initiator or the responder can choose the next pattern from a selection of two or three. Gradually the number of choices can be widened. This is one way to progress gradually from prearranged to free sparring.

In this sequence, as soon as Y responds, X pushes aside Y's blocking hand with the left hand, moves the back leg forward and pushes Y with both hands in a pattern known as Fierce Tiger Pushes Mountain *(figure 11.2b)*. X's initial attack is a feint move known as a lead: the real intention is not to punch Y, but to lead Y to respond so that X can swiftly move forward to push Y backwards.

This is a good opportunity for Y to use a kick. Y pulls the right leg back to avoid the momentum of X's push, uses both hands to separate X's arms and gives a left thrust kick. This pattern is a frontal version of Cross-hands Thrust-kick, which is executed from a side in the Simplified Tai Chi Set. If the timing is correct, the kick will hit X just at the time when X's own attack has completed its full journey. This is an example of the Tai Chi Chuan idea of 'starting later, arriving earlier' – you start your attack later than your opponent does, but your attack arrives just when the latter's is spent.

X quickly brings the right leg back into a Unicorn Step and simultaneously swings a right fist at Y's shin in an exotic Shaolin pattern called Dark Dragon Wags Tail *(figure 11.2c)*. Y lowers the kicking leg to avoid being hit, guards against X's swinging fist with the left hand, and strikes X's head with the right palm, in the Tai Chi pattern called High Patting Horse *(figure 11.2d)*.

X makes a left about turn and 'threads' the left hand (ie moves it as if pulling a needle and thread upwards) in a pattern called Golden Dragon Plays with Water *(figure 11.2e)*. Y must be careful that X's threading hand does not strike Y's face; if it attempts to, an effective counter is Green Dragon Shoots Out Pearl, sweeping away the 'threading' attack with one hand, and striking the attacker with the other.

After 'threading', X moves his left leg forward and attacks with a right straight punch, to which Y responds by warding off *(figure 11.2f)*. Thus, this sequence ends with a right straight punch countered with a right ward off, which is the way all the sequences we have studied so far start. This has the advantage later, when you are more familiar with these combat sequences, of enabling you to use this ending as the start of another sequence without any break. This is one way of progressing from prearranged to free sparring. Another occurs when the same pattern, such as Green Dragon Shoots Out Pearl, is found in more than one sequence; you can then use this pattern to switch into other sequences.

This progression from prearranged to free sparring or real combat should be gradual and methodical. If they practise properly, martial arts students can fight well using the techniques, tactics and skills that they have learnt; otherwise they are likely to fight wildly, like small children.

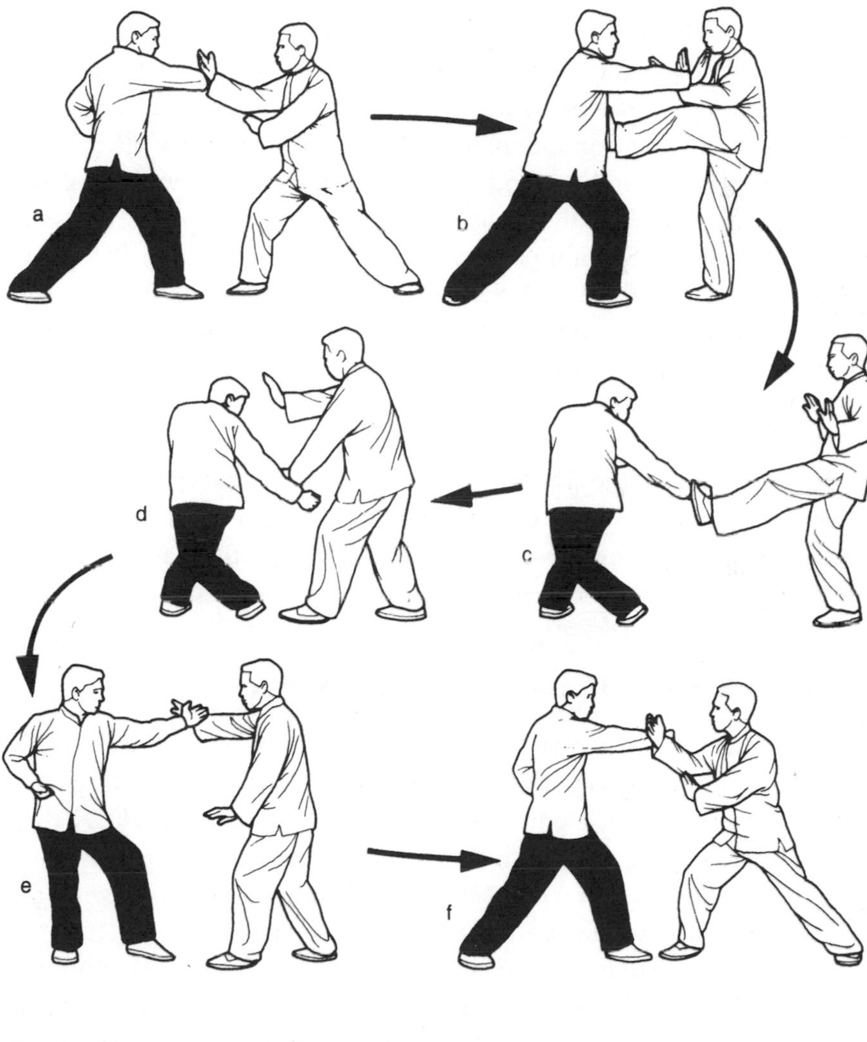

Fig 11.2 Countering a pushing attack

Sequence 7 Pull Horse – Thrust Kick

X attacks with a typical right straight punch, and Y responds as usual with *peng (figure 11.3a)*. X immediately moves forward and pushes Y, as in the previous sequence *(figure 11.3b)*. But now Y uses a different, gentler, counter: sinking down to neutralize the pushing momentum, 'threading' the hand to move X's arms to the right, then pushing both palms forward to close up X, using the pattern Like Sealed As If Closed *(figure 11.3c)*.

X turns both body and stance to the left, grips Y's wrist with the left hand and Y's elbow with the right, and pulls Y forward, using a pattern known as Pull Horse Back to Stable *(figure 11.3d)*. To avoid falling forward, Y moves the right leg diagonally forward to the right, crosses both arms in front and separates them, thus releasing X's hold. Y simultaneously kicks at X's chest or abdomen with the left heel *(figure 11.3e)*.

X moves the left leg back and deflects Y's thrust kick with a graceful 'threading' movement of the right palm, helped by an appropriate sway of the body, using a Shaolin pattern called Travelling Dragon Plays with Water *(figure 11.3f)*. Following the 'threading' movement, X moves forward with the left leg and thrusts the left palm at Y's throat *(figure 11.3g)*. Y brings the kicking leg back, and wards off X's thrusting palm with a *peng* technique.

This sequence, like others, illustrates the principle of yielding. When an opponent pushes, the Tai Chi Chuan exponent absorbs the pushing momentum by withdrawing, then pushes back to close up the opponent's arms. When the opponent pulls, instead of resisting, the Tai Chi Chuan exponent moves forward following the pulling momentum.

Sequence 8 Eagle Claw – Shoulder Strike

Instead of attacking with a right straight punch as in other sequences, X closes Y's guarding hands with the right hand, ie pushes the front guarding hand against the back one so that Y cannot counter-attack. X then strikes Y's throat with a left palm thrust in a pattern known as Poisonous Snake Shoots Venom *(figure 11.4a)*. Nevertheless, Y responds with the usual right *peng* technique at a right Bow-arrow Stance.

As soon as Y responds, X makes a small anti-clockwise circle with the left hand so that, having been 'outside' Y's *peng*, it is now 'inside'. The inserted diagram in *figure 11.4a* shows this simple but important technique. X simultaneously moves the front leg a step forward, still in a left Bow-arrow Stance, but closer to Y, and strikes the latter's chest with a

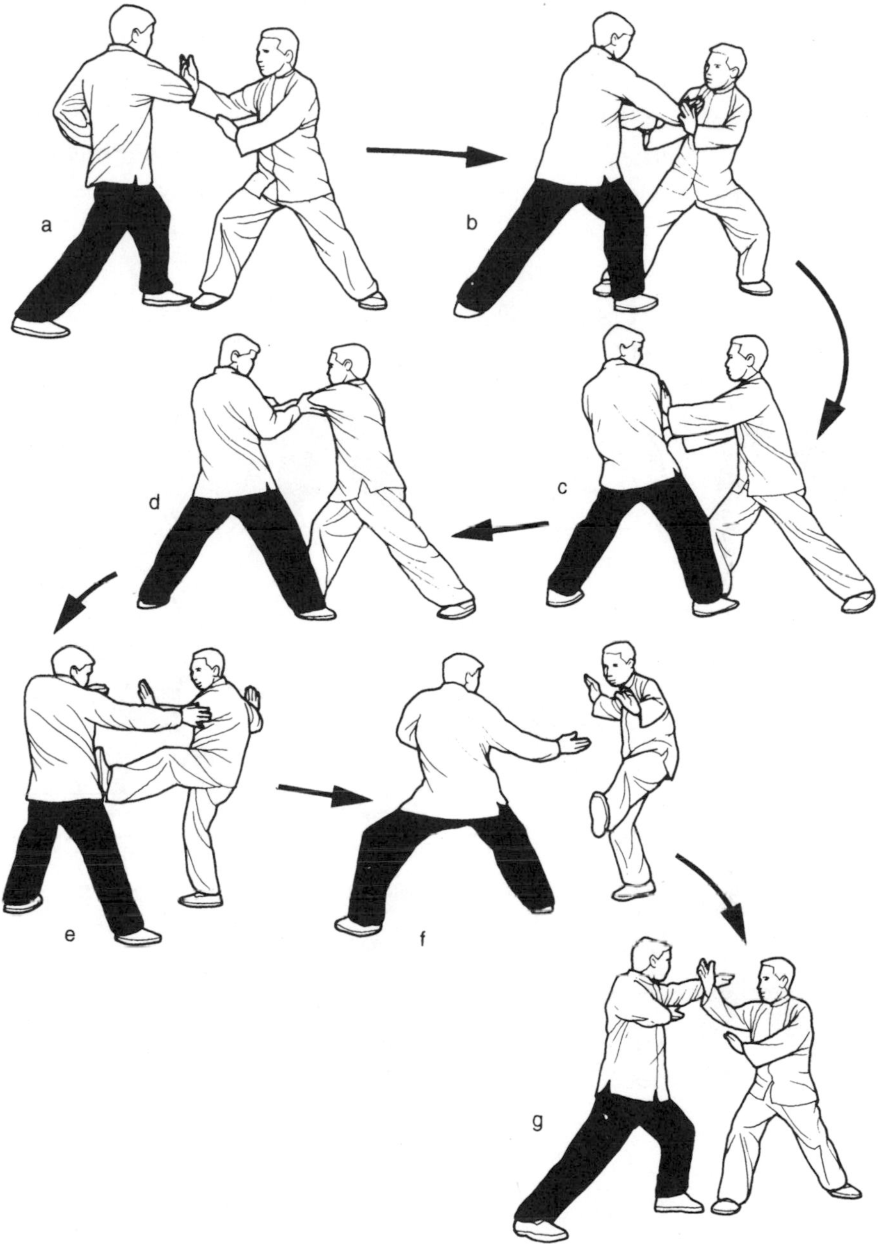

Fig 11.3 Countering a pulling attack

vertical punch. X's initial attack is therefore a lead, leading Y to respond so that X can instantly continue with the vertical punch, hopefully before Y can recover from the first defence. But if Y fails to respond to the lead, it becomes a real attack.

Y moves the front right leg back to a right Unicorn Step, intercepts and pushes aside X's punch with the left hand *(figure 11.4b)*, moves the left leg forward to a left Bow-arrow Stance, and also strikes X with a vertical punch *(figure 11.4c)* using the pattern Move–Intercept–Punch. X sinks into a Horse-riding Stance and grips Y's right wrist with the right

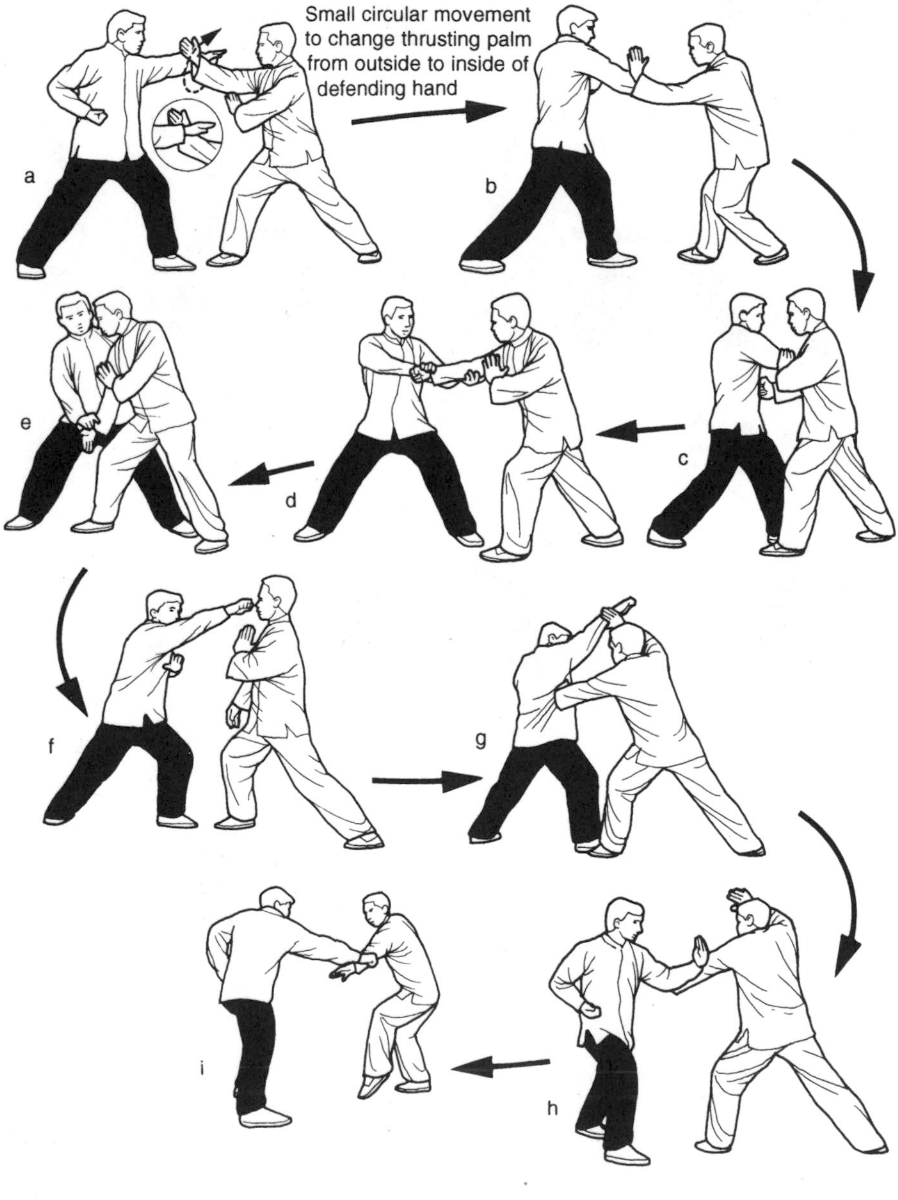
Small circular movement
to change thrusting palm
from outside to inside of
defending hand
a
b
c
d
e
f
g
h
i

Fig 11.4 Countering a gripping attack

hand and Y's right elbow with the left hand in a pattern called Old Eagle Catches Snake *(figure 11.4d).*

Y relaxes that arm, moves the left leg diagonally forward close to X then, using the left leg for anchorage, shoots the body forward to strike at X's chest with the right shoulder, *(figure 11.4e).* X quickly moves the left leg back to avoid the shoulder strike, and counter-attacks with a leopard punch (formed by making the fist with the knuckles of the second joints instead of at the third joints as in a normal fist), using the pattern Angry Leopard Charges at Fire *(figure 11.4f).* So here, both X and Y are using the advanced striking tactic of 'no defence, direct counter-attack'.

Y brings the right leg back to a right Unicorn Step to dodge X's attack, uses the right hand to lift X's right leopard punch, moves the left leg forward to a low left Bow-arrow Stance, and strikes X with the left palm in the pattern called Dodge Then Extend Arm – all in one swift, smooth movement *(figure 11.4g).* This is the tactic of 'defence–cum–counter-attack'.

X takes a small step diagonally to the right with the right leg and blocks Y's attack with the left palm, in a pattern called Asking the Way at Bow-arrow *(figure 11.4h).* Making sure that Y is not up to some trick or other, X turns left into a sideways left Bow-arrow Stance and strikes out with a right punch to Y's ribs, in a pattern called Fierce Tiger Charges at Gate. This is the tactic of 'first defence, then counter-attack'.

Y springs diagonally to the right, turns left and observes X with White Crane Flaps Wings *(figure 11.4i).* Then both combatants return to their poise patterns.

In this sequence, all the three categories of attacking tactics are used. Because both X and Y are advanced exponents, they use the tactics of 'no defence, direct counter-attack'. But when they realize that the other is also a good fighter, they find it safer to use the more elementary tactics of 'defence–cum–counter–attack' and 'first defence, then counter-attack'.

It is a basic tenet of all styles of Chinese kungfu that exponents must first ensure that they are safe from injury, before they think of attacking an opponent. When masters fight, a single blow can seriously injure or kill. So you will not find genuine kungfu exponents exchanging a lot of blows, charging wildly without thought of retreat, or using high kicks where vital sex organs are exposed – except on the very rare occasions when such methods may be necessary in special situations.

Sequence 9 Taming Tiger – Flying Diagonally

In this combat sequence, X initiates the attack by gripping Y's front guarding hand, with the pattern Catching With a Tiger Claw *(figure 11.5a)*. Y responds with Repulse Monkey *(figure 11.5b)*. The circular turning of Y's left hand releases X's grip, and Y's right palm strikes X's face.

X brings the left leg back to avoid Y's strike and grips Y's right wrist with another Tiger Claw, moving forward to a right Bow-arrow Stance for better positioning *(figure 11.5c)*. Y relaxes the right arm and follows the forward momentum of X's right hand by changing his left Four-six Stance to a left Unicorn Step. Then, continuing X's momentum, Y makes a circular turn and moves the right arm up, thus releasing X's grip as well as pushing X's arm away and up. Continuing the movement gracefully, Y moves the left leg forward to a left Bow-arrow Stance and strikes X's ribs or chest with the left palm, using the pattern Dodge, Then Extend Arm *(figure 11.5d)*. This description is quite long, but with practice all these movements should be completed in a split second. This pattern also illustrates the Tai Chi Chuan principle 'before advancing, first retreat', and the tactic of 'following the opponent's momentum'.

X grips Y's left wrist with the left hand, and presses down hard at Y's left elbow *(figure 11.5e)*. This pattern, which is meant to break the opponent's arm or dislocate his elbow, is known as Lohan Tames a Tiger.

The technique for overcoming this Taming Tiger attack is surprisingly simple, despite the fact that many martial artists claim that both the attack and its defence are impossible in practice. In combat between kungfu masters it is not uncommon because it is efficacious and comparatively easy to execute. Many students, however, are unable to use it, either because they do not know about it or because they have not practised enough to acquire the necessary skills (especially accuracy, power and speed) to execute it effectively. But if you practise sufficiently – and correctly – you will be able to use *all* the techniques described in these combat sequences with ease.

To overcome Taming the Tiger, Y moves the right leg a little to the left, at the same time subtly turning the whole left arm in a small arc in a clockwise direction, with the movement issuing from his shoulder; this will neutralize X's attack as well as preparing for the spiral-force counter-attack that immediately follows *(figure 11.5f)*.

Without any break in movement, Y moves his or her front leg in between X's legs, with the left shoulder close to X's body; with a twist of

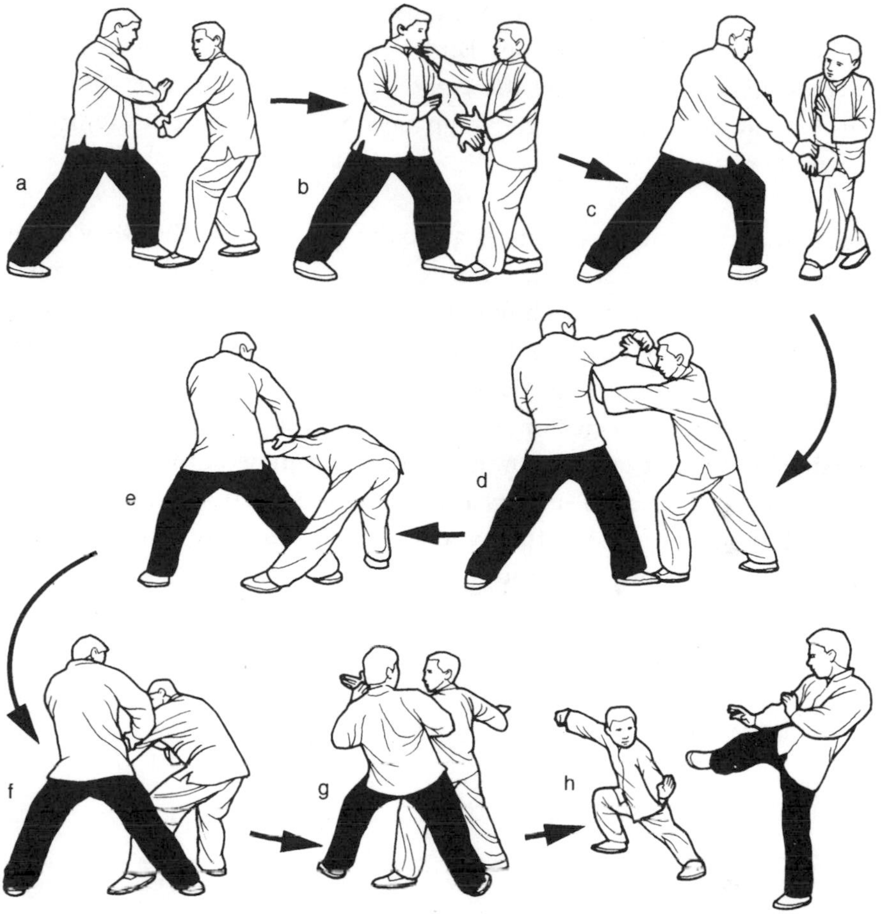

Fig 11.5 Flying Diagonally from Taming the Tiger

the whole body, which is a continuation of previous movements, Y spreads the left arm diagonally forward and upward, sending X falling backwards, *(figure 11.5g)*. This pattern is Flying Diagonally; its movement starts from the back right leg, is controlled by the rotation of the waist, and its spiral force is manifested in the whole left arm.

As is the case with many other patterns, the description of the movements is lengthy because many fine movements are involved, which are crucial for the effective execution of this technique. If you have a good foundation in basic Tai Chi Chuan skills, these movements will come naturally and should be executed elegantly in a split second. You should also have some internal force, without which it is difficult to implement this technique effectively.

To avoid being thrown away, X moves the left leg back and launches a right side kick known as Happy Bird Hops Up a Branch *(figure 11.5h)*. Y avoids this kick by moving the right leg a step to the right side, and turns left into the pattern Single Whip Low Stance. Then both return to their poise patterns.

Although these combat sequences are basic in the sense that they form the basis for the combat applications of Tai Chi Chuan, they are quite advanced in some of their techniques. Reading the descriptions may provide insights into the depth and scope of Tai Chi Chuan as a martial art, but by itself it is of course inadequate to make you combat efficient.

As in any art, the secret of success is correct and consistent practice. You should spend at least six months practising these combat sequences before you can expect to see any reasonable results. If you are prepared to spend six years on them, then you will be on the way to becoming a master, if you are not one already.

12

Enriching Daily Life with Tai Chi Chuan

How Tai Chi Chuan Enhances Health, Work and Play

You will have a sense of tranquillity, joy and inner peace, yet you will be mentally sharp and fresh at all times.

The Chinese Concept of Health

Important though the martial aspects of Tai Chi Chuan are, if you practise it purely so as to be able to defend yourself, you will not be using your time efficiently – not only because you are unlikely to get into a fight but because there are other, faster ways of learning self-defence. In my opinion, practising Tomoi or Siamese Boxing is probably the fastest way one can learn to fight, but I nevertheless prefer Tai Chi Chuan to any other martial arts except Shaolin Kungfu because of the many other wonderful benefits it brings.

I make an exception of Shaolin Kungfu because in some ways it is superior to Tai Chi Chuan[1]. For example, while at the highest level both arts focus on training the mind, the method used in Shaolin Kungfu, known as Zen, is richer and more profound, because Tai Chi Chuan generally places more emphasis on *chi* or energy. On the other hand, many people may not be able to endure the very demanding training of Shaolin Kungfu, whereas Tai Chi Chuan training is comparatively relaxing and enjoyable.

Both Tai Chi Chuan and Shaolin Kungfu enrich our daily lives, often in ways no other arts can match. In this chapter we shall study why and how Tai Chi Chuan enhances health, work and play – three decisive factors that affect the richness of our lives.

Health is more than just freedom from clinical illness. To be truly healthy a person must also be able to sleep and eat well, be emotionally stable and mentally sound, have energy and zest for work and play, and usually be capable of enjoying wholesome sex. Someone who habitually takes sleeping pills to sleep and vitamin pills as food supplements, who becomes angry or nervous easily, who is unable to think clearly, who is often lazy or languid, and unable to lead a normal sex life, cannot be called healthy.

The difference in approach to health between the Chinese and the Westerners is well described by James MacRitchie in his interesting and informative book, *Chi Kung: Cultivating Personal Energy.*

> Now one of the peculiar things about health is that in the West nobody seems to know what it is, yet here we are with a concern that affects everybody, and which has grown to a size that constitutes an 'industry' – The Health Care Industry. In the United States at least (and probably most other places) it is second in size only to the Defence Industry and the annual expenditure on health is around 750 billion dollars a year. That is three-quarters of a trillion dollars.
>
> The first thing one might conclude from these figures is that people are incredibly healthy in the US. They are not. They are nowhere near as healthy as the Chinese, and comparatively the Chinese have nothing at all. However the most astonishing and absurd thing, given these numbers, is that:
>
> *In the West we do not have a*
> *measurable definition of health*
>
> There is no medical text book which defines the state of health. There is no monitoring process for when, and how much, we are healthy. We only know when we are unhealthy, because then something is wrong. The working definition of health in Western medicine is when you are not ill...
>
> In China, this whole proposition is reversed. They simply turn it around. When someone is ill they ask the simple question 'Why is this person not healthy?'
>
> Perhaps we should take just a moment or two to look at the Chinese definition of health. Their definition of health is understood in terms of the ENERGY SYSTEM, because the energy system is of a slightly different and 'higher' level than the flesh and blood and bones. The energy system functions as a 'control system' or 'blueprint' for the body. It lays down the basic framework. The hierarchical sequence of control and influence is as follows:

> ENERGY/CHI → BLOOD → CELLS → TISSUES → ORGANS → FUNCTIONS → RELATIONSHIPS → THE WHOLE
>
> So if the basic level of your energy/control-system/blueprint is out of order then you are likely to get sick.[2]

MacRitchie's succinct observations show why all the health factors mentioned at the start of this chapter, such as sleeping well, being emotionally stable and having a zest for work and play, are inter-related. This explains why the mechanistic, reductionist treatment of illness is unsatisfactory, why conventional Western medicine is unable to establish the causes of such diseases as hypertension, asthma, rheumatism, ulcers, diabetes and cancer, and, on a positive note, why patients often report having had these so-called incurable diseases cured by alternative means like practising Chi Kung and Tai Chi Chuan.

Energy and Chinese Medicine

The basis of all Chinese health care and medicine is *chi* or energy. All Chinese medical practices – including herbalism, acupuncture, massage therapy, external medicine, traumatology and Chi Kung therapy – are directed towards correcting energy disharmony. If the energy flow is disharmonious it will affect the normal, healthy working of each successive hierarchical level mentioned by MacRitchie and manifest as a disorder of the body (and mind). Treatment, therefore, needs to be holistic and aimed at the root cause. If we treat a diseased liver only at the level of the organ, for example, its disordered tissues or cells may cause the same disease to recur, or it may manifest as disorders in other parts of the body. In Chinese medicine we do not treat the liver or its tissues and cells; we treat the whole person at its basic *chi* level.

If a cancer patient consults a Chinese physician, the physician will not describe the patient as suffering from cancer, because in traditional Chinese medicine, cancer does not exist! There is a modern Chinese term for cancer – *ai* – but it is not a traditional Chinese medical term; it is a modern term translated from English.

How, then, would a Chinese physician describe the illness of a cancer patient? He or she would describe the illness – any illness – not from the perspective of its symptoms at a localized site, but from the perspective of the whole person in relation to the root causes at the basic energy level. In determining the causes, the physician is not as concerned with what caused the illness, such as the types of carcinogens or the amount of radiation, as with what caused the patient to be unhealthy, ie why he or she failed to adjust to the carcinogens or radiation when other people did so successfully. Hence the physician may describe the disorder as stagnation of liver energy due to a blockage of the lung meridian and insufficient *chi* at the spleen system, or accumulation of heat poison at the intermediate level of the chest due to an energy blockage at the pericardium meridian. Different patients suffering from what conventional doctors may label as the same type of cancer are usually described differently by Chinese physicians, because the reasons why the patients have failed to overcome the cancer naturally are usually different.

Although these descriptions may not make sense to those who only view illness from the conventional Western medical paradigm, to the Chinese physician they are meaningful and concise, often describing the causes, location and developmental stage of the disease. More importantly, these descriptions never sign any death warrants; in fact, if the causes of the disease, such as the energy blockage or poisonous heat described above, are eliminated, the patient will recover without ever knowing that they suffered from cancer!

It may surprise someone who is used to being told that cancer is often fatal and incurable, that it can be relieved. Even more surprising, perhaps, is that according to Western cancer experts, we all have cancer thousands of times during our lives, yet we cure ourselves without knowing about it.

Why then do some people develop cancer – or any other disease for that matter? According to Chinese medical thought, it is because certain parts of their body (which includes the mind, as the mind and body are always treated as one unity in Chinese medicine) have failed to function as they should, and this failure is due to disharmonious energy flow. The *Nei Jing* or *Internal Classic of Medicine*, considered to be the most authoritative text in Chinese medicine, advises that if your vital energy flows harmoniously in your meridians, then illness simply cannot occur. If, because of your Western perspective on health, you find this statement difficult to accept, reflect on the fact that this view, more than any other, is responsible for maintaining the health of the largest population of the world for the longest period of history. It has also enabled me, as a Chi Kung grandmaster, to help relieve many patients of their cancers and other so-called incurable diseases like asthma, diabetes, hypertension, ulcers, insomnia and sexual inadequacy.[3]

Translated into conventional medical terms, harmonious *chi* flow means that the feed-back system, defence system, immune system, regenerative system, hormonal system, transport system and all other body systems are functioning naturally. If harmful microbes enter our body, our defence system will provide the necessary antibodies to kill or inhibit them and our transport system will flush them out of our body. If there is wear and tear, or if there is a harmful deposition of toxic waste in the body, such as acid eating into the stomach or cholesterol forming in the blood vessels, our regenerative system will repair the wear and tear or the hormonal system will produce the necessary hormones or chemicals to neutralize the toxic waste. If we are emotionally or mentally stressed, our body will marshal the necessary systems to flush out the negative emotions and rest the mind.

These life processes are occurring in every one of us every moment of our lives. It is only when people's energy system fails, as when what the Chinese call the defence and protection energy fail to reach the 'heat evil' or microbes, that they have to take antibiotics. It is only when their organ energy fails to work properly that they need to have part of a damaged organ cut out, or take a drug to dilate their blood vessels. It is only when some related meridians are so blocked that their negative emotions cannot be flushed out or their heart energy is insufficient to nourish their mind, that they have to take tranquillizers, antidepressants or undergo psychotherapy.

The Effects of Tai Chi Chuan on Health

As the root cause of illness is blockage of energy flow, the logical remedy is to clear the blockage. Of the numerous therapeutic approaches to clearing energy blockage, such as herbalism, acupunture, massage, external medicine and physiotherapy, practising Chi Kung is the most direct and effective for curing chronic illness and illness where the causes are difficult to define, like hypertension, rheumatism, depression and cancer. But what has all this to do with Tai Chi Chuan? Everything, because Tai Chi Chuan when practised correctly is a complete set of Chi Kung itself, although generally it is more significant in promoting health than in curing illness.

In this respect, Tai Chi Chuan is superior to Shaolin Kungfu. Apart from the higher levels which not many students reach, in much of Shaolin Kungfu training, Chi Kung and mind development are trained separately from set practice, whereas in Tai Chi Chuan training, Chi Kung and mind development are incorporated into set practice right at the beginning. This was an extremely useful innovation by Zhang San

Feng when he evolved Tai Chi Chuan from Shaolin Kungfu. Instead of having to train in Shaolin Kungfu, Chi Kung and Zen – the three arts that are of greatest benefit to the enhancement of health, work and leisure – he put them together as one unified art. But of course if you practise Tai Chi only as dance, you will only obtain the benefits that are generally associated with dance, such as flexibility, elegance and relaxation. You are unlikely to gain those benefits, like radiant health, vitality and mental clarity that are characteristic of genuine Tai Chi Chuan training.

Promoting harmonious energy flow and attaining a heightened state of mind, which are excellent for combat efficiency as well as for enabling all our body systems to function properly, are the two cardinal features of Tai Chi Chuan. If you have practised the art for many years but have never experienced them, then you have definitely missed some of its best benefits.

What are the signs that indicate that you have attained harmonious energy flow and a heightened state of mind? When you have achieved a high level of energy control, you can usually feel the energy flow yourself and channel the energy wherever you wish. If you channel it to your palms, for example, they can be very powerful even if you have never practised against a sandbag. You will also solve any health problems you may have – complaints like colds, fever, bodily pain, depression, nervousness and anxiety will never bother you. You will eat and sleep well, and enjoy your work as much as your play.

When you have attained a heightened state of mind, you will have a sense of tranquillity, joy and inner peace, yet you will be mentally sharp and fresh at all times. Your emotional and mental dimension will have widened and deepened, and the sort of pettyness with which many people are preoccupied, like gossip and envy will appear very childish. You will be amazed at the depth and clarity with which you perceive and solve problems which appeared formidable before. And your friends will also feel the calmness and confidence that you inspire.

If you think this is too good to be true, just remember that these are qualities which all true masters exhibit. They were not born with them; they earned them from dedicated practice in great arts like Shaolin Kungfu and Tai Chi Chuan. They have generously recorded their methods so that you too can follow and benefit from them if you are ready to practise them conscientiously.

More Energy for Work and Play

In some ways the distinction between work and play is subjective. The general view that work is something we have to slog at for a living and play is what we engage in for fun is not always valid. Many industrialists today go to work because they enjoy it rather than as a means of earning a living, while some professional sportspeople dislike what they do. When you try to do Lifting Water 200 times with your legs trembling as you stand in your stance, you might call Tai Chi Chuan work, but later, when this training brings a sense of tranquillity with internal energy flowing inside your body, and experience what the Tai Chi Chuan master Xu Zhi Yi describes as 'a deep taste of pleasure', you will probably call it play. So we shall look at the effects of Tai Chi Chuan on work and play together because the same factors are applicable in both.

Irrespective of whether you work or play in an office or on a sports field, for yourself or an employer, with zest or reluctance, you need energy. Without energy, physical or mental or both, no work or play can ever be done. For most people, energy is derived from the air they breathe and the food they eat. Although many people may not realize it, according to the discoveries of Chi Kung or energy masters, the air they breathe gives about four times more energy than the food they eat. Still fewer are aware that energy masters can actually tap energy directly from the cosmos! But if you practise Tai Chi Chuan consistently, especially the Infinite Ultimate Stance and abdominal breathing, you too can develop this ability. Even in ordinary people, cosmic energy from the environment is constantly being exchanged with vital energy in the body.

Not many people, however, pay much attention to these two essential sources of energy, despite the frequent outcries against pollution in the air and junk food on the market. The Chinese approach towards health, as suggested by MacRitchie's quotation earlier, is to ask not why the air and food we take in are substandard, but why we cannot make the best use of what air and food we can get. So, instead of climbing a mountain once a while to breathe fresh air, and take factory-produced vitamins to supplement our diet, the Chinese approach is to improve the respiratory and digestive systems so that, like the Tai Chi principle of minimum force against maximum strength, we can get the most from the air and food on which we have to exist every day.

Tai Chi Chuan serves this function very well; a common comment from students is that their breathing has become slower and deeper, and their appetite has improved. Slower and deeper breathing is a logical result of breath control when performing Tai Chi Chuan sets or combat sequences, as well as of Tai Chi Chi Kung training. The appetite becomes better because the harmonious energy flow derived from Tai Chi Chuan practice harmonizes the digestive and other body systems.

Those who are trying to lose weight will have a bonus if they practise Tai Chi Chuan: their improved digestive system will turn whatever they eat into energy and not into mass – unless that is what their body naturally needs. More energy from improved respiratory and digestive systems, of course, means better work and play. Sportspeople at international level will find the ability to breathe slowly and deeply even when they are engaged in fast, vigorous movements particularly useful – and it is a skill that is necessary for Tai Chi Chuan combat. If they can tap energy from the cosmos, as the masters can do, they may have that extra edge over their opponents which is crucial in international competition.

A Healthy Body and a Relaxed Mind

Two other factors affecting our work and play are our physical body and mind. It may seem trite to say that a healthy body and a relaxed mind make us more effective in work and play, but it is astonishing how little attention is actually paid to this simple truth. Tens of thousands of dollars are spent by companies, sports organizations and states on medical bills when workers or sportspeople become sick or injured, and more is spent on holidays and recreational facilities to help them wind down when they have become over stressed – not to mention the cost of absenteeism. But how many spend any money on *maintaining* physical, emotional and mental health, such as by employing masters to teach them genuine Tai Chi Chuan? It is heartening to note that insurance companies in Germany now pay their clients to learn Tai Chi Chuan and Chi Kung, but they are the exception.

Tai Chi Chuan is without doubt an excellent way to promote physical, emotional and mental health. Even people who learn it only as a dance form report noticeable benefits, as is evident from the widespread popularity of the dance aspects. This will give you an idea of how much more benefits genuine Tai Chi Chuan can provide. Its greatest benefits are not found in its external form but in its internal significance, especially in its energy and mind aspects. As the master Hao Yue Yu advises at the very start of his Tai Chi Chuan treatise, *Tai Chi Chuan Set Practice and Combat Sequences*, 'The significance of Tai Chi Chuan lies not in its form but in its energy flow, not in the external but in the internal.' This statement applies to health as well as to combat.

We are familiar with the typical image of a business executive who has to take a number of pills to keep his or her blood pressure, cholesterol level, nervous tension and other complaints under control. But most people do not realize that many top-class sportsmen and women, despite their unquestionable fitness, are actually unhealthy! Top-class gymnasts, for example, have serious arthritis problems, professional golfers suffer from back pain, and international footballers endure internal injuries which are often left untreated. But worse than their physical illness is the tremendous emotional stress these people have to endure – probably more than business executives in the so called rat-race. It is not uncommon, for instance, to find jittery athletes, literally biting their finger-nails between competitions or matches, because of the tension induced by the uncertainty of their situation.

Tai Chi Chuan is a wonderful art for helping executives, sportspeople and others involved in high-pressure activities to overcome their pressing problems. Even if a manager thinks only of profit and not of the welfare of the people who work for him or her, it is still worth providing genuine Tai Chi Chuan training for them. It provides the physical and emotional health we all need. The harmonious energy flow which results from Tai Chi Chuan practice helps prevent illness or injury, and speeds recovery. It is well known that sportspeople in China recover from injuries much faster than other athletes; the secret is Chi Kung therapy, the effect of which can be obtained from practising Tai Chi Chuan. One can imagine how much money a team can save if a valuable player recovers in three days instead of six in the middle of an international tournament.

Unlike in the West, where maintaining health is treated separately from curing illness, in the Chinese view health and illness lie along the same continuum, because conceptually at one end energy flow is harmonious, while at the other it is disorderly. So the *chi* flow effect of Tai Chi Chuan training prevents you from being sick if you are already healthy, and cures you of your illness if you are not. *Chi* flow is the crucial feature of Tai Chi Chuan: it is found in every facet of its training. If you practise it for some time but do not experience *chi* flow, it is time to examine your training methods.

In addition to maintaining health and curing illness, Tai Chi Chuan contributes to mental development – the wonderful effect of the second characteristic of the training, attaining a heightened state of mind. There is no doubt that mental freshness and clarity produce better results in every aspect of our lives. It may be useful to note the difference between mental clarity and mental knowledge. Like the difference between skills and techniques in Tai Chi Chuan combat, one concerns quality and the other quantity. Tai Chi Chuan helps to improve the quality of the mind so that we can better apply whatever knowledge, mental or practical, we can acquire.

Every movement in Tai Chi Chuan is an occasion for mind training: when one makes a move, one's mind is in the movement; when one regulates one's breathing, the mind is focused to direct *chi* to flow where one desires. And at all times, especially when one is engaged in sparring or fighting, one has to be perfectly relaxed. The skills of mental concentration, mental control and relaxation developed in Tai Chi Chuan training can be rewardingly transferred to our daily lives.

The techniques of meditation practised in advanced Tai Chi Chuan can also be applied to daily life. A business executive, for example, may go into meditation and review a business project in a state of heightened consciousness. A top-class sportsman or woman may go into meditation and imprint upon the subconscious mind the techniques needed in his competition. This method, in fact, was the standard approach used, usually without being aware of its psychological labelling, by Tai Chi Chuan and other kungfu masters to enhance combat efficiency. The masters would go over selected combat sequences while in a state of flowing meditation so that the sequences would 'sink into their heart'; when they were engaged in real combat, they let the sequences flow spontaneously. This explains why their fighting movements were so fast and accurate, and how they could make split–second life or death decisions.

Hence, Tai Chi Chuan enhances our work and play by decisively improving the three most basic contributing factors for their success or otherwise, namely energy, body and mind. They are so basic that, ironically, most people overlook them, and concentrate on extrinsic factors like acquiring the latest techniques, motivating talks, and threats or incentives to influence performance. No one denies the usefulness of these extrinsic factors, but if someone does not have sufficient energy, is sick or is mentally stressed – situations which are not uncommon nowadays – the extrinsic factors may actually have adverse effects.

Vital energy, good health and mental freshness are important factors, affecting every aspect of our daily lives. It is interesting to compare the difference in approach between the West and the Chinese in attaining them. To improve energy levels, for example, people in the West employ methods like running and carrying weights. From the Chinese viewpoint this is confusing function with substance, or effect with cause. Seeking to increase energy levels in this way involves trying to improve the cause by working on its effect. In Tai Chi Chuan the approach is reversed; we strengthen the substance, and as a result its function improves. In other words, by increasing one's energy level, one can not only run and carry weights better, but also improve one's performance in other areas where energy is involved.

The methods used to increase energy level in Tai Chi Chuan training include improving breathing habits to produce a better exchange of fresh air and toxic waste, storing accumulated energy at energy fields in the body, clearing meridians to promote harmonious energy flow, loosening and strengthening body tissues and organs to adjust to the new energy level, and attaining a heightened state of mind for better energy control. By any standard, energy management has been developed to a very sophisticated and high level in Tai Chi Chuan.

This advanced aspect of energy flow in Tai Chi Chuan makes it an excellent system for promoting health. Unlike typical Western methods of health care like physical exercise, diet control and food supplements which manifest the mechanistic and reductionist philosophy of conventional Western medicine, the Tai Chi Chuan approach is holistic, looking after not only the physical but also the emotional and mental health of its practitioners. Practising this art, therefore, makes life rewarding and wholesome.

The other principal aspect of Tai Chi Chuan in its contribution to enriching life is its mind training. It is sobering to reflect that while our education system pays a great deal of attention to putting knowledge into our heads, it does not actually provide many techniques for training the mind. Many people find it hard to concentrate, to visualize or even just to relax. In Tai Chi Chuan, if it is practised properly, mind training assumes a central role. One of the first lessons Tai Chi Chuan students learn is to relax, and they have to relax throughout if they want their practice to be meaningful. Being mindful of their movements and visualizing energy flowing to appropriate places are two basic skills that they develop every time they practise Tai Chi Chuan.

Increasing our energy level and harmonizing our energy flow, enhancing our physical, emotional and mental health, and promoting a heightened state of consciousness, explain why and how Tai Chi Chuan can enrich our lives. They also provide useful criteria for measuring how much we have benefited from this wonderful art.

13

Wudang Tai Chi Chuan

Attaining Cosmic Reality Through Tai Chi Chuan

When you are suddenly awakened to the great cosmic truth that you do not have a physical body but are actually a boundless flow of energy in unity with the energy of the cosmos, you will have achieved the highest aim of Tai Chi Chuan.

Tai Chi Chuan and Spiritual Development

Many people know that at its highest level the Wudang martial art leads to spiritual fulfilment irrespective of one's religion, but few understand why and how this is possible. The Wudang Tai Chi Chuan presented here offers a glimpse of this possibility.

Wudang Tai Chi Chuan is reputed to have been invented by Zhang San Feng in the 13th century. The set illustrated in this chapter is based on the one presented by two Wudang masters, Pei Xi Rong and Li Chun Sheng. Pei Xi Rong is descended from a distinguished line of Wudang masters, and has contributed much to our present understanding of Wudang Kungfu. The two masters say:

> In performing the set, the movements should be extended (not cramped up), the forms graceful and agile, with force flowing continuously without a break, like flowing water. When you have completed one sequence, you should continue to the next so that your movements flow without end, complementing hard and soft aspects. Use your body to lead your arms, use will-power to lead your energy flow, and use energy flow to move your body. Your practice should be slow, graceful and harmonious. When you perform any patterns, use circular movements and internal spiral force. Your movement should be made according to the endless flow of vital energy in your meridians, so that vital energy and blood are spread over all organs and parts of the body, to attain the aim of internal strength and external power.[1]

So, when you practise this Wudang Tai Chi Chuan set, you must not use mechanical strength, nor must you perform each pattern or sequence in a staccato manner. The whole set flows like water without a break. At a very advanced stage, the body movements are not caused by muscles, but by flowing energy, which in turn is directed by the mind. This is the transcendental or spiritual level of Tai Chi Chuan. At an even higher level, when you are suddenly awakened to the great cosmic truth that you do not have a physical body but are actually a boundless flow of energy in unity with the energy of the cosmos, you will have achieved the highest aim of Tai Chi Chuan. However, advanced Tai Chi Chuan should only be practised under the supervision of a master.

The Patterns of Wudang Tai Chi Chuan

As in Shaolin Kungfu, Wudang Tai Chi Chuan patterns are poetically named in four characters each. The linguistic and cultural differences between Chinese and English often result in the poetry being lost and the meaning being distorted when these names are translated from one language to another. So, if you find some of them odd or awkward, the fault lies in my translation and not in the original names.

The Wudang Tai Chi Chuan set consists of 108 patterns and is divided into eight sections. Students who are familiar only with Yang-style Tai Chi Chuan will be surprised to find that both the names and the forms of Wudang Tai Chi Chuan patterns are very different. Indeed they are closer to Shaolin Kungfu than to the image of Tai Chi Chuan most people have. The names of the Wudang Tai Chi Chuan patterns are as follows.

Section 1

1 One Chi of Void
2 Two Aspects of Yin-yang
3 Turning of Cosmos
4 Beginning of Transformation
5 Riding Horse to Ask the Way
6 Left and Right Blocking
7 Four Primary Movements
8 Fire Cannon Towards Sky
9 Golden Tortoise Reveals Back
10 Two Saints Transmit Tao
11 Gorilla Pulls Rope
12 Single Bee Buzzing at Ear
13 Wind Through Sleeves
14 Fire Cannon Towards Sky
15 Lion Opens Mouth
16 Green Dragon Presents Claw
17 Turn Round to Origin

Section 2

18 Old Dragon Wags Tail
19 Wild Horse Charges at Stable
20 White Snake Pulls Grass
21 Turning Yin-yang
22 Push Clouds to Observe Sun
23 Cloud Dragons Show Elbow
24 Big Boss Ties Up Elbow
25 Single Bee Buzzing at Ear
26 Black Tiger Snatches Heart
27 Following Wind Pushing Fan
28 Carry Tiger Push Mountain
29 Turn Round to Origin

Section 3

30 Dark Dragon Draws Water
31 Wild Horse Charges at Stable
32 Liu Jin Presents Melon
33 Big Boss Removes Helmet
34 Turning Yin-yang
35 Investigate Cave at Mountain Side
36 Gorilla Washes Face
37 Crow Spreads Wings
38 Din Jia Clears the Way
39 Wind Through Sleeves
40 Tortoise and Snake Fighting
41 Golden Bird Brushes Eyebrow
42 Jade Girl Threads Shuttle
43 Golden Cockerel Spreads Wings
44 Turn Round to Origin

Section 4

45 Turn Wrist Single Thrust
46 Cross Hand Wash Fists
47 Er Lang Carries Mountain
48 Use Sickle to Cut Grass
49 Fierce Tiger Rushes at Prey
50 Use Sickle to Cut Grass
51 Bringing a Running Horse
52 Dark Dragon Wags Tail
53 Big Bird Circles Round Flowers
54 Turn Round to Origin

Section 5

55 Reduce Body Change Shadow
56 Flying Duck Leaves Group
57 Swallow Skims Water
58 Turn Stream Reverse Sea
59 Wind Through Sleeves
60 Dark Dragon Wags Tail
61 Dark Phoenix Faces the Sun
62 Fast Horse Raises Hooves
63 Wild Horse Charges at Stable
64 Reverse Pulling a Boat
65 Turn Rudder of Boat
66 Black Bear Opens Mouth
67 Oriole Nibbles Seed
68 Black Bear Presents Claw
69 Use Sword to Cut Fish Head
70 Turn Round to Origin

Section 6

71 Dark Dragon Wags Tail
72 Swarm of Bees Rising to Top
73 Tame Tiger at Low Stance
74 White Snake Shoots out Venom
75 Thousand Tons Press Ground
76 Hold Horse Raise Spear
77 Seven Stars to Ground
78 Black Bear Sways Shoulders
79 Black Bear Turns Paw
80 Black Bear Rotates Paw
81 Golden Cockerel Slants Wings
82 Carry Void Focus on Unity
83 Single Bee Buzzing at Ear

84 Lion Turns Body
85 Pine Tree Stands High
86 Turn Round to Origin

Section 7

87 Wild Horse Charges at Stable
88 Horizontal Cloud at Purple Summit
89 Turn Back Swing Fist
90 Parrot Flies Through Forest
91 Change Flowers on Tree
92 Golden Cockerel Slants Wings
93 Lion Plays with Ball
94 Dark Dragon Spins Around Body
95 Golden Snake Circles Willow
96 Turn Round to Origin

Section 8

97 Guard Left and Right
98 Lion Charges at Ball
99 Thrice Threading the Palms
100 Swallow Spreads Wings
101 Yellow Dragon Emerges from Cave
102 Rotate Palms Like Whirlwind
103 Crow Flying Across Valley
104 Thunder at Southern Cliff
105 Heaven Pillar Welcomes Sun
106 Clapping Palms Like Whirlwind
107 Gracefully Receiving the Way
108 Returning to Cosmos at Wudang

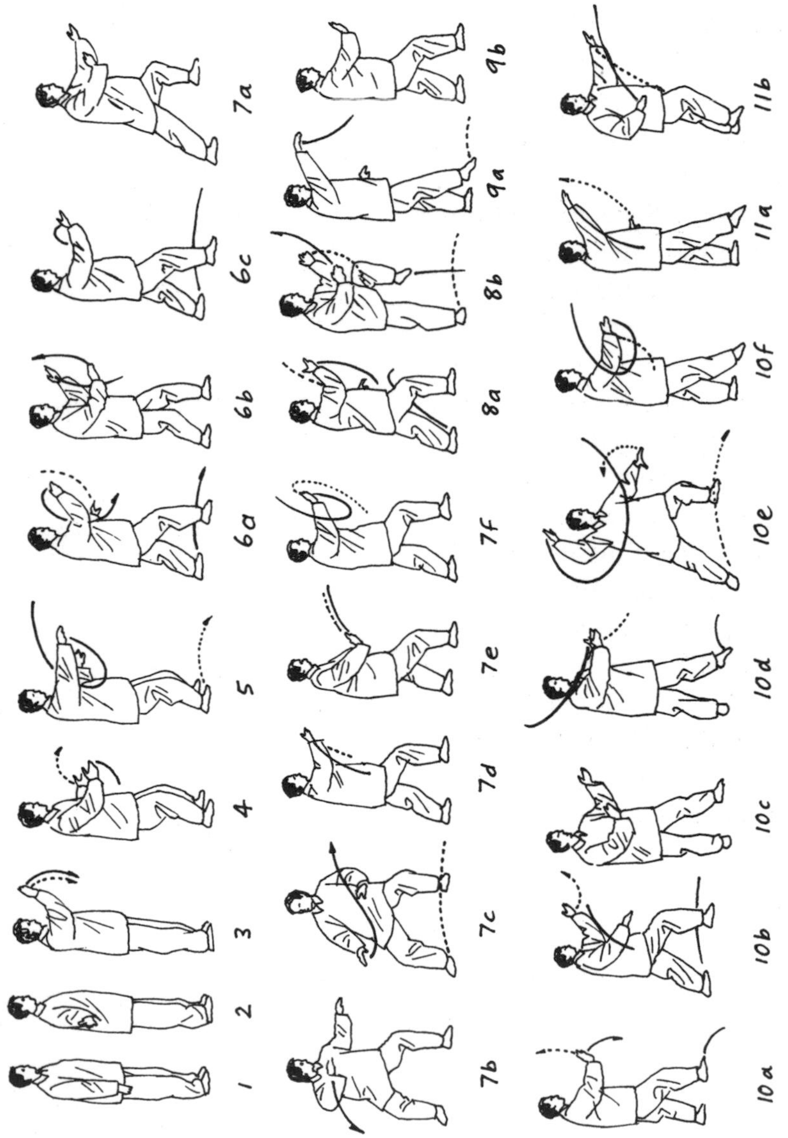
1
2
3
4
5
6a
6b
6c
7a
7b
7c
7d
7e
7f
8a
8b
9a
9b
10a
10b
10c
10d
10e
10f
11a
11b

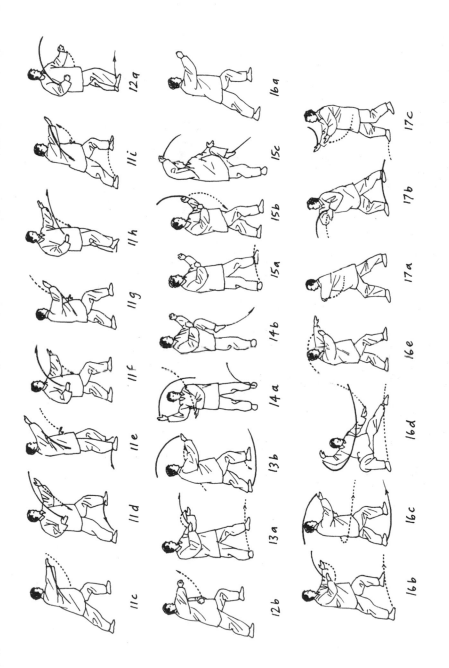

Fig 13.1 Wudang Tai Chi Chuan – Section 1

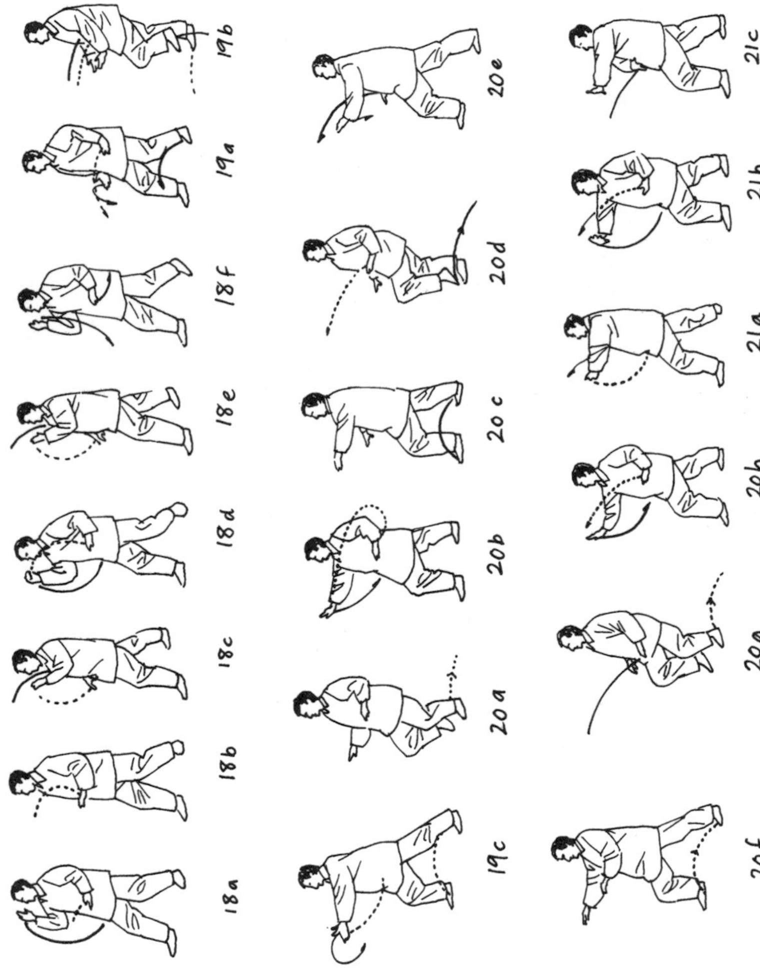
18a
18b
18c
18d
18e
18f
19a
19b
19c
20a
20b
20c
20d
20e
20f
20g
20h
21a
21b
21c

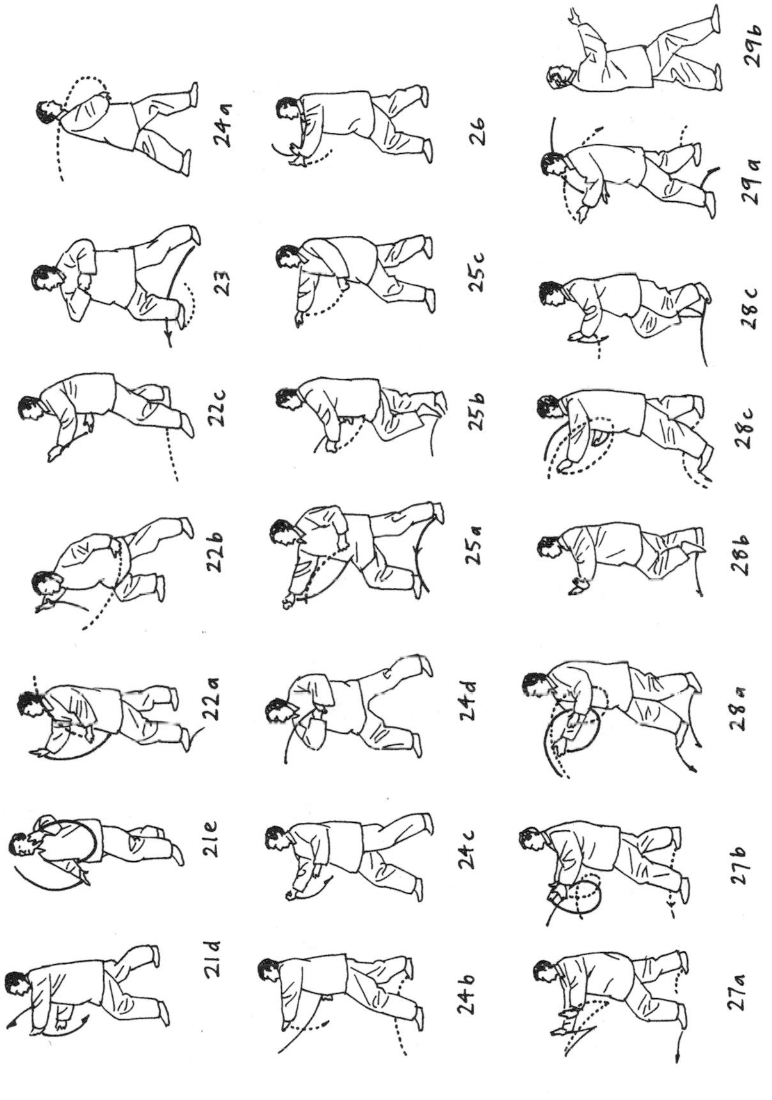

Fig 13.2 Wudang Tai Chi Chuan – Section 2

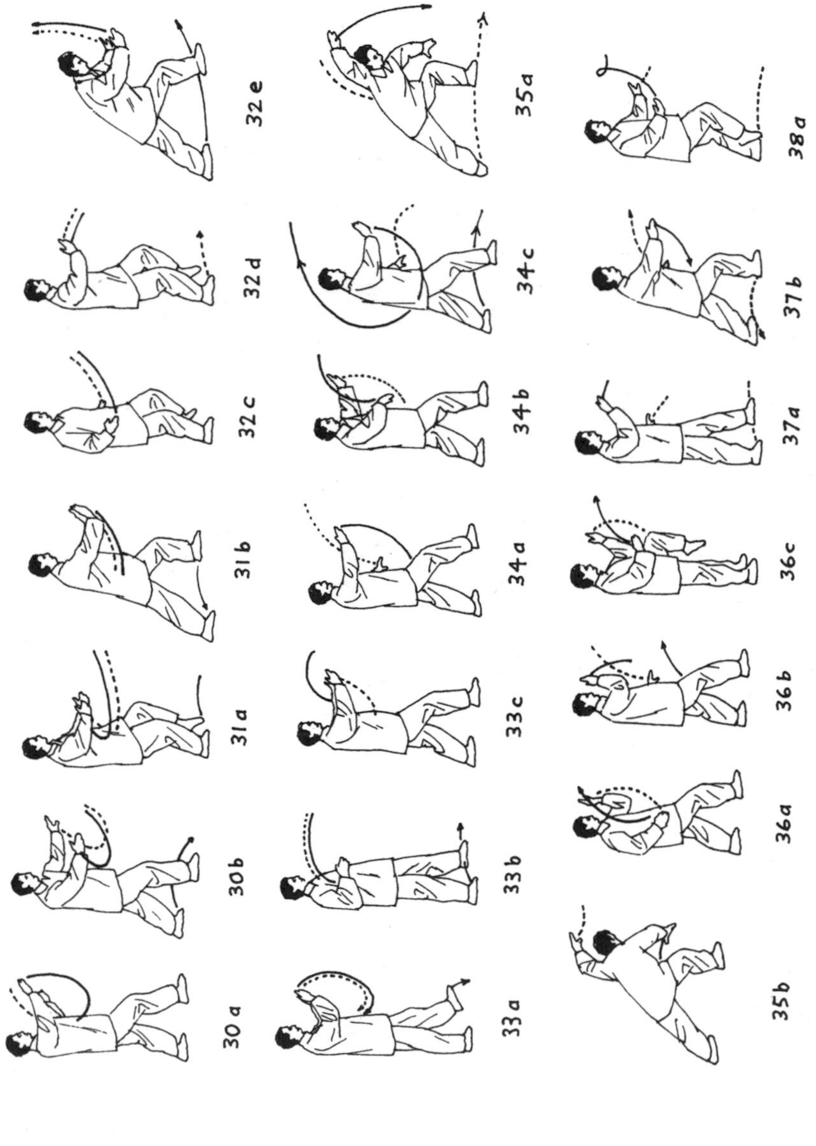
30 a
30 b
31 a
31 b
32 c
32 d
32 e
33 a
33 b
33 c
34 a
34 b
34 c
35 a
35 b
36 a
36 b
36 c
37 a
37 b
38 a

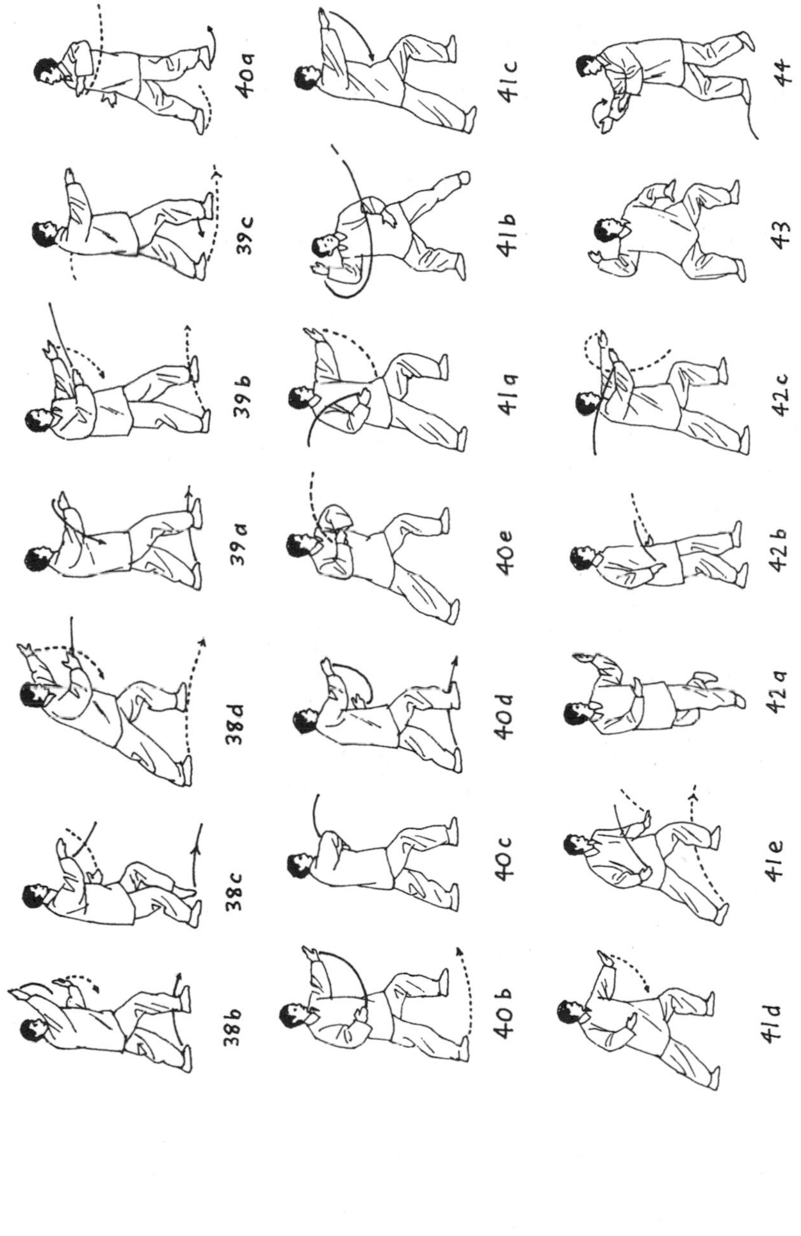

Fig 13.3 Wudang Tai Chi Chuan – Section 3

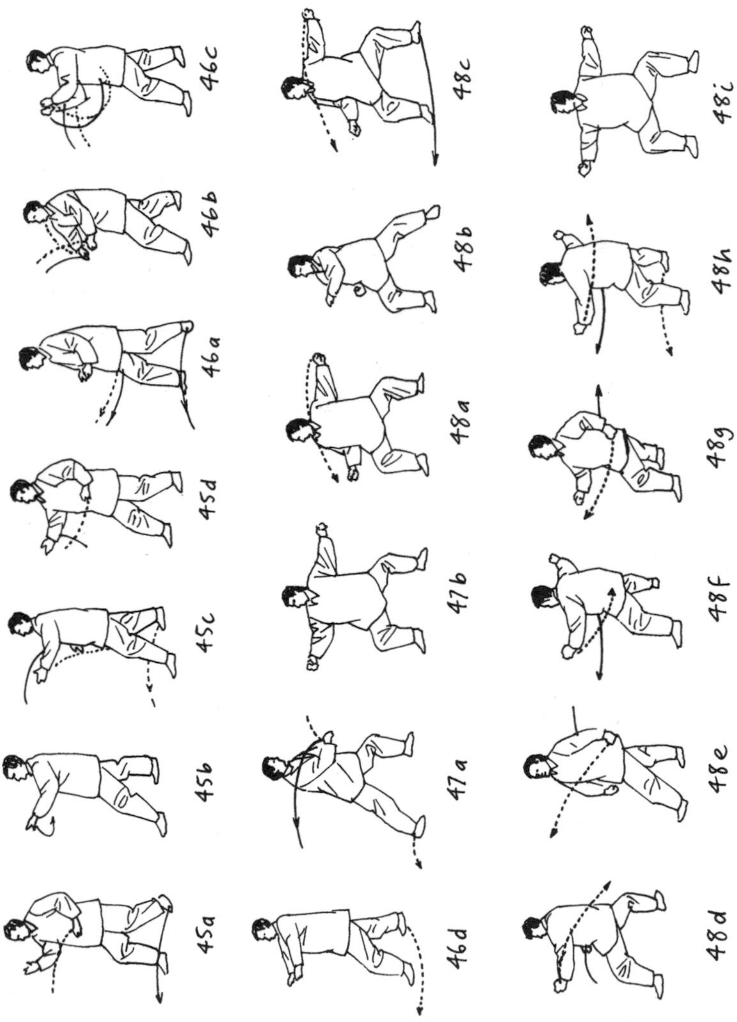
45a
45b
45c
45d
46a
46b
46c
46d
47a
47b
48a
48b
48c
48d
48e
48f
48g
48h
48i

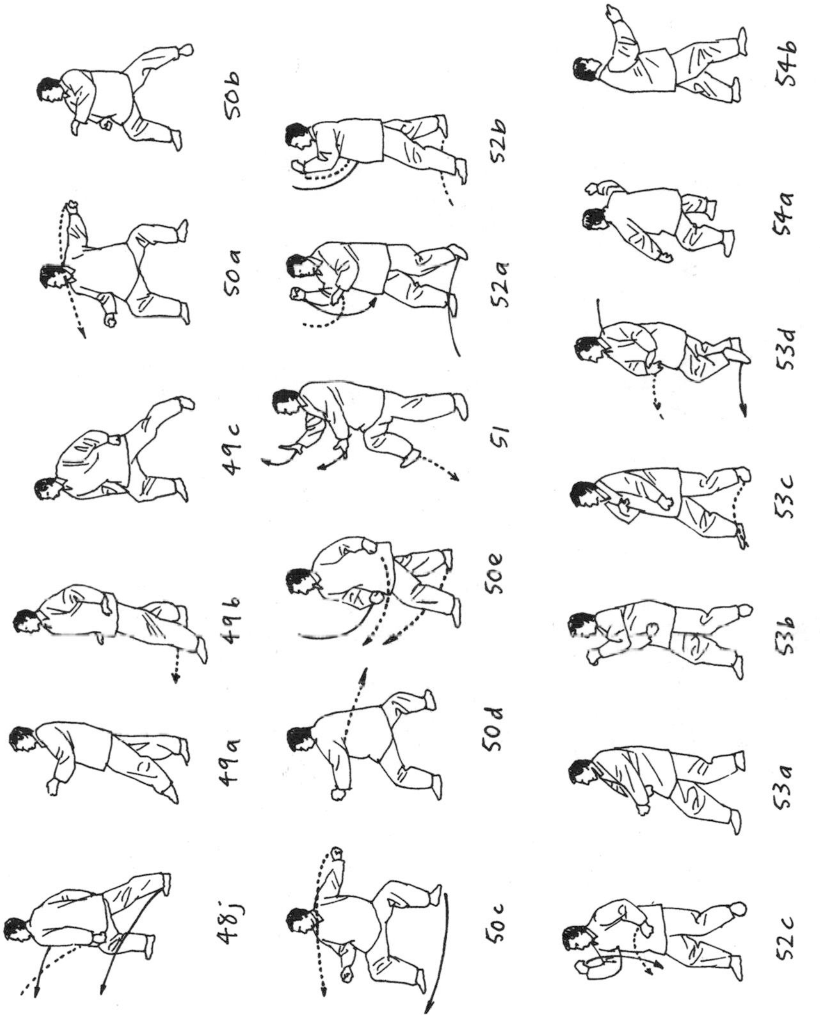

Fig 13.4 Wudang Tai Chi Chuan – Section 4

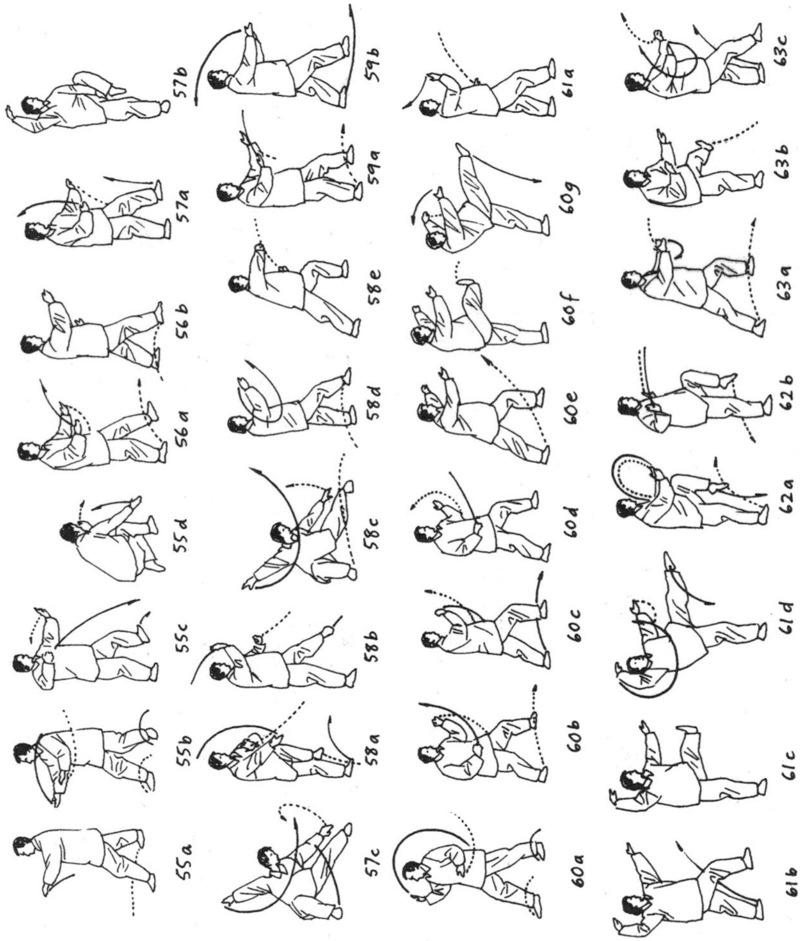
55a
55b
55c
55d
56a
56b
57a
57b
57c
58a
58b
58c
58d
58e
59a
59b
60a
60b
60c
60d
60e
60f
60g
61a
61b
61c
61d
62a
62b
63a
63b
63c

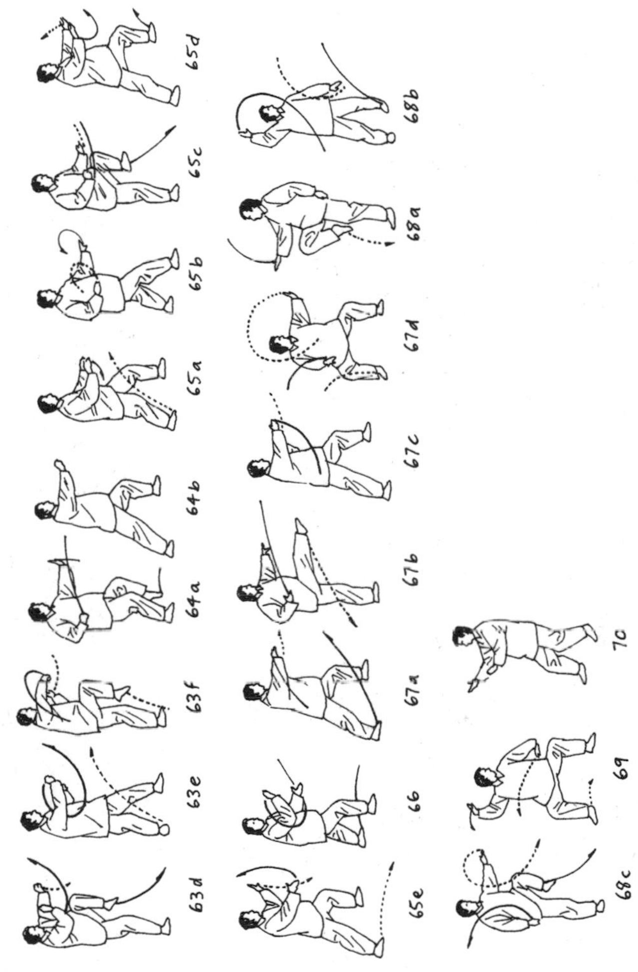

Fig 13.5 Wudang Tai Chi Chuan – Section 5

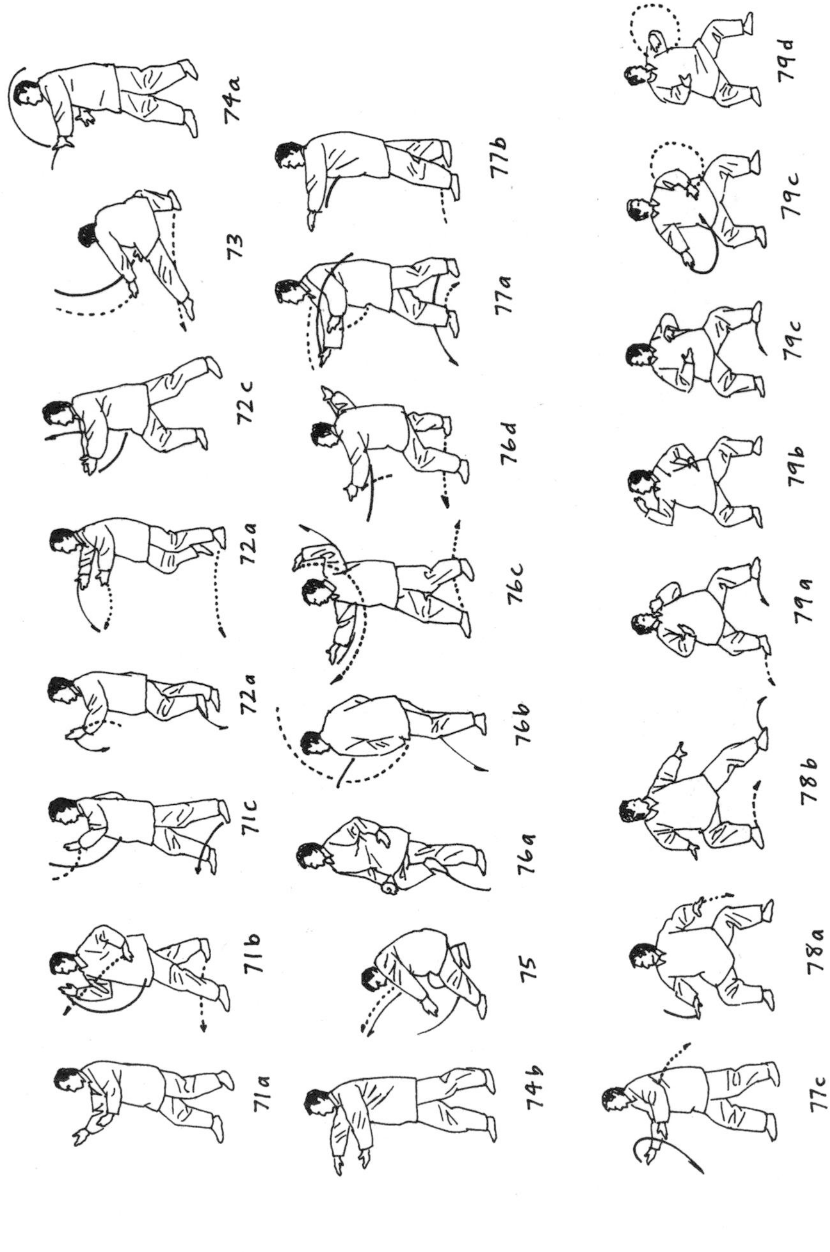
71a
71b
71c
72a
72a
72c
73
74a
74b
75
76a
76b
76c
76d
77a
77b
77c
78a
78b
79a
79b
79c
79c
79d

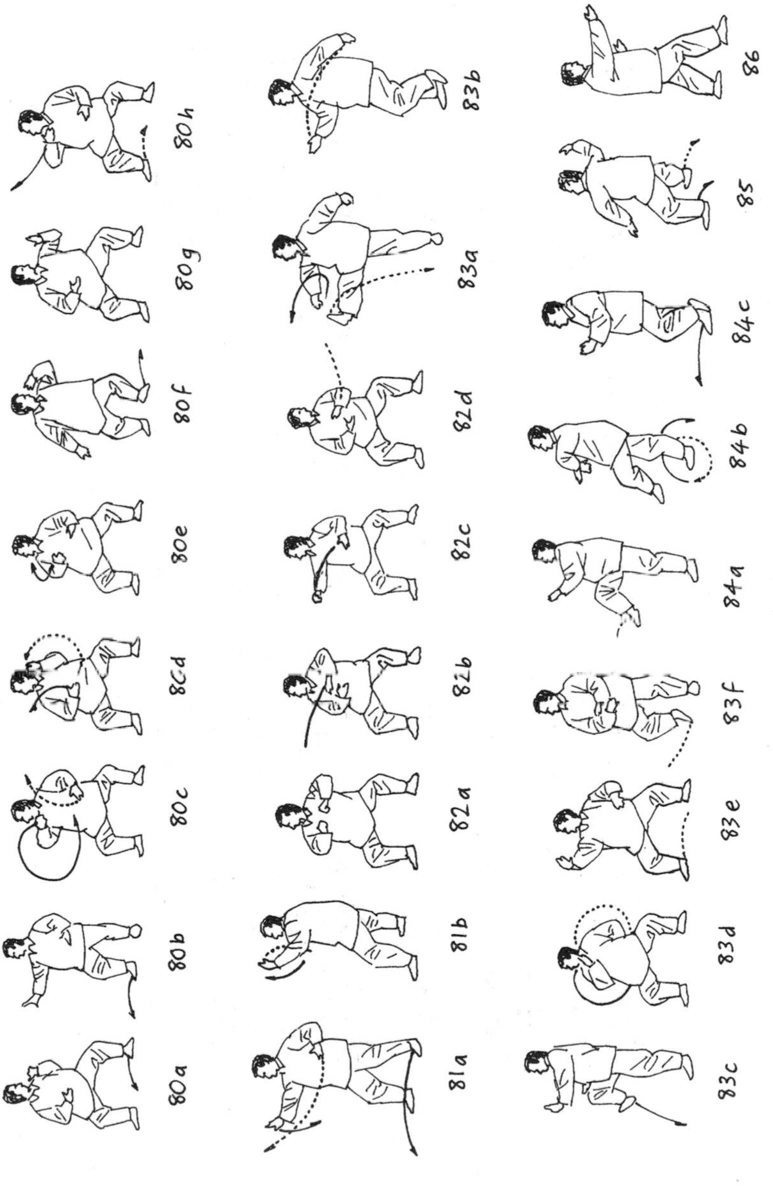

Fig 13.6 Wudang Tai Chi Chuan – Section 6

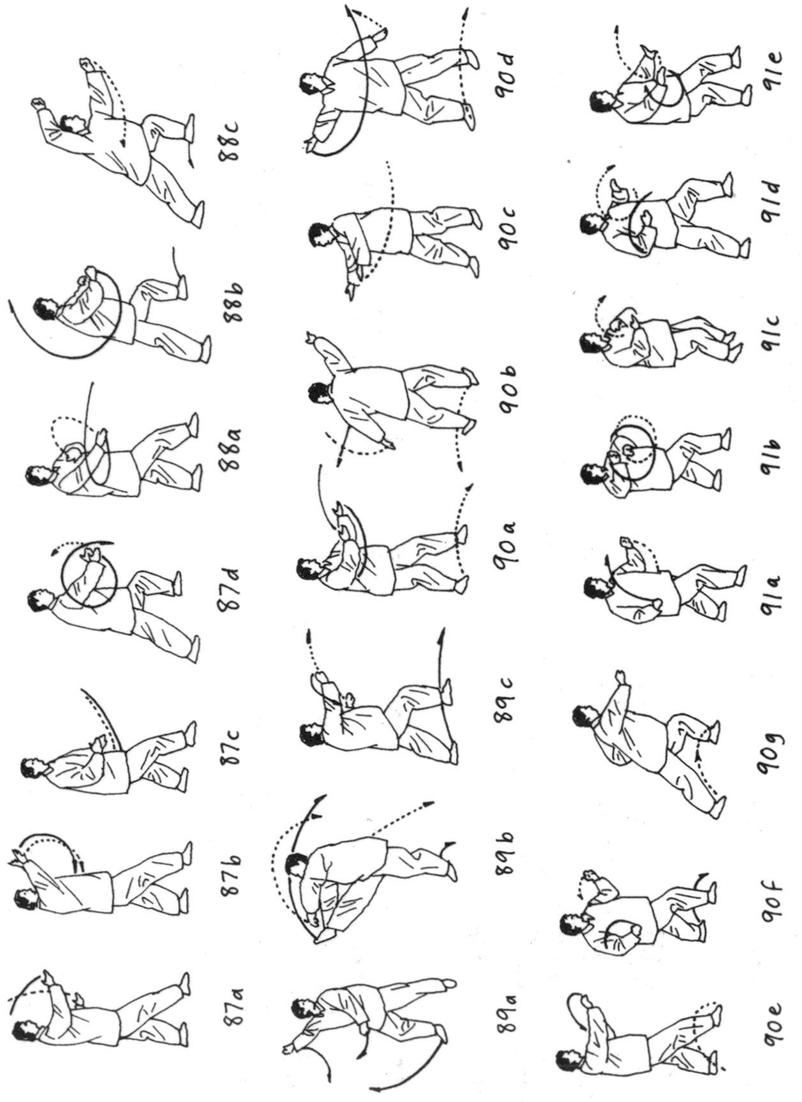
87a
87b
87c
87d
88a
88b
88c
89a
89b
89c
90a
90b
90c
90d
90e
90f
90g
91a
91b
91c
91d
91e

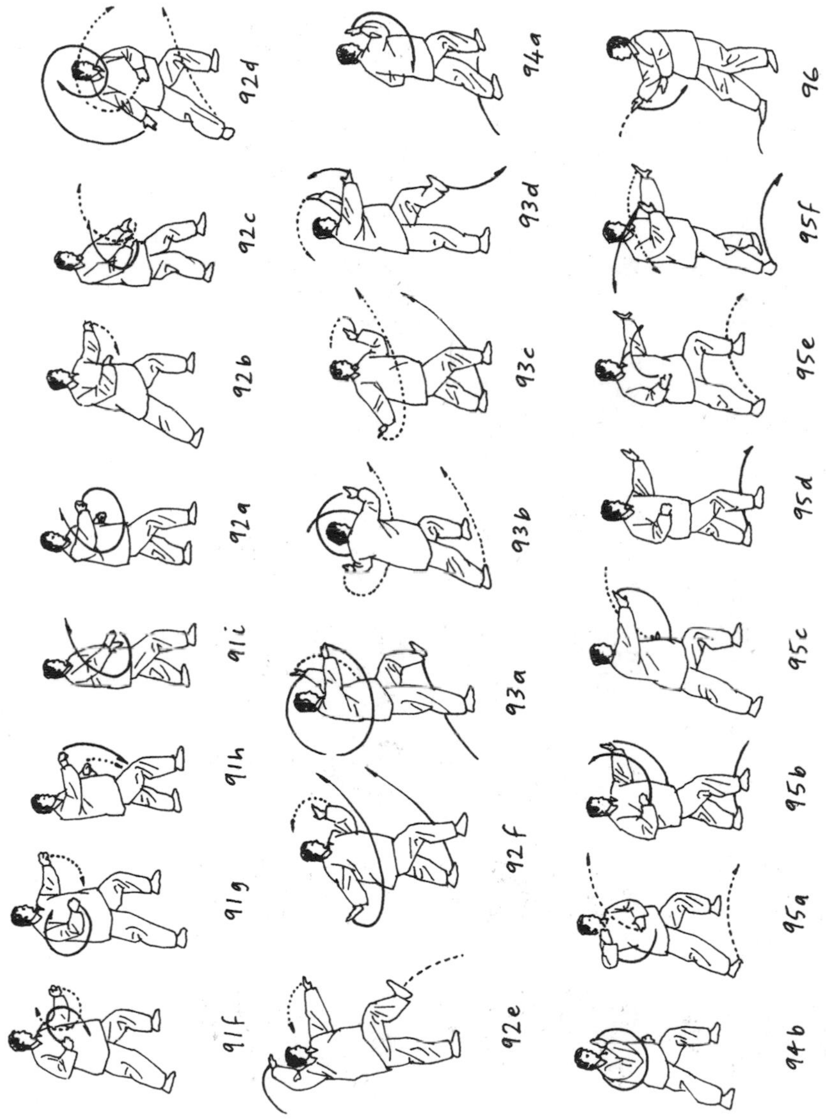

Fig 13.7 Wudang Tai Chi Chuan – Section 7

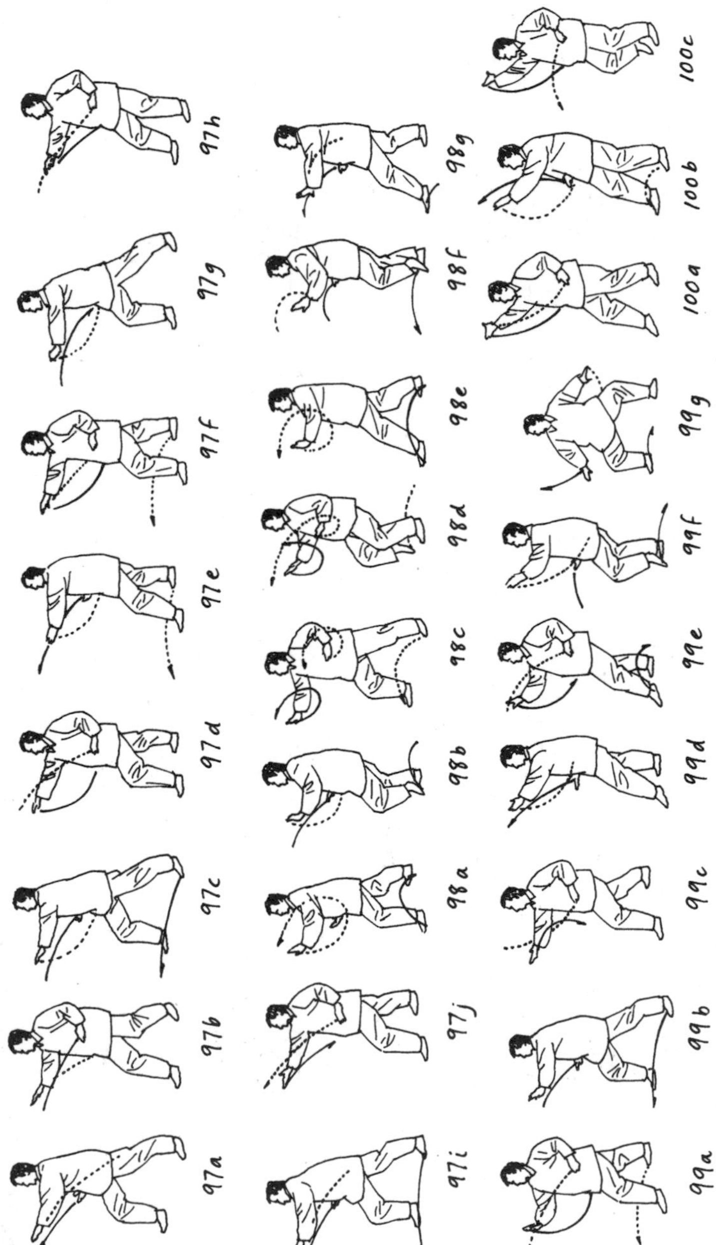
97a
97b
97c
97d
97e
97f
97g
97h
97i
97j
98a
98b
98c
98d
98e
98f
98g
99a
99b
99c
99d
99e
99f
99g
100a
100b
100c

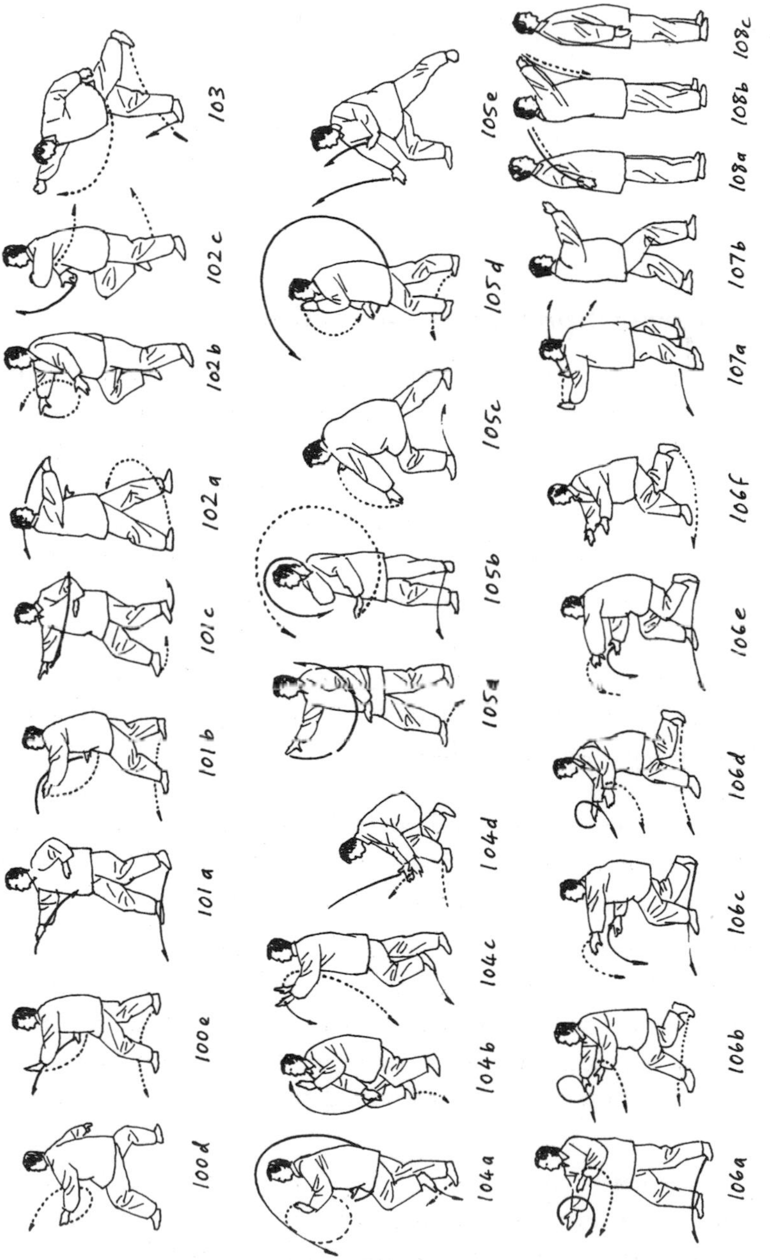

Fig 13.8 Wudang Tai Chi Chuan – Section 8

14

Chen-style Tai Chi Chuan

Tai Chi Chuan of the Hard and Fast

Of all the various Tai Chi Chuan styles, the Chen style is best known for its martial aspects.

Transition from Spirituality to Health

Those who want to study the transition of Tai Chi Chuan from its Shaolin origins through Wudang Kungfu to its present form as represented by its most popular style, Yang-style Tai Chi Chuan, will find Chen-style Tai Chi Chuan interesting. It is also of great significance to martial artists, for of all the various Tai Chi Chuan styles, the Chen style is best known for its martial aspects. It closely resembles Shaolin Kungfu in its demonstration. It was developed by Chen Wang Ting (c1600–80).

The set illustrated in this chapter is based on the one standardized by the national *wushu* committee of China, and presented by Gu Liu Xiang and Shen Jia Zhen. The two masters list the eight characteristics of Chen-style Tai Chi Chuan as follows:[1]

1. Tai Chi Chuan trains mind and energy. When practising the set, use will-power to direct energy flow so that 'when will-power arrives, energy arrives; when energy arrives, internal force arrives'.
2. The body and limbs should be stretched to their furthest reach, and be withdrawn with ease. This effect can be attained by channelling energy to the top of the head as well as focusing it at the *dan tian*, holding the chest in and extending the back, dropping the shoulders and elbows, loosening the waist and hips, rounding the thighs and bending the knees.
3. Spiral movement is the essence of Tai Chi Chuan, and the resultant force is known as 'cocoon-spinning force' or *chan si jing* in Chinese. To attain cocoon-spinning force, one must relax the whole body, involve every part in continuous movement and focus the mind and energy.

4 The concept of 'apparent' and 'solid' is very important in Tai Chi Chuan; if it is correctly put into practice, one can conserve a lot of energy. In seeking harmony between 'apparent' and 'solid', the body must be upright and balanced, and the top and bottom of the body must be co-ordinated.

5 'Once moved, all move' is an important tenet in Tai Chi Chuan. It means that once you make a movement, your whole body, including your mind and energy flow, is involved in the movement. Your external bodily movement and internal *chi* flow should be co-ordinated so that your internal force flows without interruption.

6 Movements in Tai Chi Chuan are continuous, without any break, so that they constitute one endless flow of energy. In set practice, you should not stop at a pattern after its completion, but flow to the next one.

7 At the initial stage you should be as 'soft' as possible. This involves relaxing the mind, loosening the body and not using any strength at all. Then through mind focussing, energy flow and spiral movement, you become 'hard' or forceful. The force is not mechanical, but the result of internal power. Then you can be 'hard' or 'soft' according to need.

8 You should initially practise Tai Chi Chuan slowly. Slow performance is necessary to generate internal energy flow as well as to notice and correct faults in body movements and balance. When you have attained a reasonable standard in internal force and correct movements, you should increase your speed. However, not all patterns are to be performed fast; some, like those used to generate internal energy flow or to redirect the opponent's momentum, should be performed slowly.

The Patterns of Chen-style Tai Chi Chuan

The original set consists of 83 patterns, but there are many repetitions, and these have been removed in the revised set presented here, leaving only 54:

1 Infinite Ultimate Stance
2 Immortal Pounds Mortar
3 Lazy to Roll Sleeves
4 Six Seal Four Close
5 Single Whip
6 Immortal Pounds Mortar

7 White Crane Flaps Wings
8 Towards Swamp Throw Step
9 Slantingly Throw Step
10 Cover Hand Thrust Punch
11 White Crane Flaps Wings
12 Close Body Punch
13 Leaning with the Back
14 Green Dragon Emerges from Water
15 Double Pushing Hands
16 Twice Changing Palms
17 Fist Below Elbow
18 Reverse Rolling of Biceps
19 Retreat to Press Elbow
20 Circling the Middle
21 Dodge, Then Through the Back
22 Six Seal Four Close
23 Single Whip
24 Cloud Hands
25 High Patting Horse
26 Right Snap Kick
27 Left Snap Kick
28 Thrust Kick
29 Strike the Ground
30 Turn Round Double Kick
31 Strike Tiger
32 Whirlwind Kick
33 Thrust Kick
34 Guard Hand to Punch
35 Catch and Strike
36 Carry Head Push Mountain
37 Thrice Changing Palms
38 Front Pattern
39 Back Pattern
40 Wild Horse Spreads Mane
41 Double Stamp Legs

42 Jade Girl Threads Shuttle
43 Sway Leg Drop Fork
44 Golden Cockerel Stands Solitary
45 Cross-hands Sway Lotus
46 Punch to Abdomen
47 White Monkey Presents Fruit
48 Earth Dragon
49 Seven Stars
50 Retreat to Ride Tiger
51 Turn Round Doubly Sway Lotus
52 Cannon Punch
53 Immortal Pounds Mortar
54 Infinite Ultimate Stance

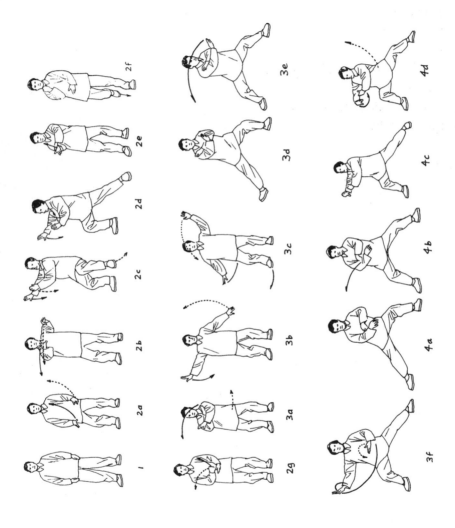
1
2a
2b
2c
2d
2e
2f
2g
3a
3b
3c
3d
3e
3f
4a
4b
4c
4d

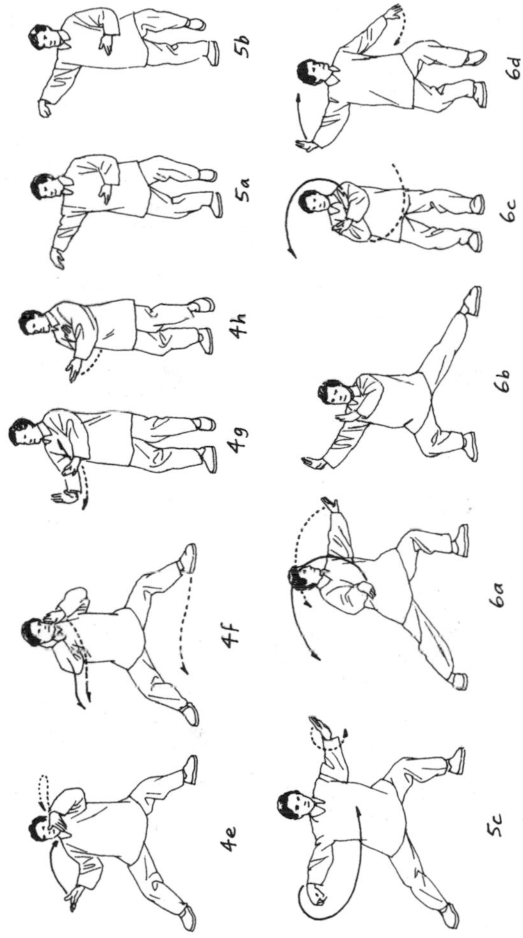

Fig 14.1 Chen-style Tai Chi Chuan (1)

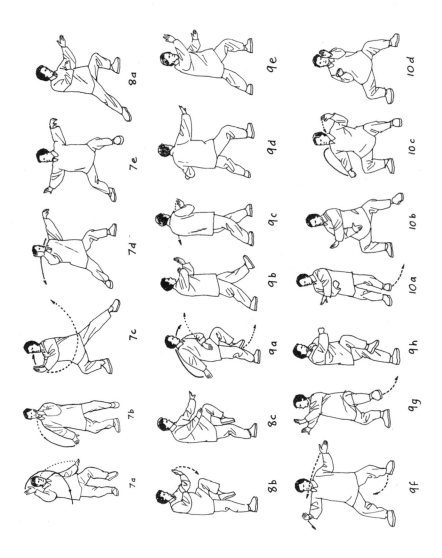
7a
7b
7c
7d
7e
8a
8b
8c
9a
9b
9c
9d
9e
9f
9g
9h
10a
10b
10c
10d

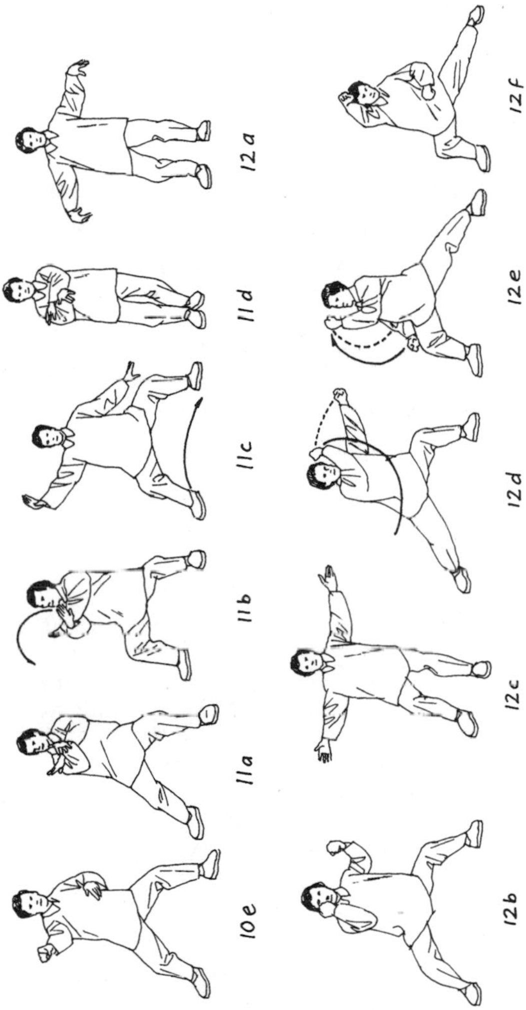

Fig 14.2 Chen-style Tai Chi Chuan (2)

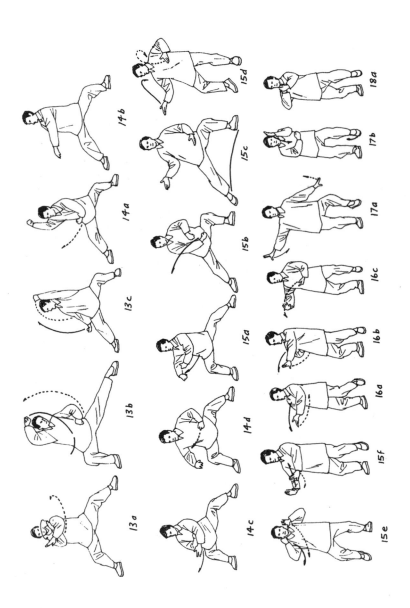
13a
13b
13c
14a
14b
14c
14d
15a
15b
15c
15d
15e
15f
16a
16b
16c
17a
17b
18a

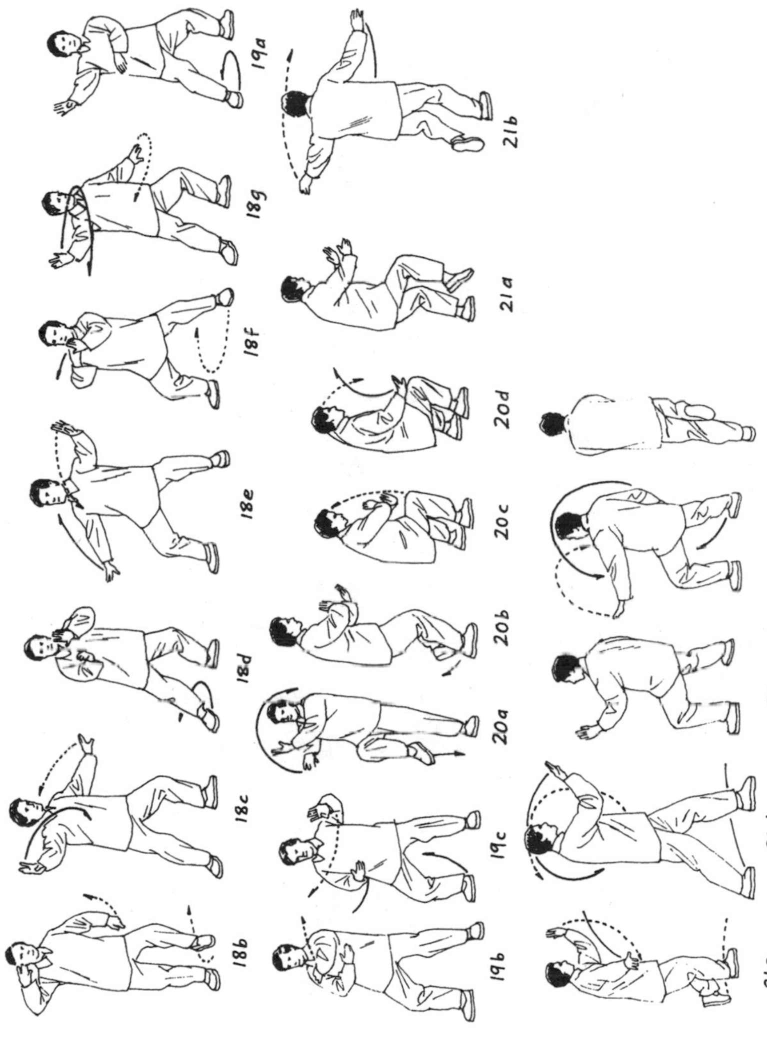

Fig 14.3 Chen-style Tai Chi Chuan (3)

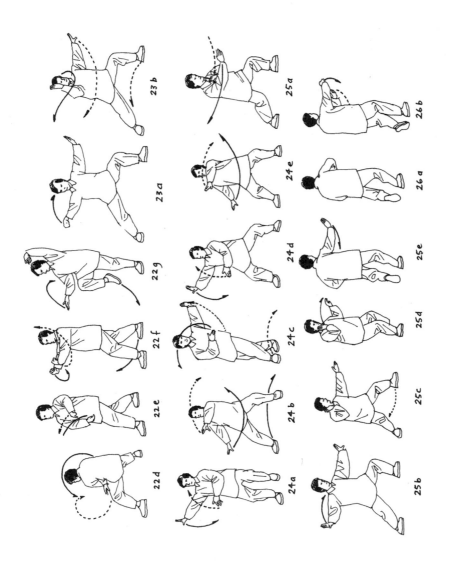

22d
22e
22f
22g
23a
23b
24a
24b
24c
24d
24e
25a
25b
25c
25d
25e
26a
26b

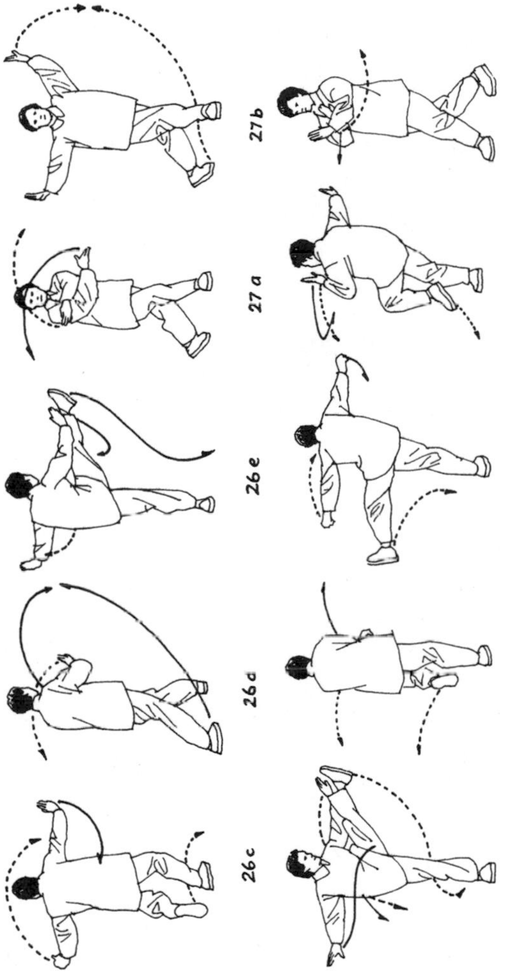

Fig 14.4 Chen-style Tai Chi Chuan (4)

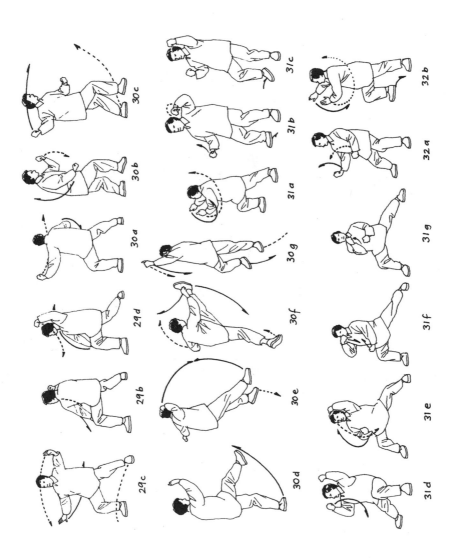
29c
29b
29d
30a
30b
30c
30d
30e
30f
30g
31a
31b
31c
31d
31e
31f
31g
32a
32b

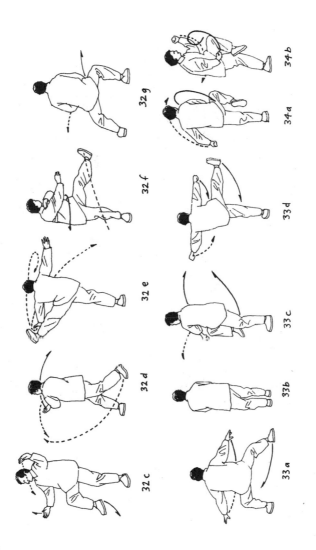

Fig 14.5 Chen-style Tai Chi Chuan (5)

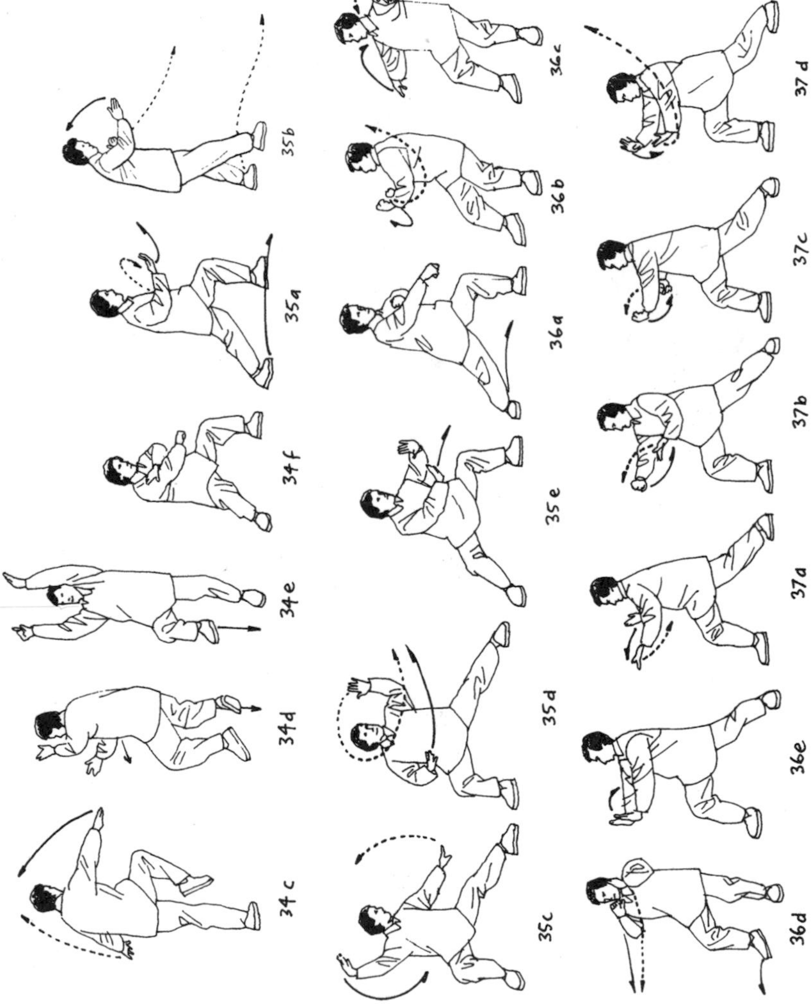
34c
34d
34e
34f
35a
35b
35c
35d
35e
36a
36b
36c
36d
36e
37a
37b
37c
37d

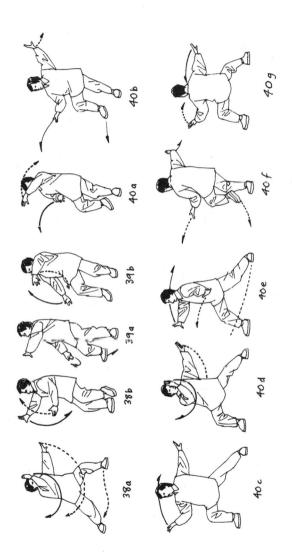

Fig 14.6 Chen-style Tai Chi Chuan (6)

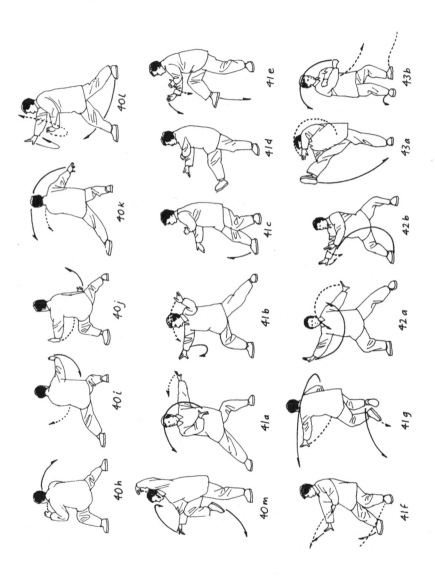
40h
40i
40j
40k
40l
40m
41a
41b
41c
41d
41e
41f
41g
42a
42b
43a
43b

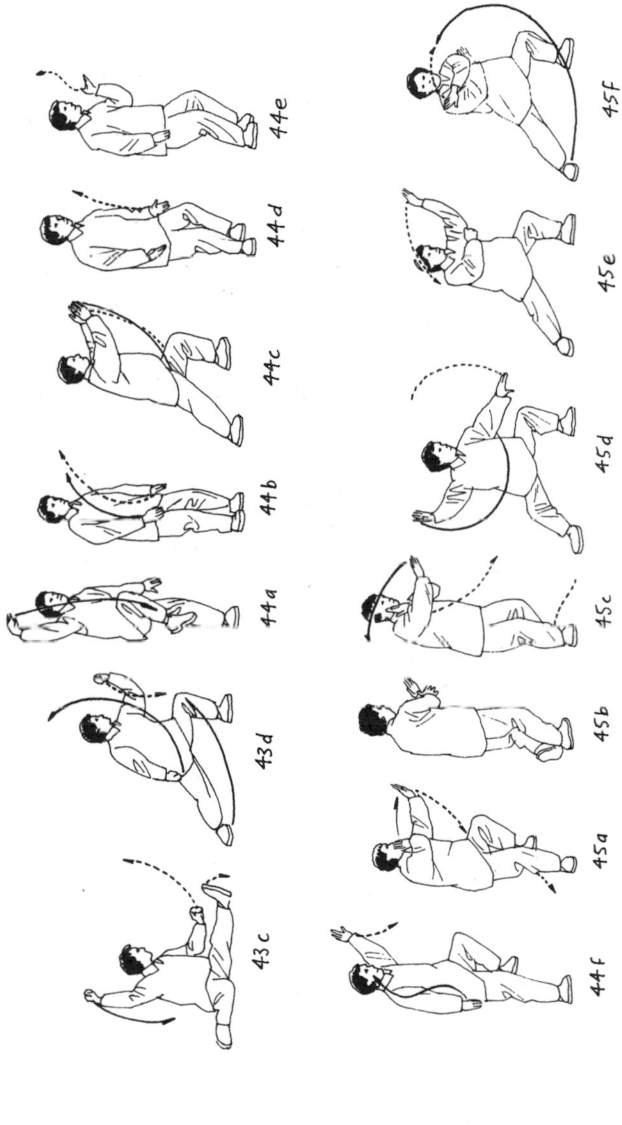

Fig 14.7 Chen-style Tai Chi Chuan (7)

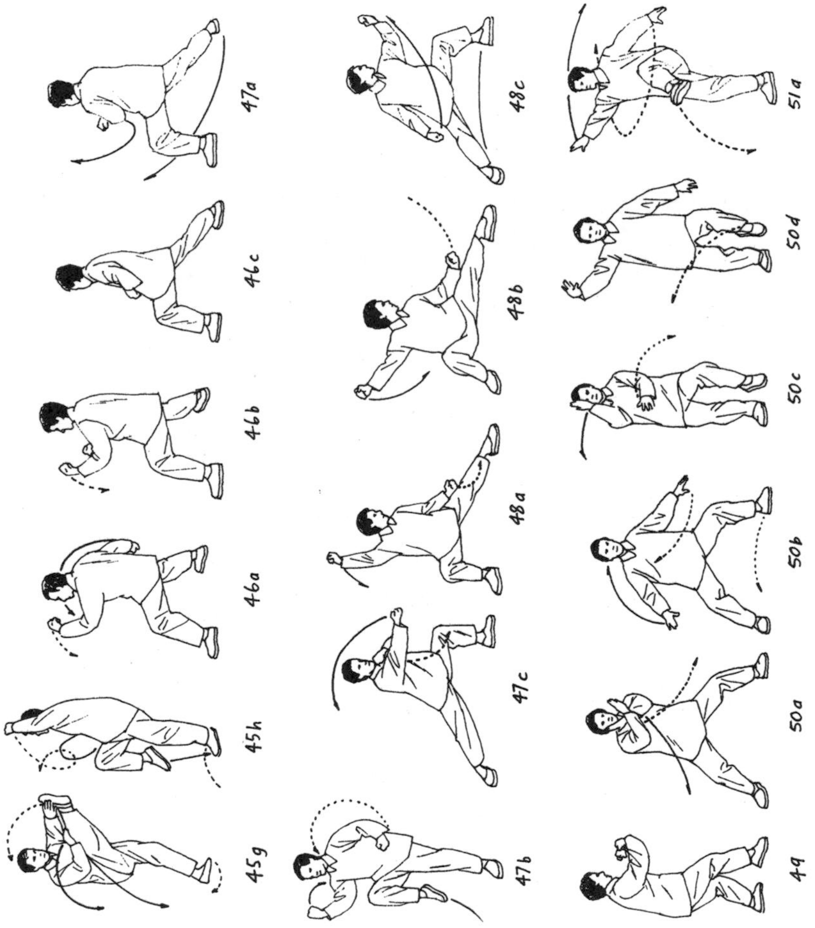

45g 45h 46a 46b 46c 47a 47b 47c 48a 48b 48c 49 50a 50b 50c 50d 51a

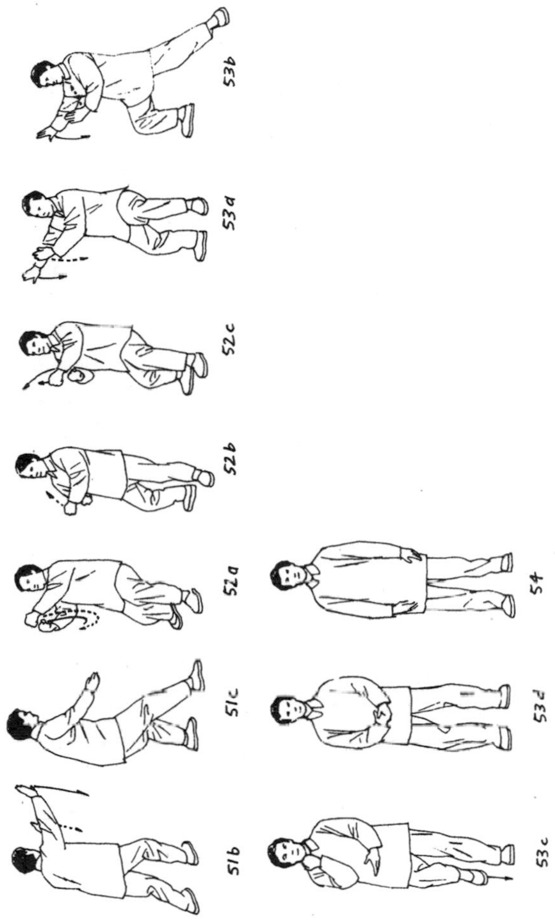

Fig 14.8 Chen-style Tai Chi Chuan (8)

15

Yang-style Tai Chi Chuan

Gentle, Graceful Movements for Health

Few people consistently practise Tai Chi Chuan according to the yin-yang concept. This is one reason why few people become Tai Chi Chuan masters.

The Most Widely Practised Style of Tai Chi Chuan

Of the various styles of Tai Chi Chuan, the Yang Style developed by Yang Lu Chan (1799–1872) is the most widely practised, to the extent that many people have the mistaken impression that it is the only form of Tai Chi Chuan.

The second-generation Yang master, Yang Ban Hou, summarized the essence of his art in nine poems, known collectively as the *Nine Essential Secrets of Tai Chi Chuan.* One of these poems, 'Secret of Yin-yang', which provides invaluable advice is translated below:

> Yin-yang of Tai Chi few people consistently practise.
> Hard and soft are in swallow, shoot, float and sink.
> Front or side, receive or release accordingly move.
> Movement and stillness transformation can bring.
> To generate or control, the situation will dictate.
> Dodging and advancing, in movements are found
> What lightness-heaviness and apparent-solid are.
> Lightness in heaviness do not be bound.[1]

However, not only is the rhyme and rhythm lost in the translation, the meaning is obscure to readers not familiar with the Chinese language or with Tai Chi Chuan terminology. The expanded meaning of the poem is as follows.

Few people consistently practise Tai Chi Chuan according to the yin-yang concept. This is one reason why few people become Tai Chi Chuan masters. This yin-yang concept includes the following important factors: hard-soft, swallow-shoot, float-sink, front-side, receive-release, movement-stillness, generate-control, dodge-advance, light-heavy and apparent-solid.

Being 'hard' or 'soft' applies to both techniques and force. Whenever you 'swallow', as when you shift your body back to avoid an opponent's attacking force, or whenever you 'shoot', as when you swiftly move forward to your opponent, you must be 'hard' or 'soft' according to the demands of the situation. Similarly whenever you 'float' or 'sink' an opponent, ie divert the attack upwards or downwards, you should be 'hard' or 'soft' accordingly.

Whether you face your opponent from the front or the side, and whether you receive an attack by following the opponent's momentum or release your own attack at an opportune moment, all depend on a consideration of the yin-yang balance. In the constantly changing combat situation, you must apply the principle of yin-yang in movement or stillness. For example, in your rapid movement, which is symbolized by yang, you must remain calm, which is yin; in your physical or mental stillness, you must ensure that your internal force flows endlessly.

In combat, you may take the initiative and generate a series of movements for your opponent to respond to, or you may let the opponent take the initiative and respond accordingly, seeking out any weakness so that you can counter-attack unexpectedly. The interplay of this yin-yang of generating your initiative or controlling your opponent's is dictated by the needs or opportunities of the combat situation. When an opportunity arises, irrespective of whether you are generating or controlling the movements, you may dodge the opponent's movement and attack from the side, or you may advance directly.

You must also be aware of the yin-yang of 'lightness' and 'heaviness', and of being 'apparent' and being 'solid'. For example, if your attack is 'light', ie fast, it must also be 'heavy', ie powerful. If your fast attack misses your opponent, you must let it be 'apparent', ie you need not back up a failed attack with force; but if the attack is successful, you must make it 'solid', ie back it with force. There must always be 'lightness' in your 'heaviness' so that you are not bound by your own 'heaviness'; for example, if your hands are powerful, they must also be dextrous; if your stances are stable, they must also be agile.

The Patterns of Yang-style Tai Chi Chuan

The set presented here is based on the one demonstrated by the third-generation master Yang Deng Fu, who was mainly instrumental in establishing the present form of the Yang Style. From the original 108 patterns, he shortened the set to 85 patterns by eliminating some that are repeated numerous times. The set illustrated below consists of only 70 patterns because some other repetitions are also left out.

The names of the Yang-style Tai Chi Chuan patterns are as follows:

1 Tai Chi Starting Pattern
2 Grasping Sparrow's Tail
3 Single Whip
4 Lifting Up Hands
5 White Crane Flaps Wings
6 Twist Knee Throw Step (left)
7 Playing the Lute
8 Twist Knee Throw Step (left and right)
9 Playing the Lute
10 Twist Knee Throw Step (left)
11 Move–Intercept–Punch
12 Like Sealed as if Closed
13 Cross hands
14 Carry Tiger Back to Mountain
15 Observe Fist Below Elbow
16 Repulse Monkey
17 Flying Diagonally
18 White Crane Flaps Wings
19 Twist Knee Throw Step (left)
20 Needle at Sea Bottom
21 Fan Going Through Back
22 Swing Punch
23 Move–Intercept–Punch
24 Move–Intercept–Punch
25 Grasping Sparrow's Tail
26 Single Whip
27 Cloud Hands
28 Single Whip
29 High Patting Horse
30 Right Snap Kick

31 Left Snap Kick
32 Turn Round Thrust Kick
33 Twist Knee Throw Step (left and right)
34 Plant Fist
35 Swing Punch
36 Move–Intercept–Punch
37 Right Thrust Kick
38 Strike Tiger (left)
39 Strike Tiger (right)
40 Turn Round Thrust Kick
41 Double Bees Buzzing at Ears
42 Left Thrust Kick
43 Turn Round Right Thrust Kick
44 Move–Intercept–Punch
45 Like Sealed as if Closed
46 Cross-hands
47 Carry Tiger Back to Mountain
48 Slanting Single Whip
49 Wild Horse Spreads Mane
50 Grasping Sparrow's Tail
51 Single Whip
52 Jade Girl Threads Shuttle
53 Single Whip
54 Cloud Hands
55 Single Whip Low Stance
56 Golden Cockerel Stands Solitary (right)
57 Golden Cockerel Stands Solitary (left)
58 High Patting Horse
59 White Snake Shoots out Venom
60 Turn Round Thrust Kick
61 Strike to Abdomen
62 Grasping Sparrow's Tail
63 Single Whip
64 Seven Stars
65 Turn Round Sway Lotus
66 Shoot Tiger
67 Move–Intercept–Punch
68 Like Sealed as if Closed
69 Cross Hands
70 Infinite Ultimate Stance

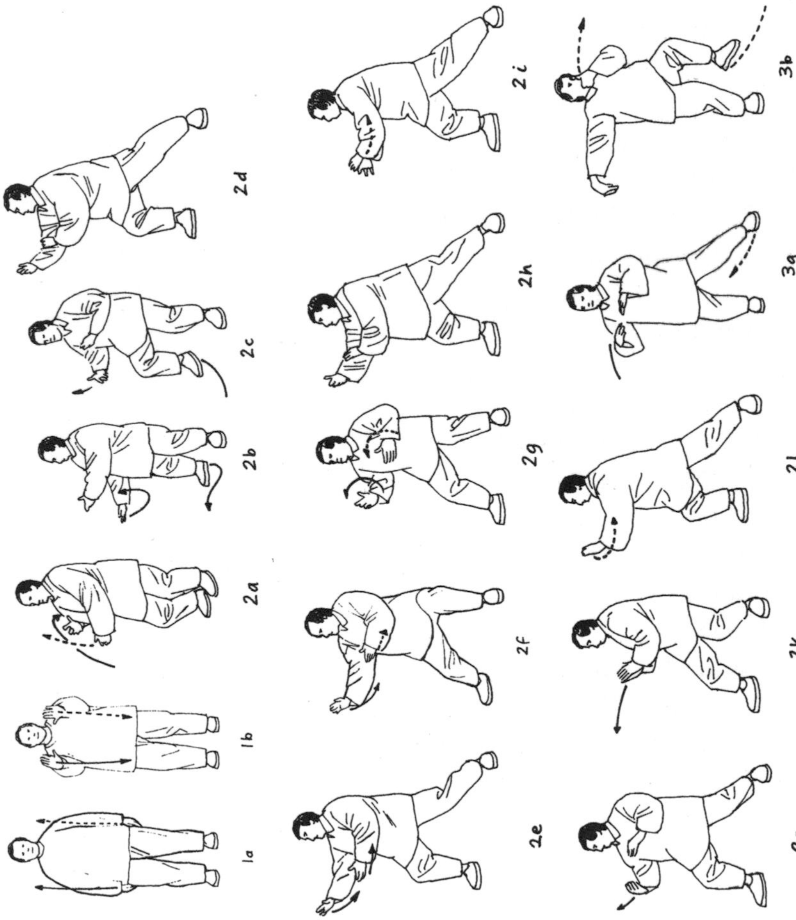
1a
1b
2a
2b
2c
2d
2e
2f
2g
2h
2i
2j
2k
2l
3a
3b

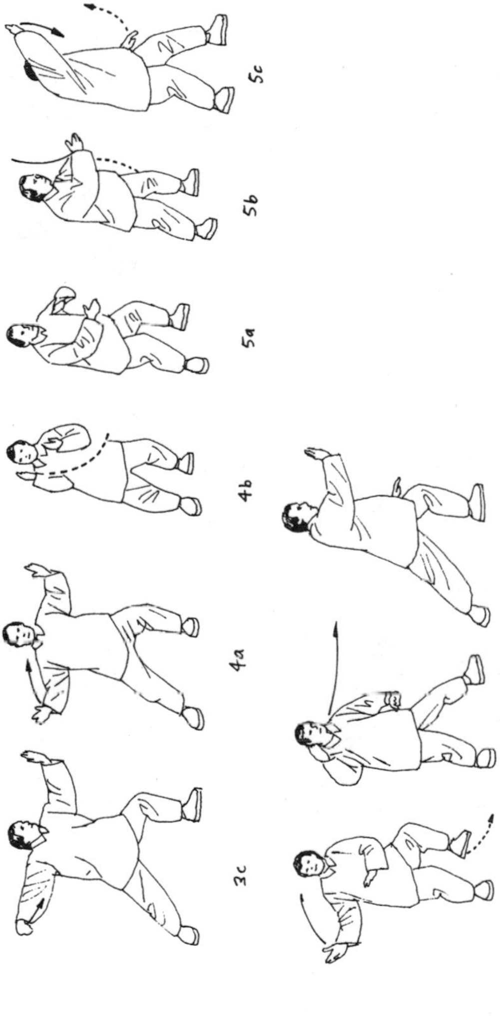

Fig 15.1 Yang-style Tai Chi Chuan (1)

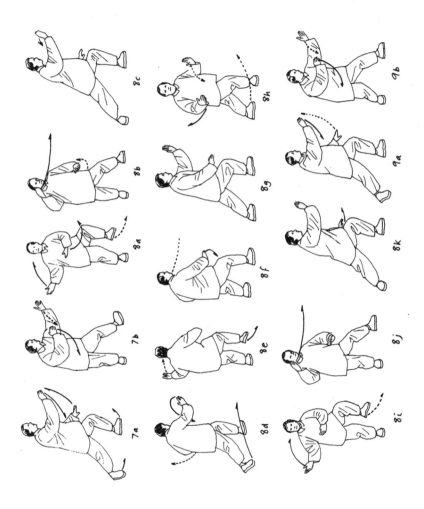
7a
7b
8a
8b
8c
8d
8e
8f
8g
8h
8i
8j
8k
9a
9b

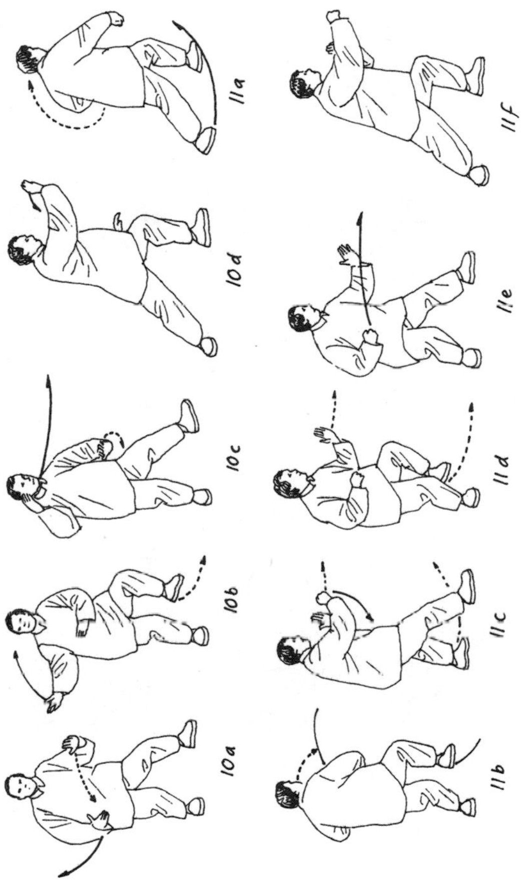

Fig 15.2 Yang-style Tai Chi Chuan (2)

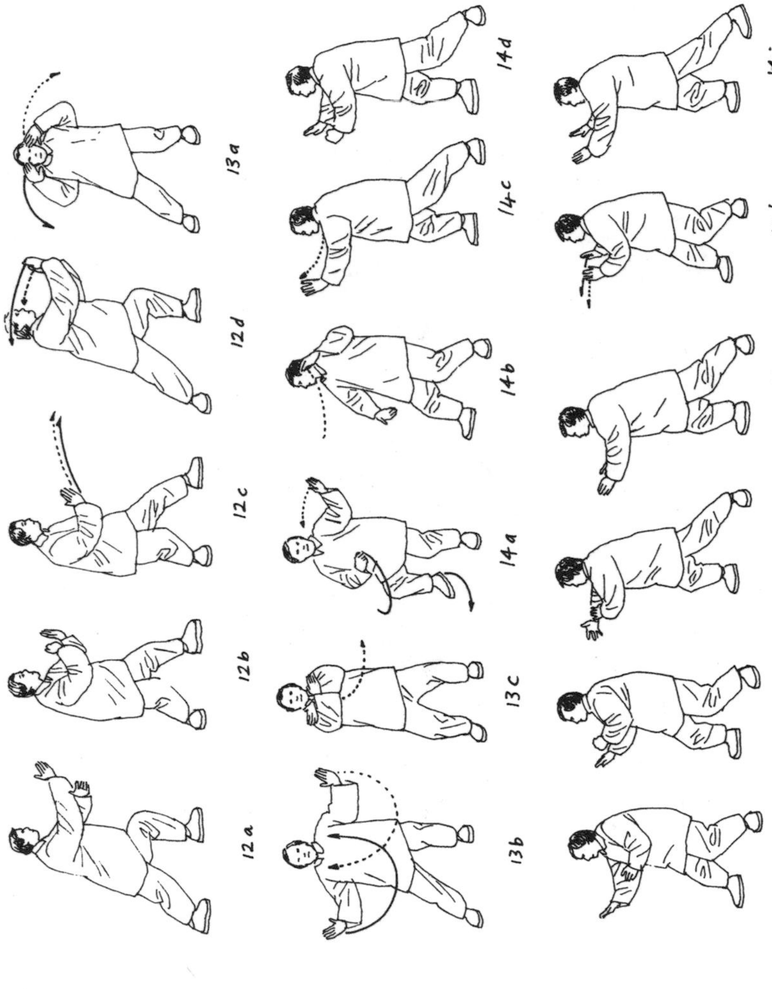

12a
12b
12c
12d
13a
13b
13c
14a
14b
14c
14d
14e
14f
14g
14h
14i
14j

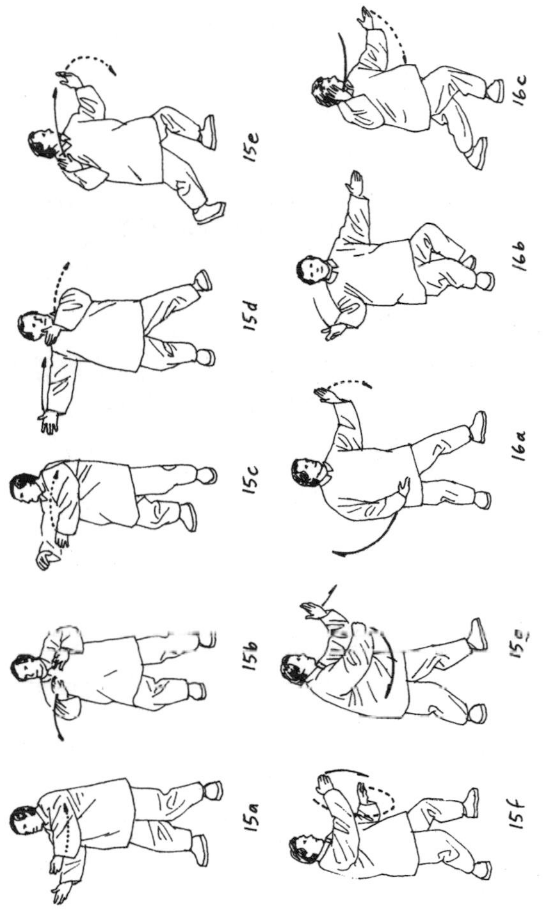

Fig 15.3 Yang-style Tai Chi Chuan (3)

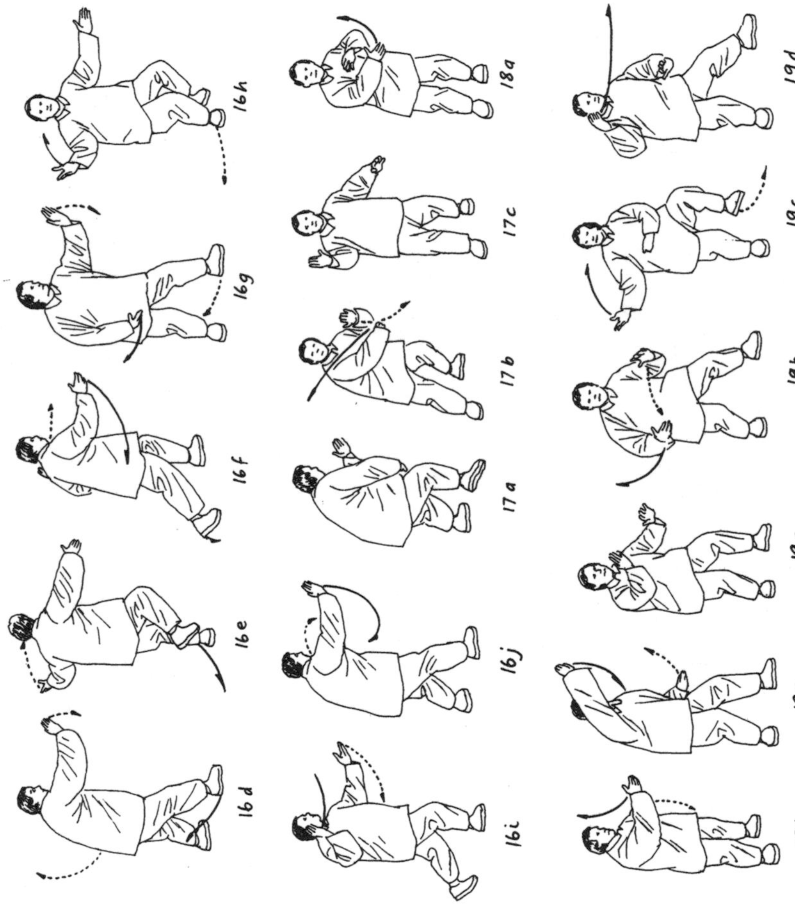
16d
16e
16f
16g
16h
16i
16j
17a
17b
17c
18a
18b
18c
19a
19b
19c
19d

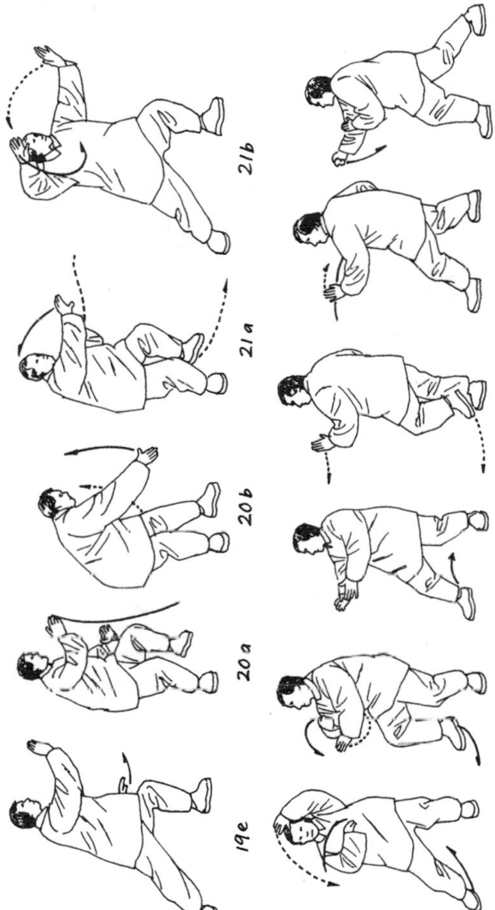

Fig 15.4 Yang-style Tai Chi Chuan (4)

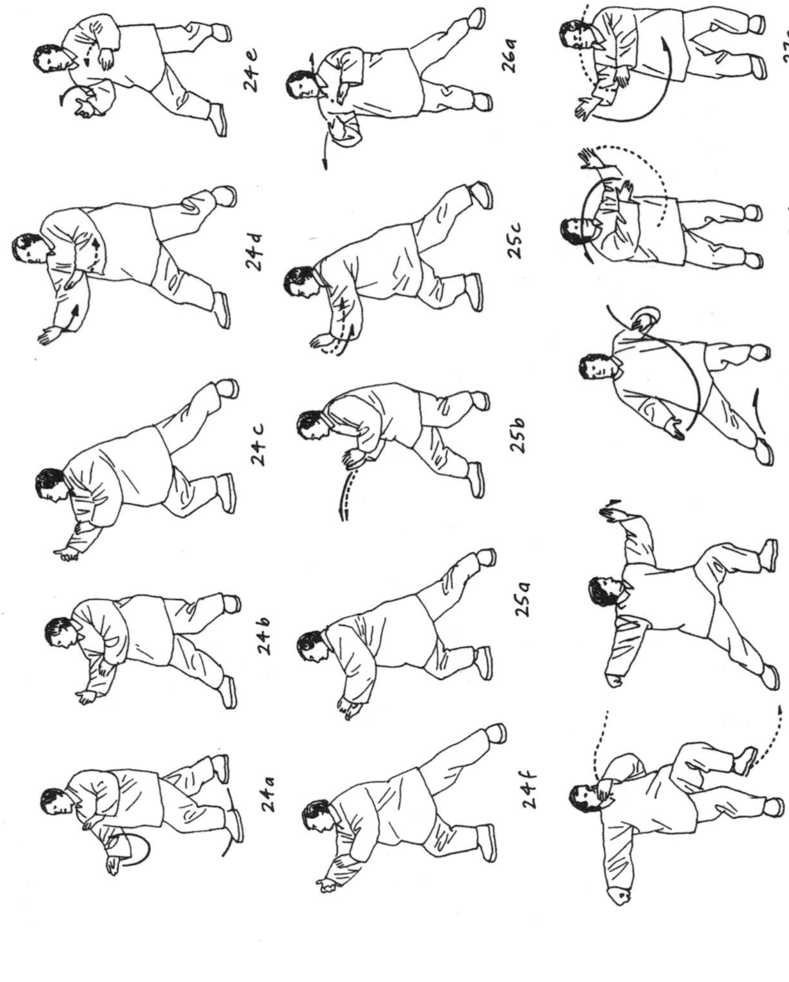

24a
24b
24c
24d
24e
24f
25a
25b
25c
26a
26b
26c
27a
27b
27c

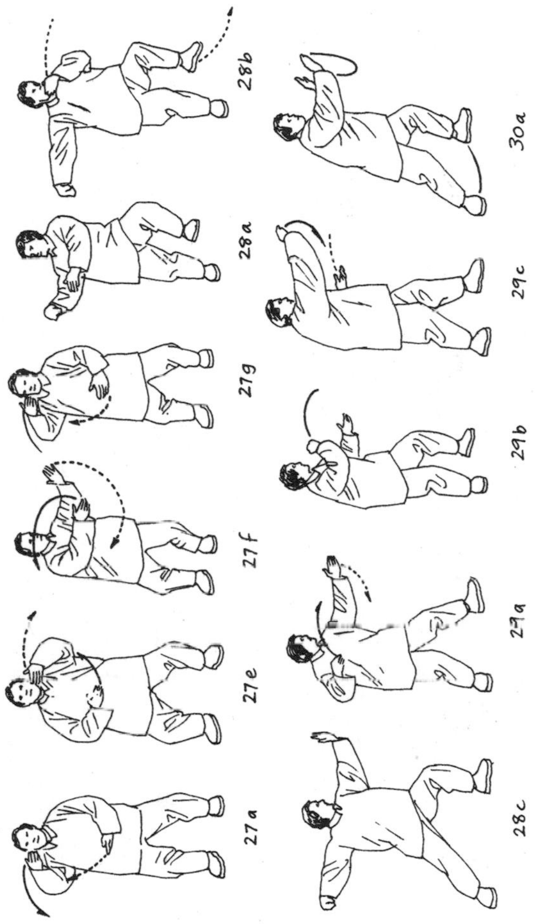

Fig 15.5 Yang-style Tai Chi Chuan (5)

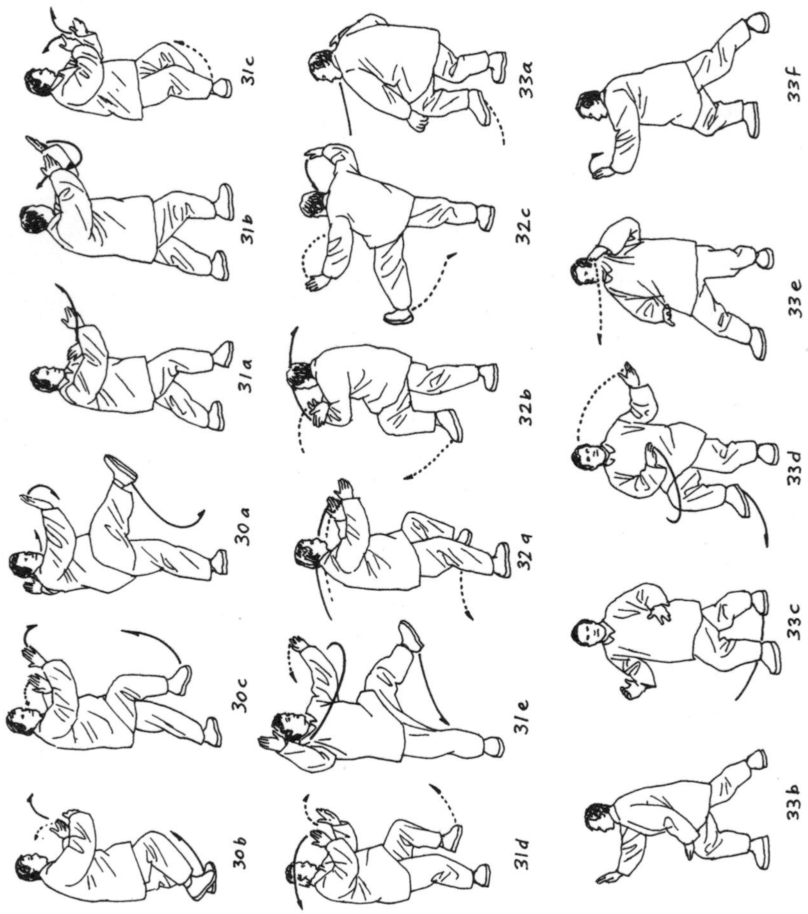
30b
30c
30a
31a
31b
31c
31d
31e
32a
32b
32c
33a
33b
33c
33d
33e
33f

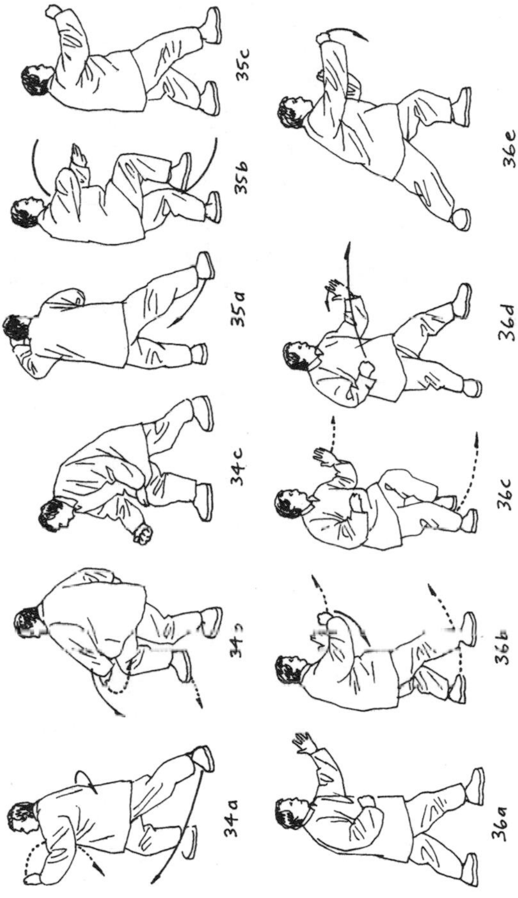

Fig 15.6 Yang-style Tai Chi Chuan (6)

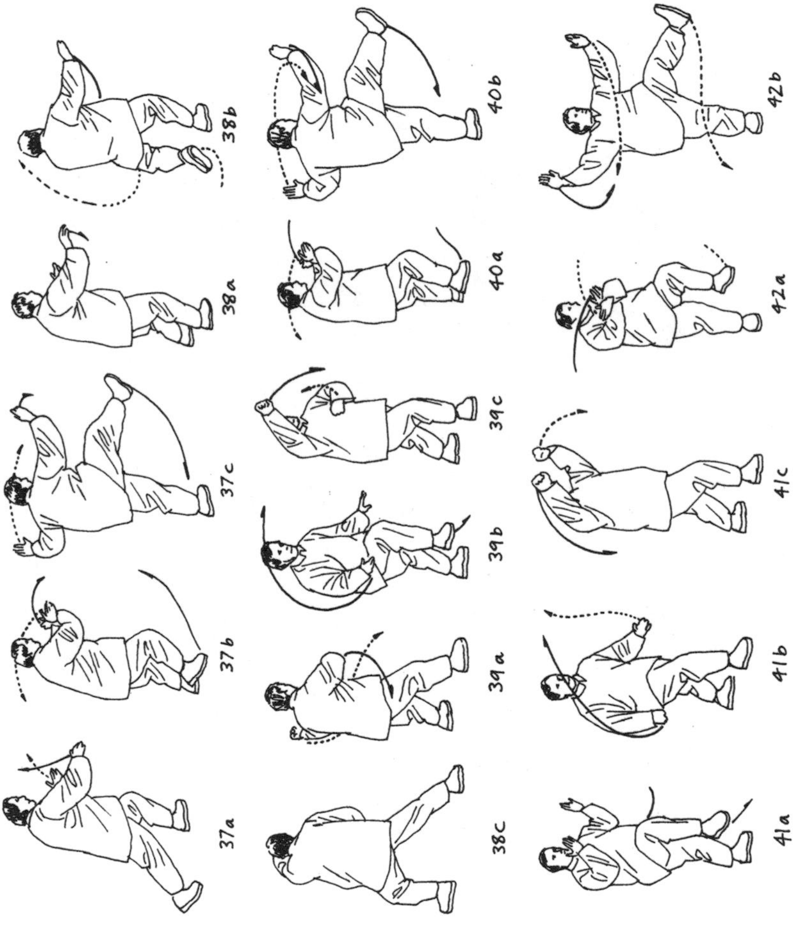
37a
37b
37c
38a
38b
38c
39a
39b
39c
40a
40b
41a
41b
41c
42a
42b

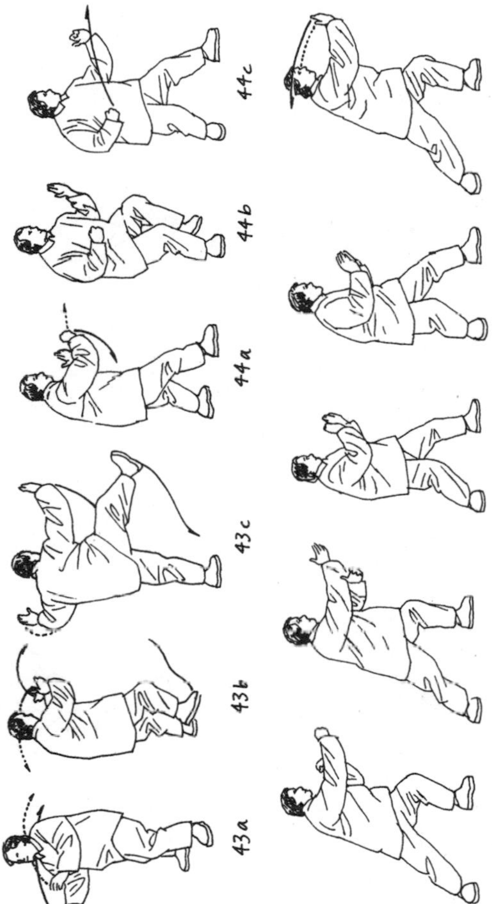

Fig 15.7 Yang-style Tai Chi Chuan (7)

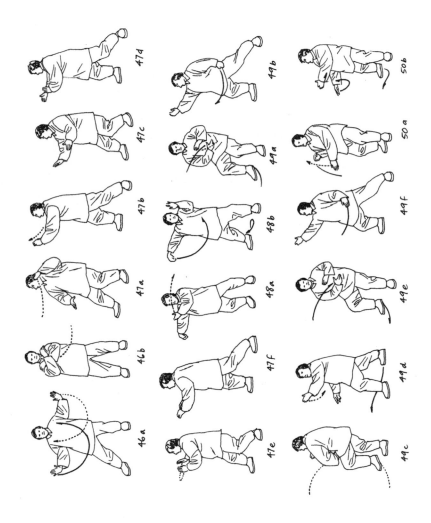
46a
46b
47a
47b
47c
47d
47e
47f
48a
48b
49a
49b
49c
49d
49e
49f
50a
50b

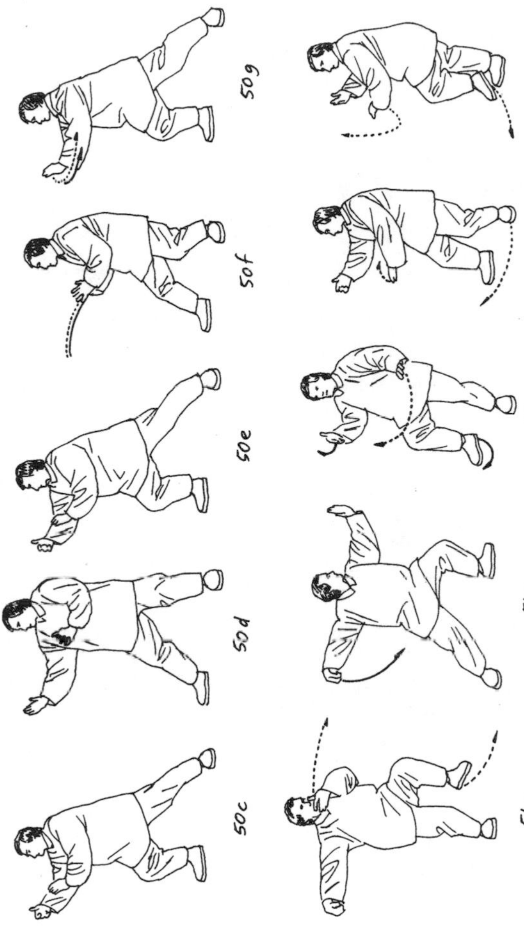

Fig 15.8 Yang-style Tai Chi Chuan (8)

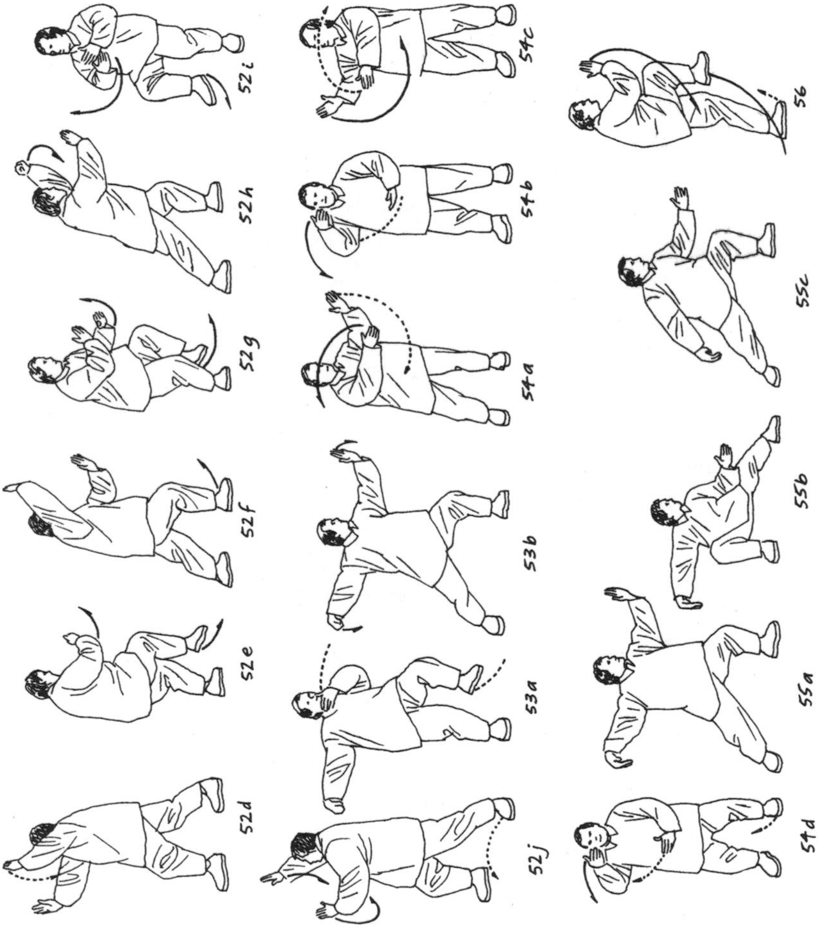
52d
52e
52f
52g
52h
52i
52j
53a
53b
54a
54b
54c
54d
55a
55b
55c
56

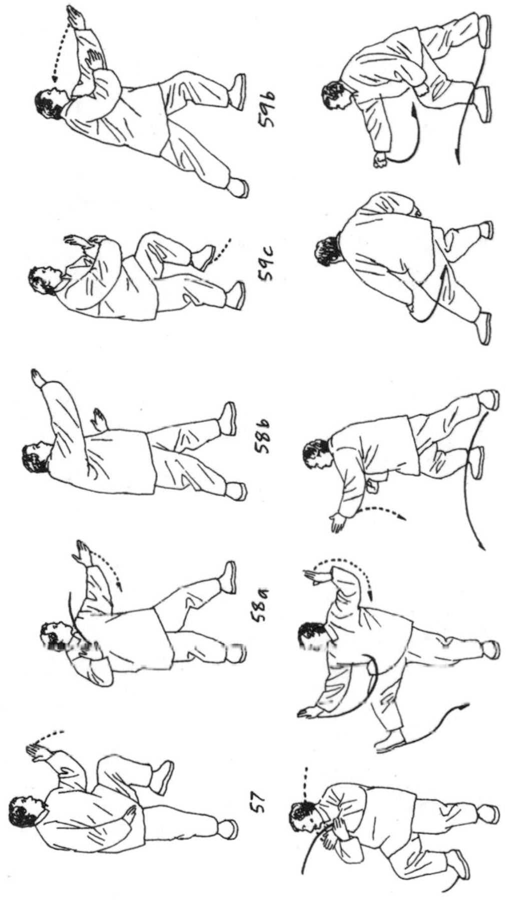

Fig 15.9 Yang-style Tai Chi Chuan (9)

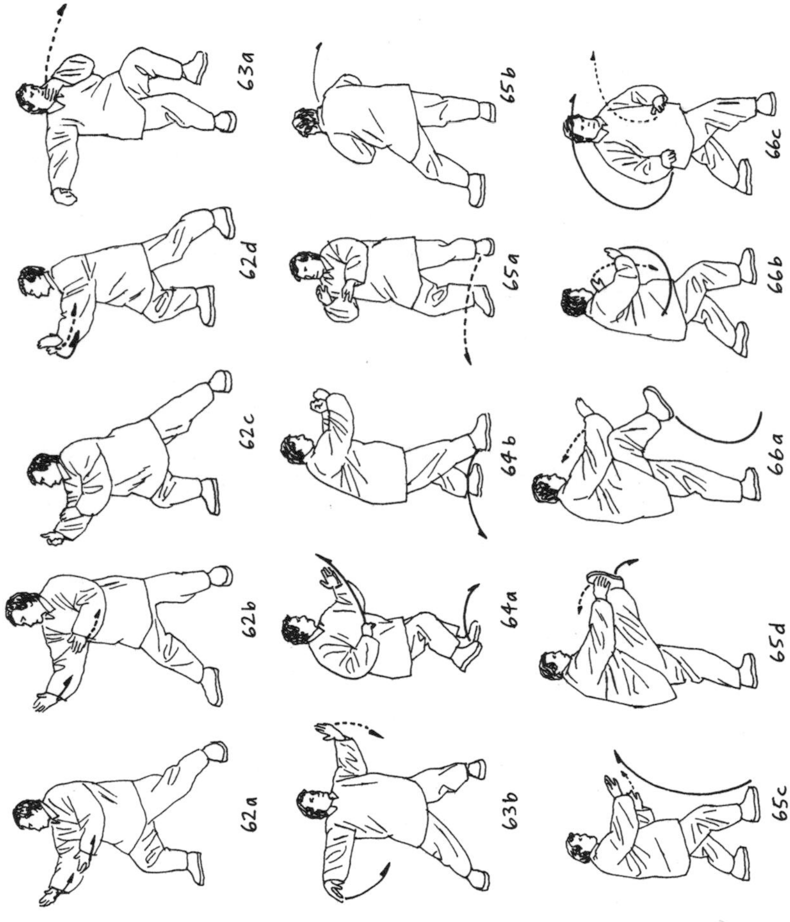
62a
62b
62c
62d
63a
63b
64a
64b
65a
65b
65c
65d
66a
66b
66c

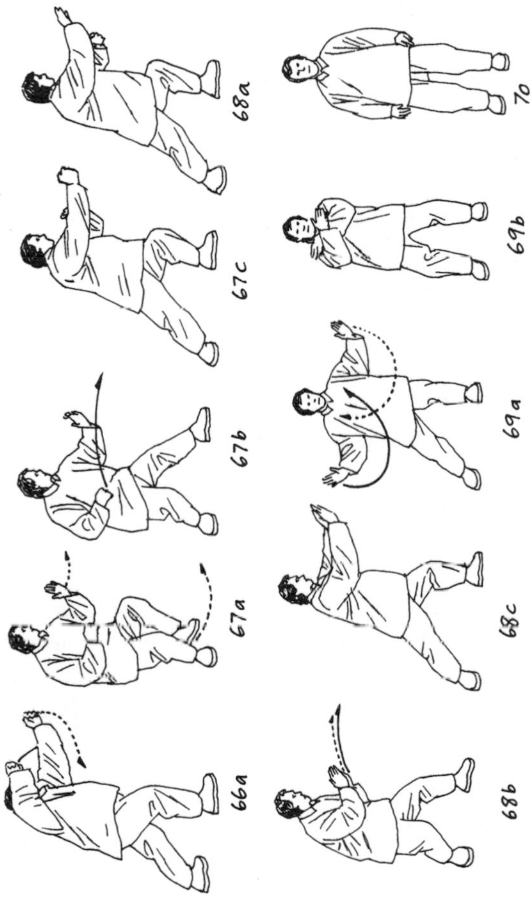

Fig 15.10 Yang-style Tai Chi Chuan (10)

16

The Wu Style of Wu Yu Xiang

Small Movements and Body Technique for Combat

The correct practice of these eight principles of 'body technique' or external form helps the exponent to enhance the internal force in his body.

External Form for Internal Power

A glance at the illustrations below may give the impression that most of the patterns in Wu-style Tai Chi Chuan are similar. This is due to the fact that, unlike the Yang Style, where the circular movements are big, the movements in Wu-style Tai Chi Chuan, while also circular, are small. The illustrations usually show the patterns at their completion and if there is not much movement, it is easy to think that one pattern is similar to another, while they may be very different in their intermittent movements.

There are two Wu Styles in Tai Chi Chuan. The style explained here was developed by Wu Yu Xiang (1812–80), who first learnt the Yang Style from Yang Lu Chan, and later the Chen Style from Chen Jing Ping.

The Wu Style is rich in literature on the philosophy and practice of Tai Chi Chuan. The following advice, entitled 'Concerning Some Personal Experience in Teaching and Practising' by the Wu Style master, Hao Shao Ru, is helpful to instructors and students alike.

1 One should always start learning Tai Chi Chuan with body technique, according to Wu Yu Xiang's eight principles of body technique, because body technique is the most fundamental. In learning body technique one should also connect the external to the internal.

2 In Tai Chi Chuan it is not possible to attain even basic requirements immediately. Thus it is helpful to progress in two stages.

3 The first stage involves the training of external form; this is learning patterns and sets, and one must pay attention to body technique. Co-ordinate the upper and lower limbs with the body, and get to a stage where the body and limbs follow the will.

4 The second stage is to train internal form, which is also called internal force. Gradually achieve the unity of will-power, energy flow and physical form. Proceed from the external to the internal, from the gross to the fine. Then there is no external and no internal, no gross and no fine, being lost in the nebulous void. Only when such a state is reached can one continually progress towards the highest summit of Tai Chi Chuan.[1]

Like all great masters, Hao Shao Ru indicates that the highest attainment in Tai Chi Chuan is not merely combat efficiency, but a return to the great void.

'Body technique' in the above quotation means the external form of Tai Chi Chuan. The eight principles of body technique taught by Wu Yu Xiang, and formalized by his distinguished disciple Li Yi Yu, are:

- Pull in the chest
- Extend the back
- Inflate the thighs
- Withdraw the ribs
- Push up the head
- Raise the anus
- Alert the energy
- Sharpen the mind[2]

The combined action of pulling the chest in and extending the back fills the upper body with internal force. 'Inflate the thighs' means the thighs are open but the knees are curved in, as in the Tai Chi Stance, as if holding a ball between the thighs. This enables the abdomen to be filled with energy. Withdrawing the ribs is done by dropping the shoulders and keeping the elbows close to the body, thus enabling the mid-body to be charged with internal force. Pushing up the head makes the exponent's posture upright. Raising the anus helps retain internal force in the abdomen. Alerting the energy and sharpening the mind are internal considerations for the external form.

The correct practice of these eight principles of body technique or external form helps you enhance internal force in your body. But you are advised not to apply these principles without a master's supervision; incorrect application may result in internal injury. Inflating the thighs and withdrawing the ribs suggest why the stances are comparatively high and narrow, and the hand movements small and close to the body, giving the style its characteristic form.

The correct body technique or external form in Wu-style Tai Chi Chuan is not aimed at physical or technical advantage, as in the case of most other martial arts, but at conserving and enhancing internal force. The above eight principles will help you to do this.

The Patterns of Wu Yu Xiang-style Tai Chi Chuan

The set illustrated here is based on the one demonstrated by the fifth-generation Wu Style master Jiao Song Mao. There are 85 patterns in the original set, but a few repeated patterns have been eliminated, giving only 78 in the revised set presented below.

1 Tai Chi Starting Pattern
2 Lazy to Roll Sleeves (left)
3 Lazy to Roll Sleeves (right)
4 Single Whip
5 Lifting Up Hands
6 White Crane Flaps Wings
7 Twist Knee Throw Step (left)
8 Playing the Lute
9 Twist Knee Throw Step (left)
10 Twist Knee Throw Step (right)
11 Move–Intercept–Punch
12 Six Seal Four Close
13 Carry Tiger Back to Mountain
14 Playing the Lute
15 Lazy to Roll Sleeves
16 Single Whip
17 Lift Up Hands
18 Palm Strike to Face
19 Observe Fist Below Elbow
20 Repulse Monkey

21 Playing the Lute
22 White Crane Flaps Wings
23 Twist Knee Throw Step
24 Playing the Lute
25 Press Down
26 Green Dragon Emerges from Water
27 Through the Back
28 Single Whip
29 Cloud-hands
30 High Patting Horse (left)
31 High Patting Horse (right)
32 Observe Fist Below Elbow
33 Jade Girl Threads Shuttle
34 Playing the Lute
35 Lifting Up Hands
36 Lazy to Roll Sleeves
37 Single Whip
38 Cloud-hands
39 Single Whip
40 Twist Knee Throw Step (right)
41 Twist Knee Throw Step (left)
42 Right Snap Kick
43 Left Snap Kick
44 Turn Round Snap Kick
45 Plant Fist
46 Double Kick
47 Taming Tiger
48 Lifting Up Hands
49 Snap Kick
50 Turn Round Thrust Kick
51 Move–Intercept–Punch
52 Six Seal Four Close
53 Carry Tiger Back to Mountain
54 Playing the Lute
55 Lazy to Roll Sleeves
56 Jade Girl Threads Shuttle
57 Single Whip
58 Low Stance
59 Golden Cockerel Stands Solitary (right)
60 Golden Cockerel Stands Solitary (left)
61 Repulse Monkey
62 Wild Horse Spreads Mane
63 Playing the Lute
64 Press Down
65 Through the Back
66 Playing the Lute
67 Green Dragon Emerges from Water
68 Cross-hands Sway Lotus
69 Punch to Abdomen
70 Lazy to Roll Sleeves
71 Seven Stars
72 Ride Tiger
73 Turn Around Sway Lotus
74 Shoot Tiger
75 Double Cannons
76 Playing the Lute
77 Lifting Up Hands
78 Infinite Ultimate Stance

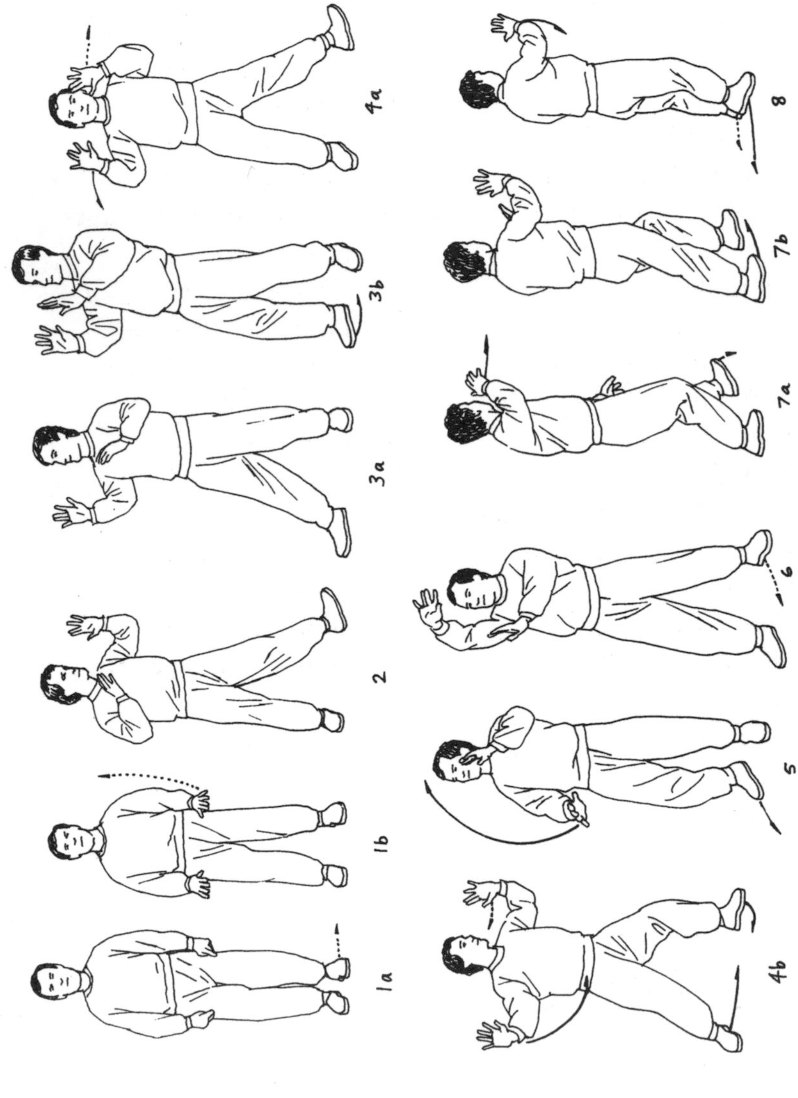
1a
1b
2
3a
3b
4a
4b
5
6
7a
7b
8

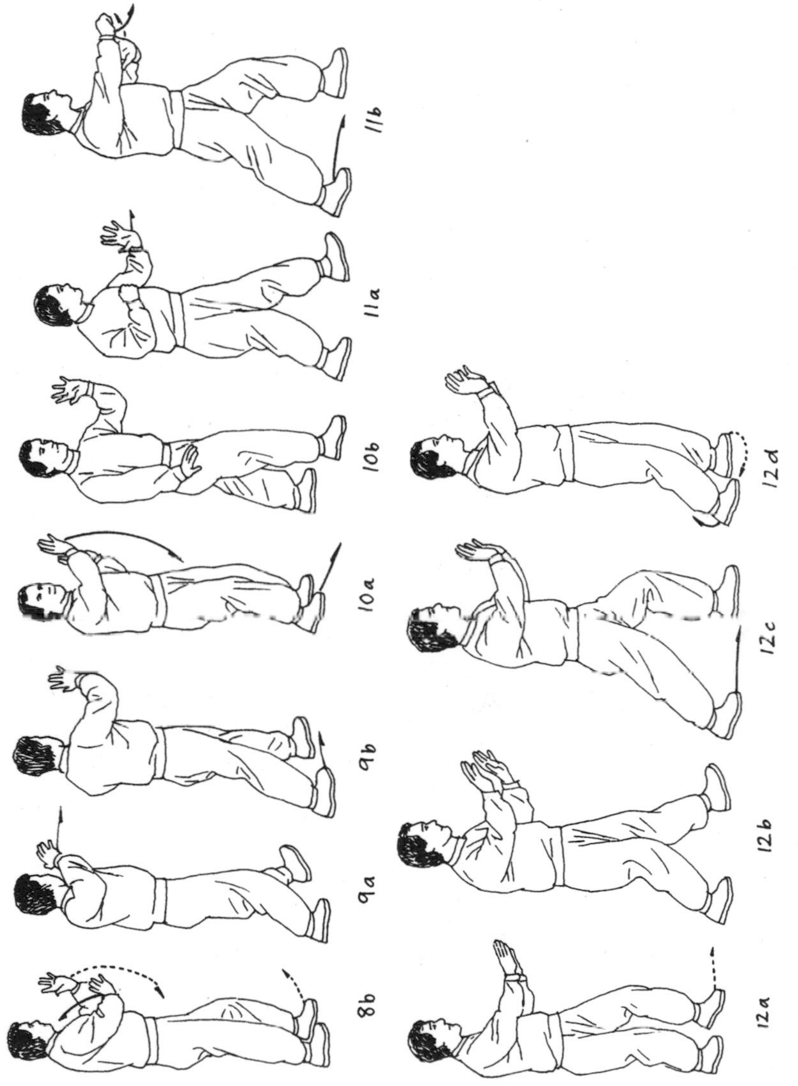

Fig 16.1 Wu Yu Xiang-style Tai Chi Chuan (1)

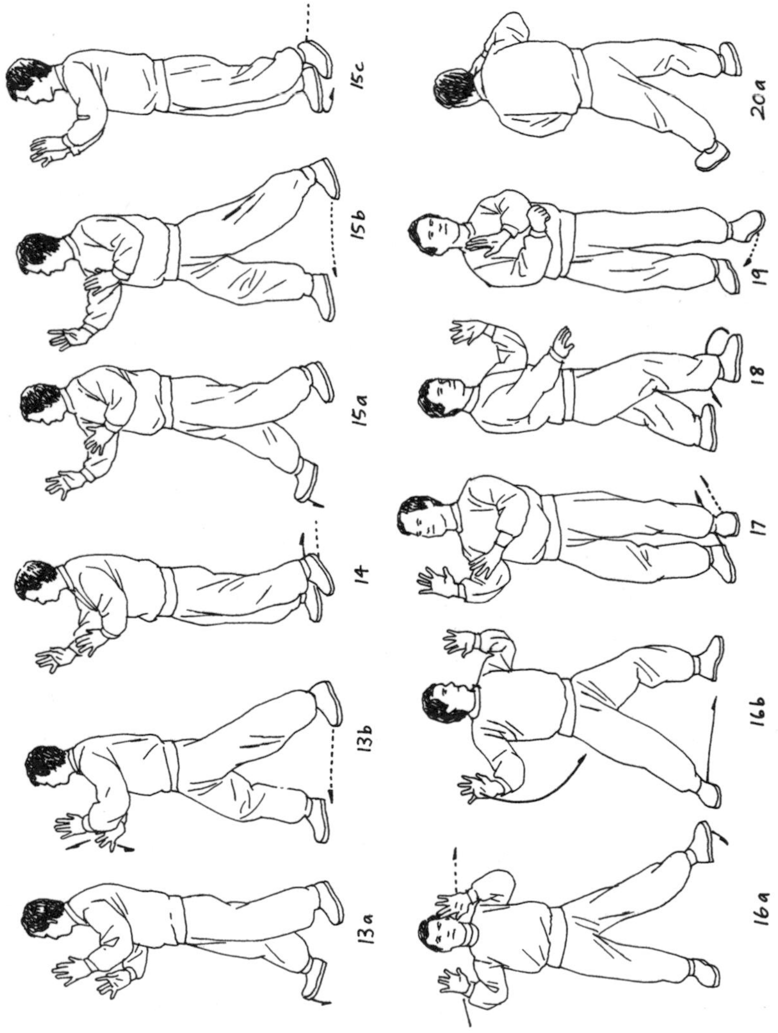
13a
13b
14
15a
15b
15c
16a
16b
17
18
19
20a

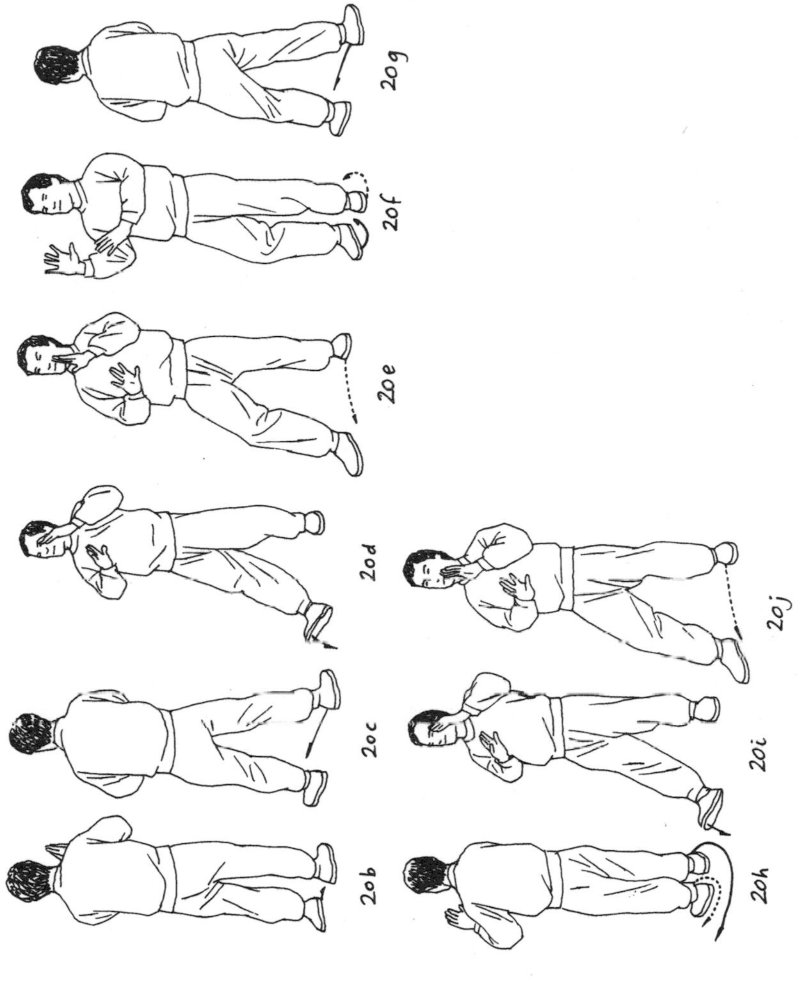

Fig 16.2 Wu Yu Xiang-style Tai Chi Chuan (2)

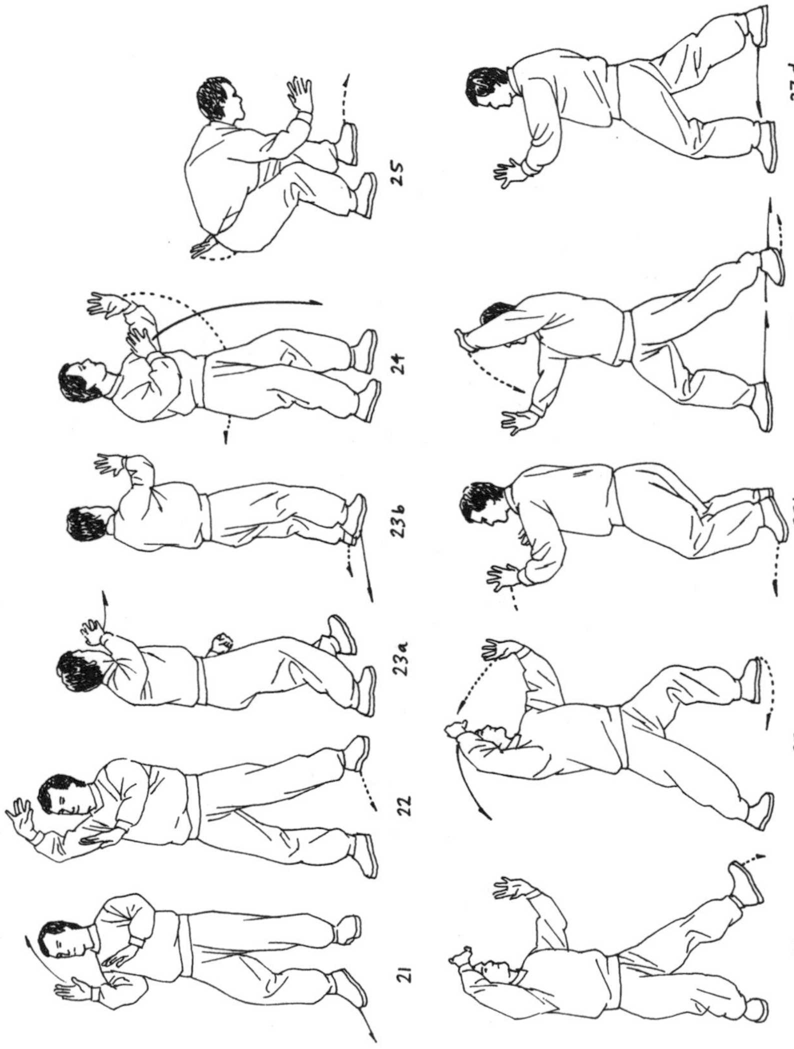
21
22
23a
23b
24
25
26
27a
27b
27c
27d

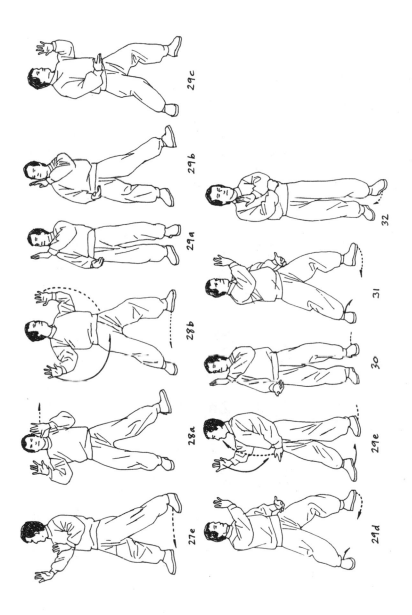

Fig 16.3 Wu Yu Xiang-style Tai Chi Chuan (3)

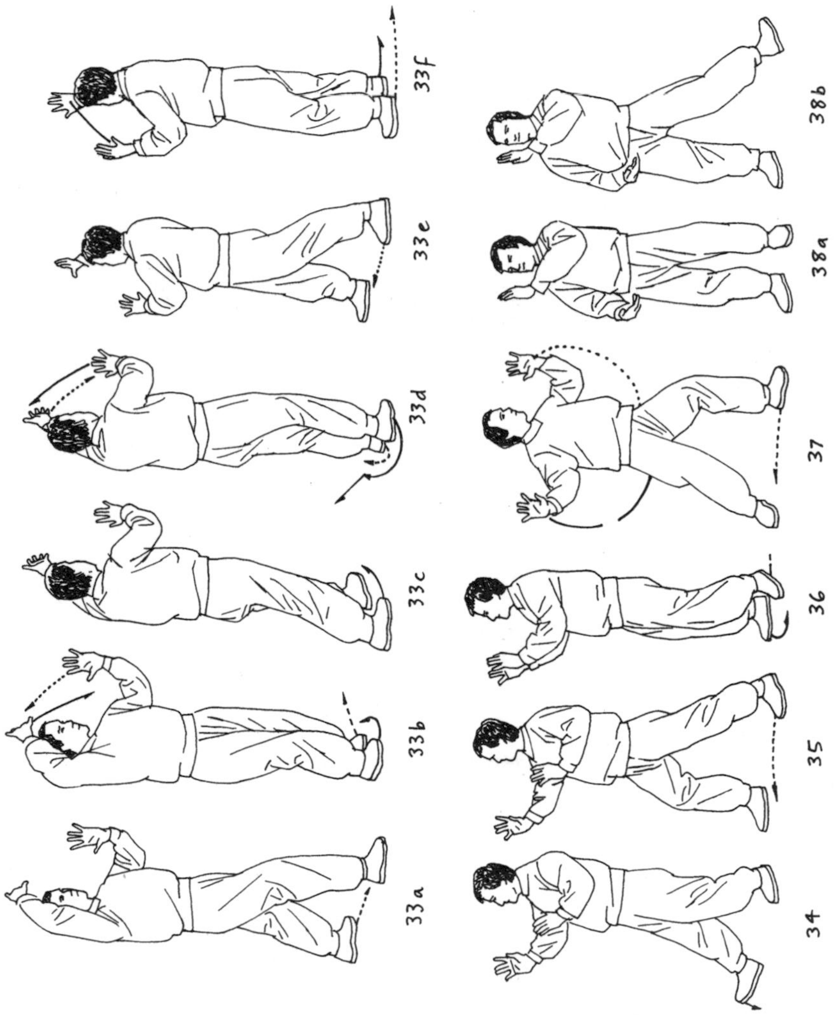
33a
33b
33c
33d
33e
33f
34
35
36
37
38a
38b

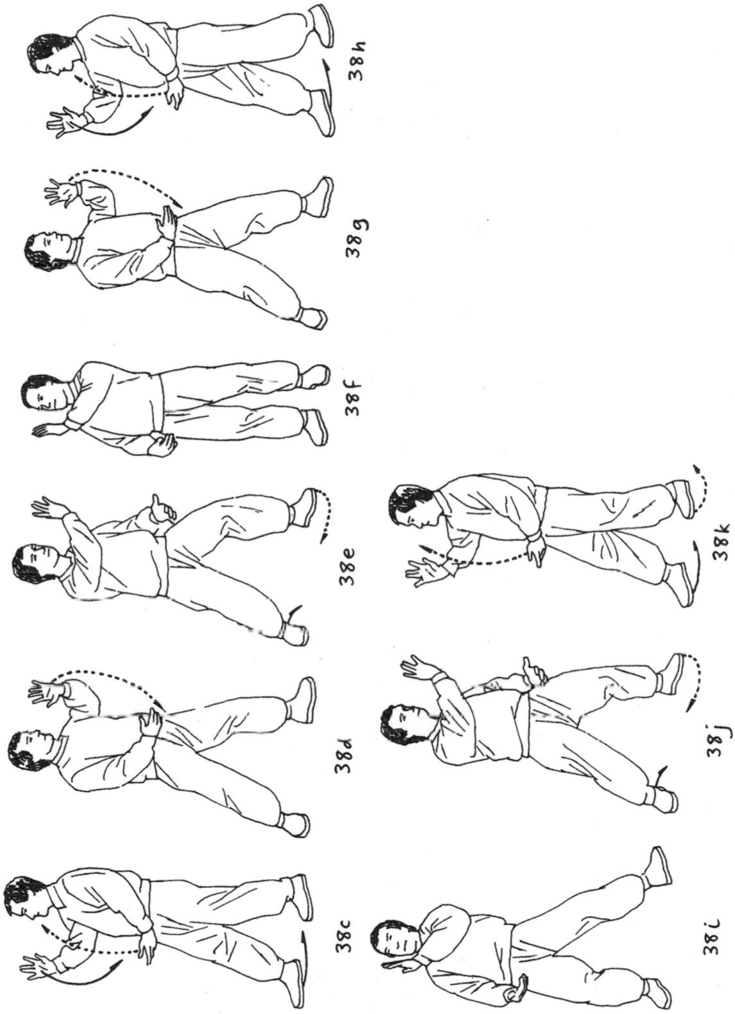

Fig 16.4 Wu Yu Xiang-style Tai Chi Chuan (4)

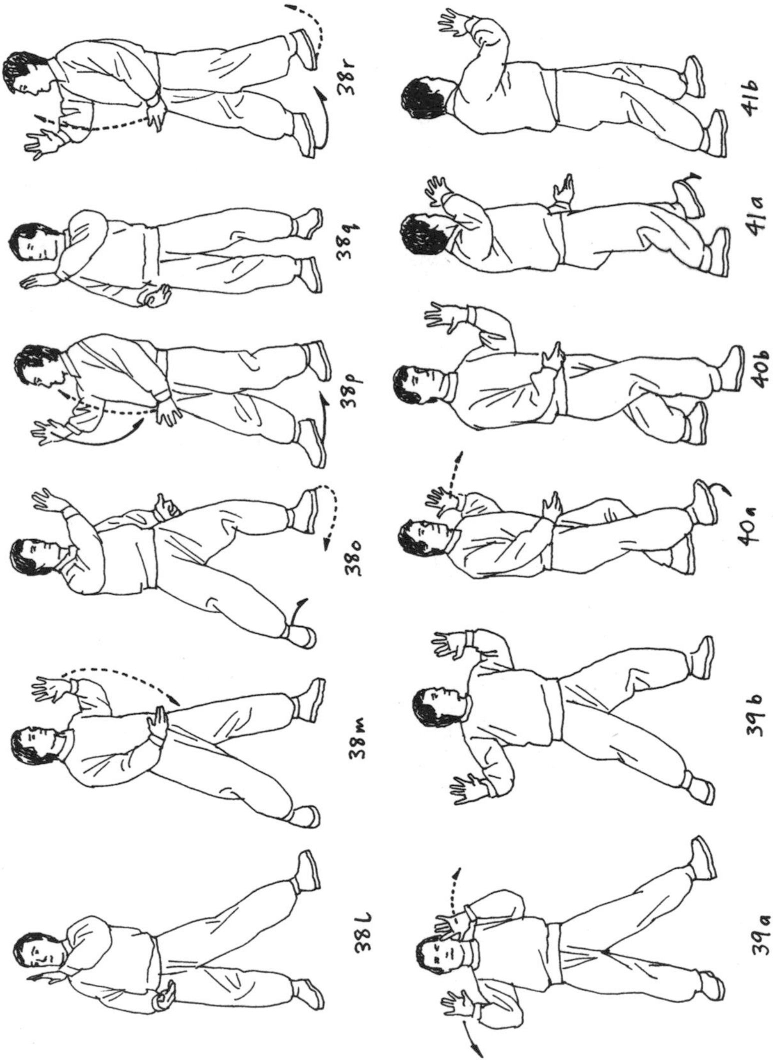
38L
38m
38o
38p
38q
38r
39a
39b
40a
40b
41a
41b

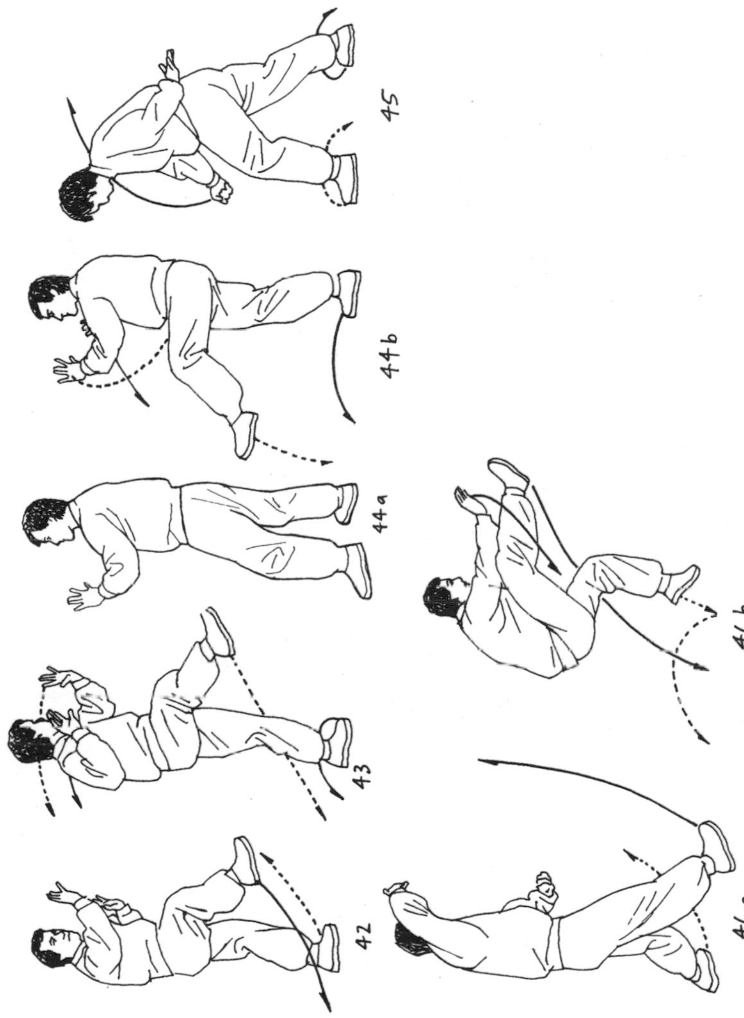

Fig 16.5 Wu Yu Xiang-style Tai Chi Chuan (5)

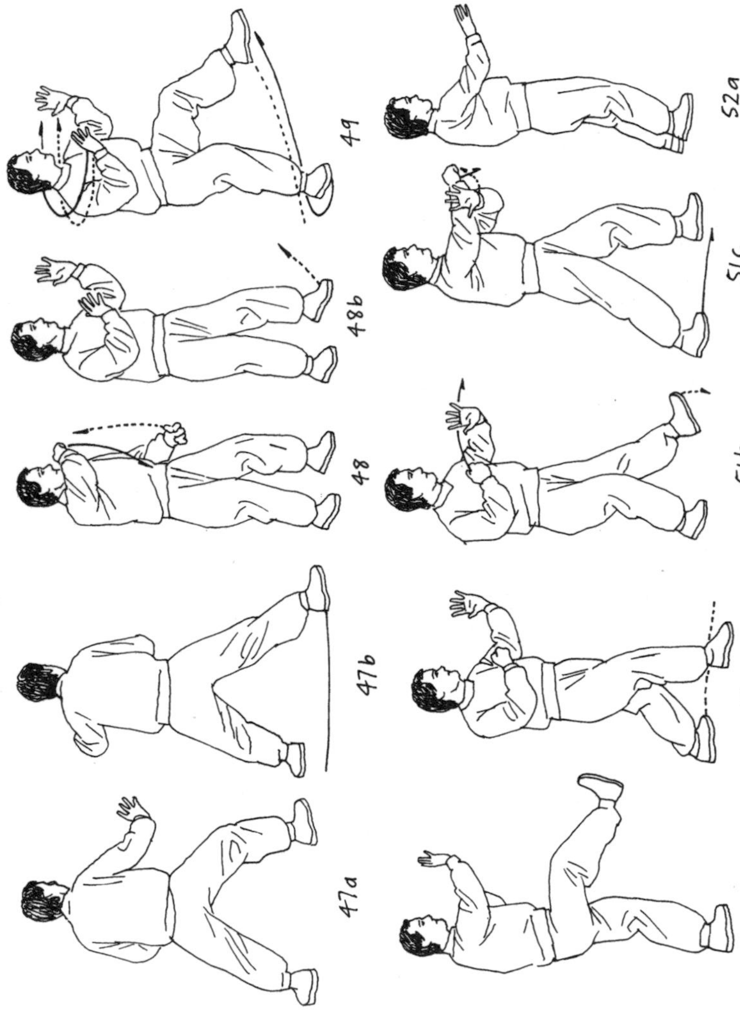
47a
47b
48
48b
49
50
51a
51b
51c
52a

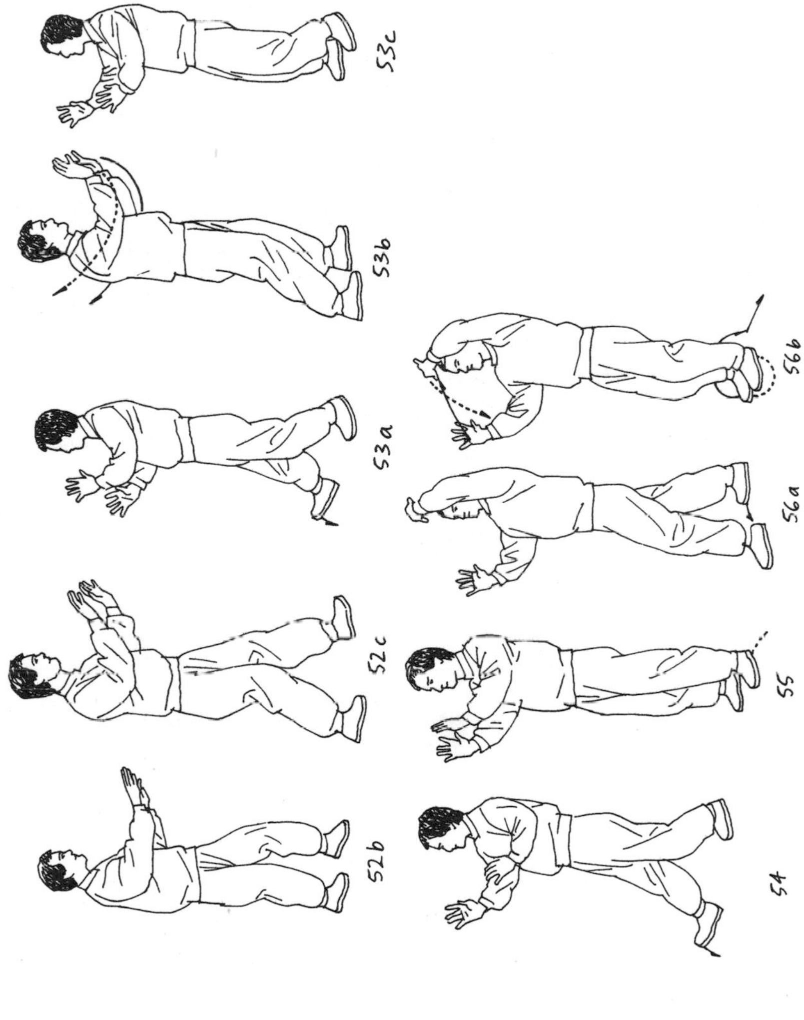

Fig 16.6 Wu Yu Xiang-style Tai Chi Chuan (6)

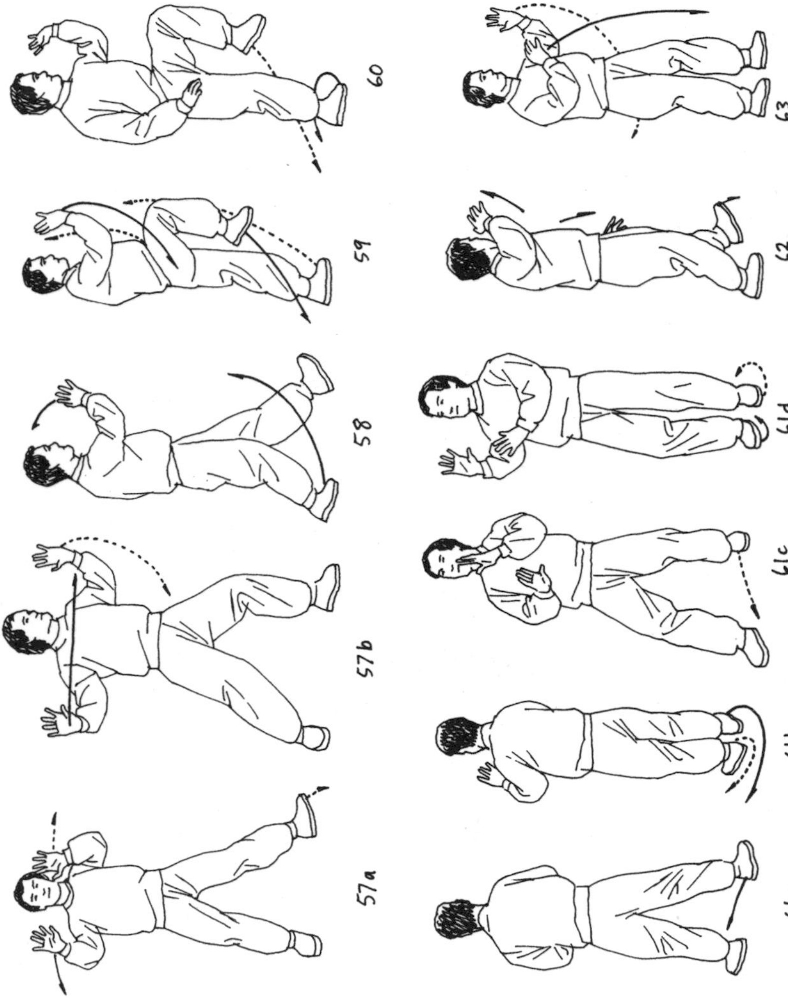
57a
57b
58
59
60
61a
61b
61c
61d
62
63

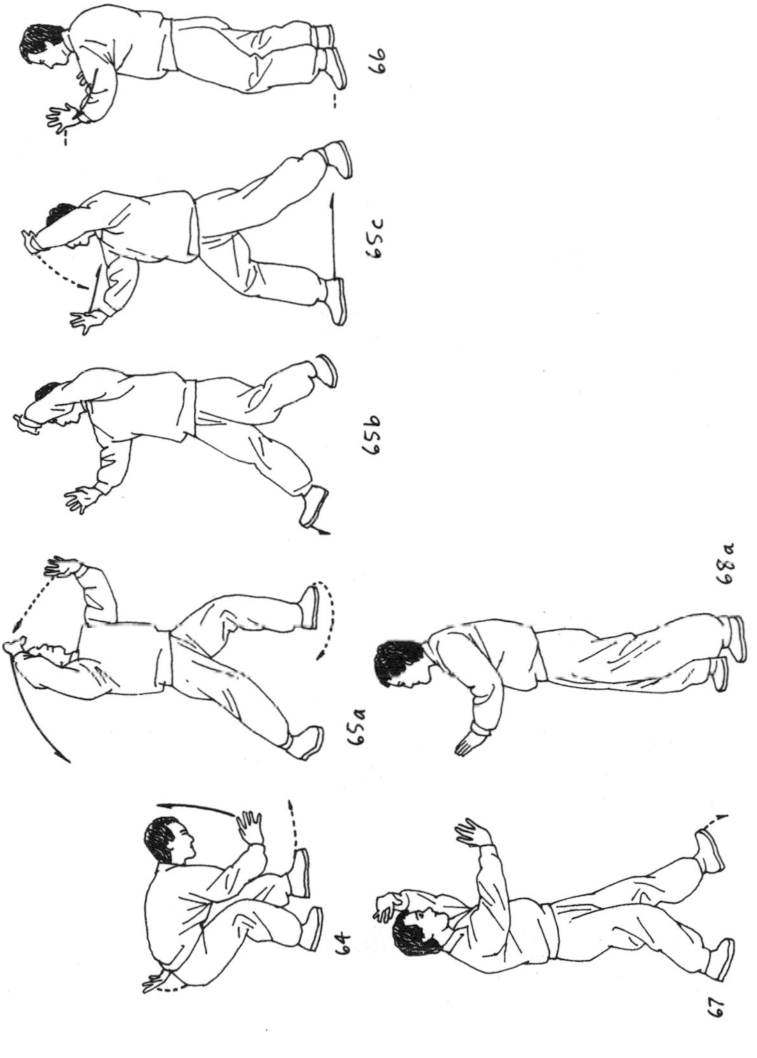

Fig 16.7 Wu Yu Xiang-style Tai Chi Chuan (7)

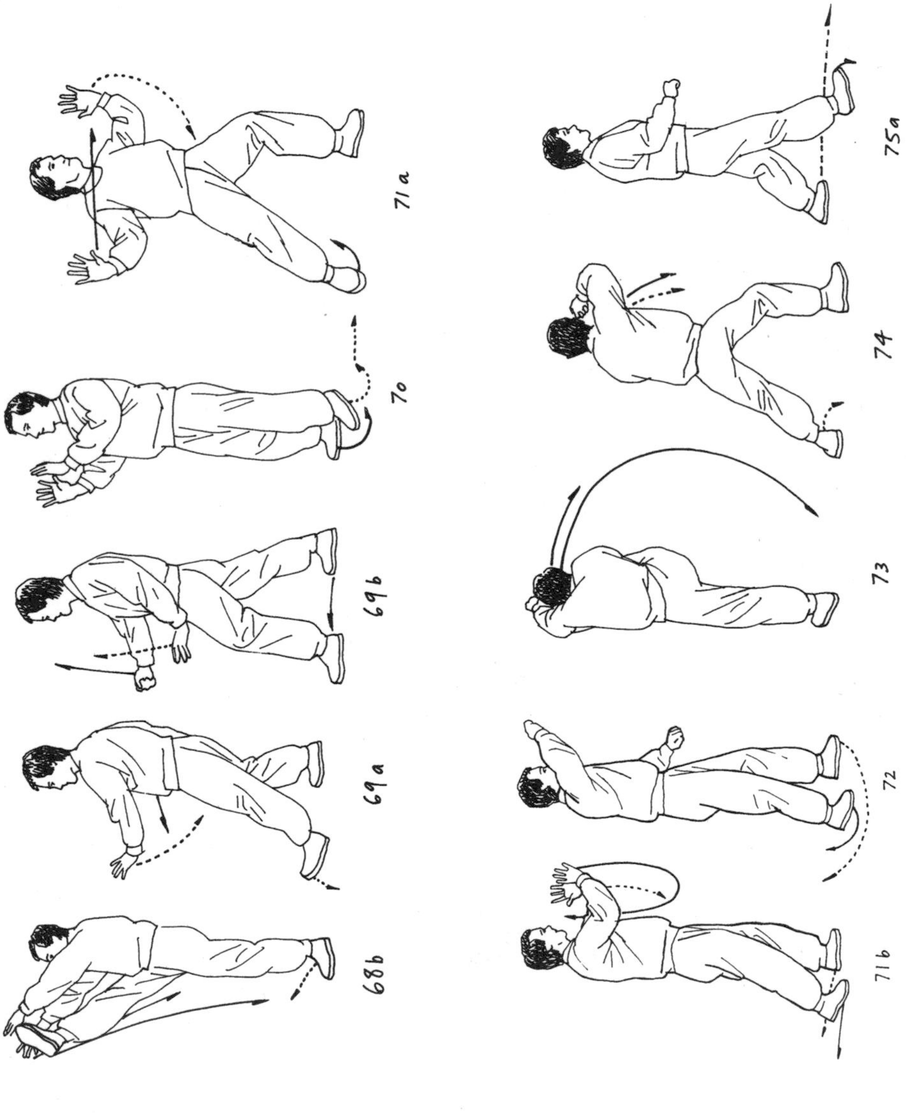
68b
69a
69b
70
71a
71b
72
73
74
75a

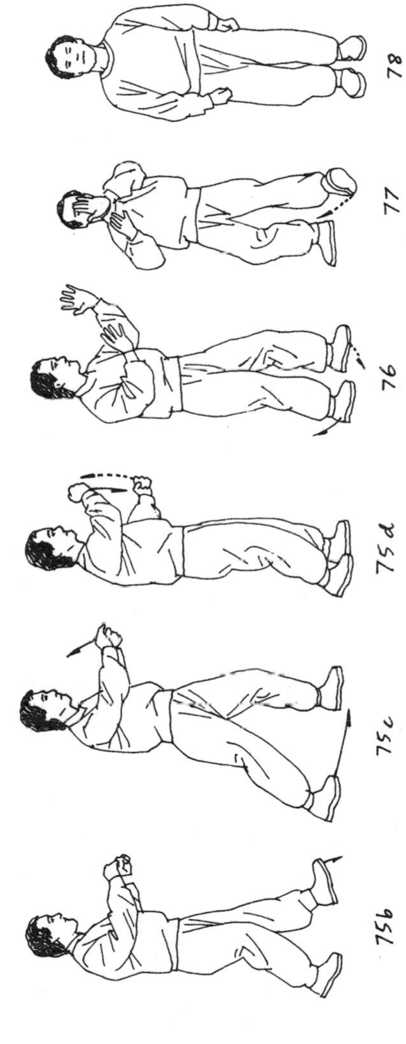

Fig 16.8 Wu Yu Xiang-style Tai Chi Chuan (8)

17

The Tai Chi Chuan of Wu Chuan You

How to Avoid Being Hurt in Combat

If properly put into practice these principles will enable you to accomplish a state of combat where even if you lose you still remain unhurt. This is obviously preferable to some arts where being hurt is inevitable even if you win.

For Health and for Combat

The second of the Wu styles of Tai Chi Chuan as explained in Chapter 3, was developed by Wu Chuan You (1834–1902), a Manchurian, who studied under Yang Ban Hou.

The third-generation master, Xu Zhi Yi, classifies the benefits of this Wu-Style under two main groups: health and combat. He lists six typical health benefits as follows:[1]

1 'Once moved, all move' is an important principle in Tai Chi Chuan training. Hence when a student practises Tai Chi Chuan, every part of the body is exercised.

2 Practising Tai Chi Chuan enables the student to eliminate irrelevant thoughts, focus the mind and create the ideal conditions for the nervous system to function properly. It has all the benefits of physical sport as well as of meditation.

3 When you have immersed yourself in the circular movements of Tai Chi Chuan, when you can differentiate the transformation of 'appearance' and 'solidness', when you can regulate your breathing, you will have had a deep taste of pleasure which will benefit both your emotional and your physical health.

4 The slow, graceful movements of Tai Chi Chuan and the principle of 'stillness in movement, and movement in stillness' help you to develop patience, tolerance and tranquillity.

5 It is suitable for the old as well as the young, the strong as well as the weak. Combat application through Pushing Hands is not risky as Tai Chi Chuan depends on using the opponent's strength.
6 A special feature of Tai Chi Chuan is that it can be practised by recuperating patients according to their different needs. The physical movements provide effective exercises for the whole body, deep breathing regulates the function of the heart and the circulation of the blood, and a focused and relaxed mind, by enhancing the nervous system, stimulates the self-regenerative and curative functions to overcome illness and promote health.

Concerning combat, Xu Zhi Yi lists the following four benefits:

1 Tai Chi Chuan uses 'soft' to overcome 'hard'. The exponent employs 'running' techniques to 'lead' the opponent's movement to failure, then applies 'sticking' techniques to exploit the advantage of gaining natural momentum for him- or herself and forcing the opponent into adverse momentum. This is possible only if the weakness of 'double heaviness' is avoided. Double heaviness is only knowing how to use 'hardness' but not 'softness'.
2 In combat, Tai Chi Chuan exponents use stillness to await motion, meaning that they will let the opponent make the first move, 'lead' the initial attack to failure and the opponent to an unfavourable position, then counter-attack at the appropriate time, manifesting the principle 'start later but arrive earlier'. Therefore, tactics that seek to rush at an opponent or to attack hastily are avoided. The Tai Chi Chuan exponent must bear in mind the following two points: attack only when you have an advantage and when, if your attack fails, your opponent will be unable to counter-attack.
3 The aim of 'using four *tahils* to overcome a thousand *katies*' can be achieved in two main ways: add my own force to my opponent's momentum, or withdraw my own force. Hence in Tai Chi Chuan force is never used against force; rather the technique is to manoeuvre your opponent into an unfavourable position then strike, following the tenet of 'the small to subdue the big'.
4 Use retreat as means of advance. Although there are countless ways of applying force successfully in Tai Chi Chuan, they can be summed up in two words: 'run' and 'stick'. 'Run' refers to minimizing the opponent's force to protect ourselves; 'stick' refers to controlling the opponent's movements after minimizing them. These two tactics are actually two aspects of the same tactic, and should complement each other.

These principles clearly show that exchanging blows wildly without any thought for one's own safety is not part of Tai Chi Chuan. If properly put into practice, they will enable you to accomplish a state of combat where even if you lose you still remain unhurt. This is obviously preferable to some arts where being hurt is inevitable even if you win.

The Patterns of Wu Chuan You-style Tai Chi Chuan

The set presented below is based on the performance by Wu Chuan You's son, Wu Jian Quan. The original set consists of 83 patterns; in the set illustrated, repeated patterns have been eliminated, leaving only 53.

1 Infinite Ultimate Stance
2 Tai Chi Starting Pattern
3 Grasping Sparrow's Tail
4 Single Whip
5 Lifting Up Hands
6 White Crane Flaps Wings
7 Twist Knee Throw Step (left and right)
8 Playing the Lute
9 Move–Intercept–Punch
10 Like Sealed As If Closed
11 Cross Hands
12 Carry Tiger Back to Mountain
13 Slanting Single Whip
14 Observe Fist Below Elbow
15 Repulse Monkey
16 Flying Diagonally
17 Lifting Up Hands
18 Needle at Sea Bottom
19 Fan Going Through Back
20 Swing Punch
21 Move–Intercept–Punch
22 Single Whip
23 Cloud-hands
24 Single Whip
25 High Patting Horse
26 Left and Right Snap Kicks
27 Turn Round Thrust Kick
28 Plant Fist

29 Move Forward Pat Horse
30 Snap Kick
31 Strike Tiger
32 Double Kick
33 Double Bees Buzzing at Ears
34 Turn Body Double Kick
35 Wild Horse Spreads Mane
36 Jade Girl Threads Shuttle
37 Single Whip
38 Lower Stance
39 Golden Cockerel Stands Solitary
40 Single Whip
41 Palm Strike to Face
42 Turn Round Cross-hands Sway Lotus
43 Punch to Abdomen
44 Lower Stance
45 Seven Stars
46 Ride Tiger
47 Palm Strike to Face
48 Turn Round Double Sway Lotus
49 Shoot Tiger
50 Palm Strike to Face
51 Swing Punch
52 Move Forward Pat Horse
53 Unity of Tai Chi

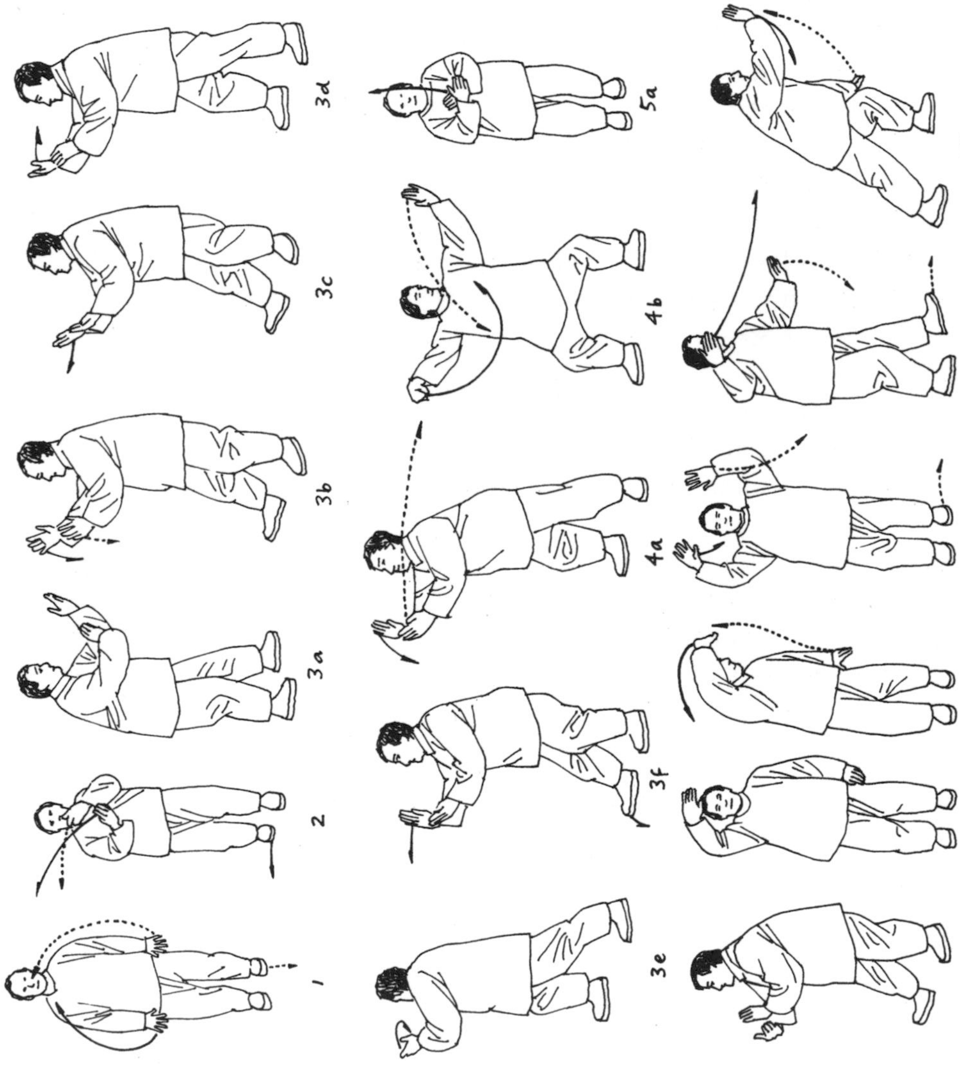
1
2
3a
3b
3c
3d
3e
3f
4a
4b
5a
5b
5c
6a
6b
7a
7b

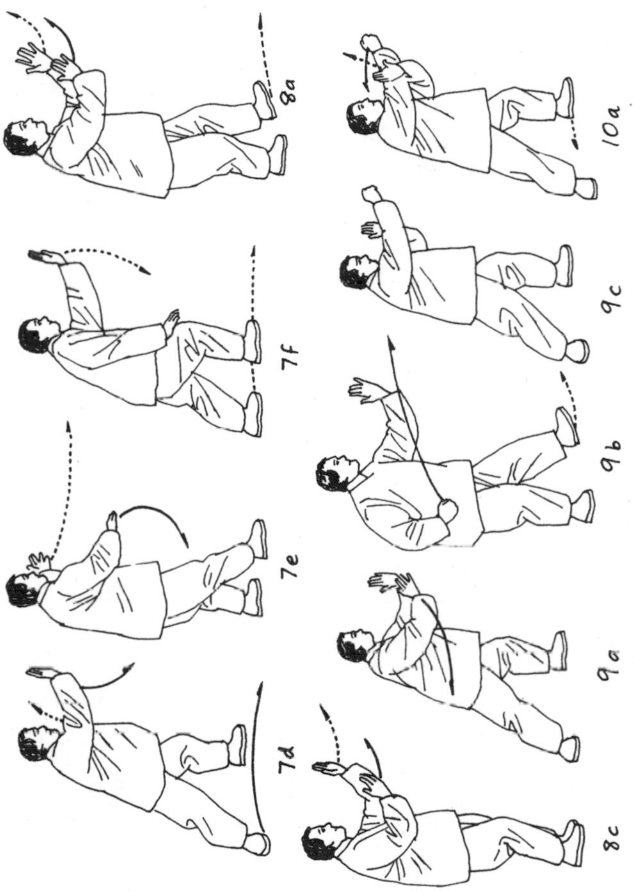

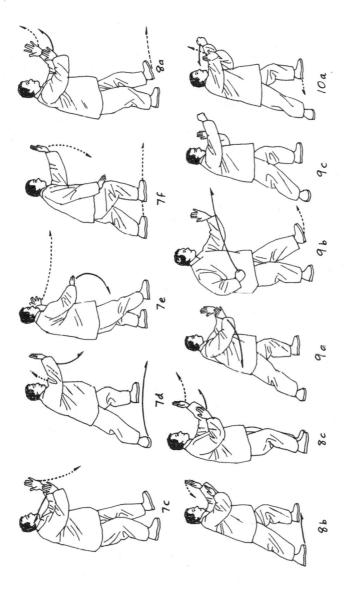

Fig 17.1 The Tai Chi Chuan style of Wu Chuan You (1)

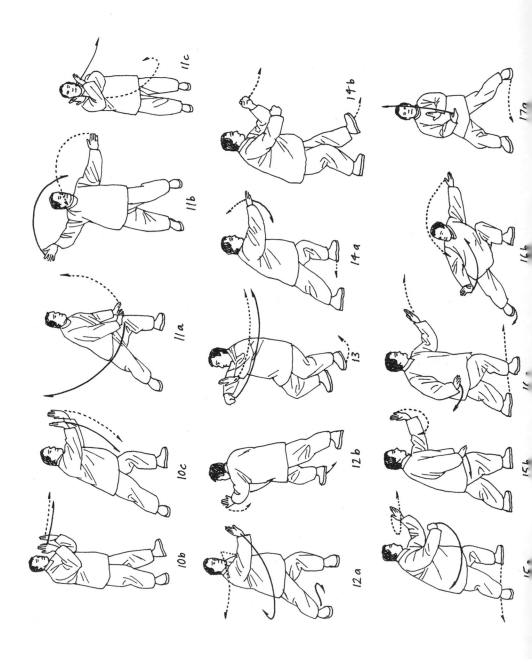
10b
10c
11a
11b
11c
12a
12b
13
14a
14b
15b
16b

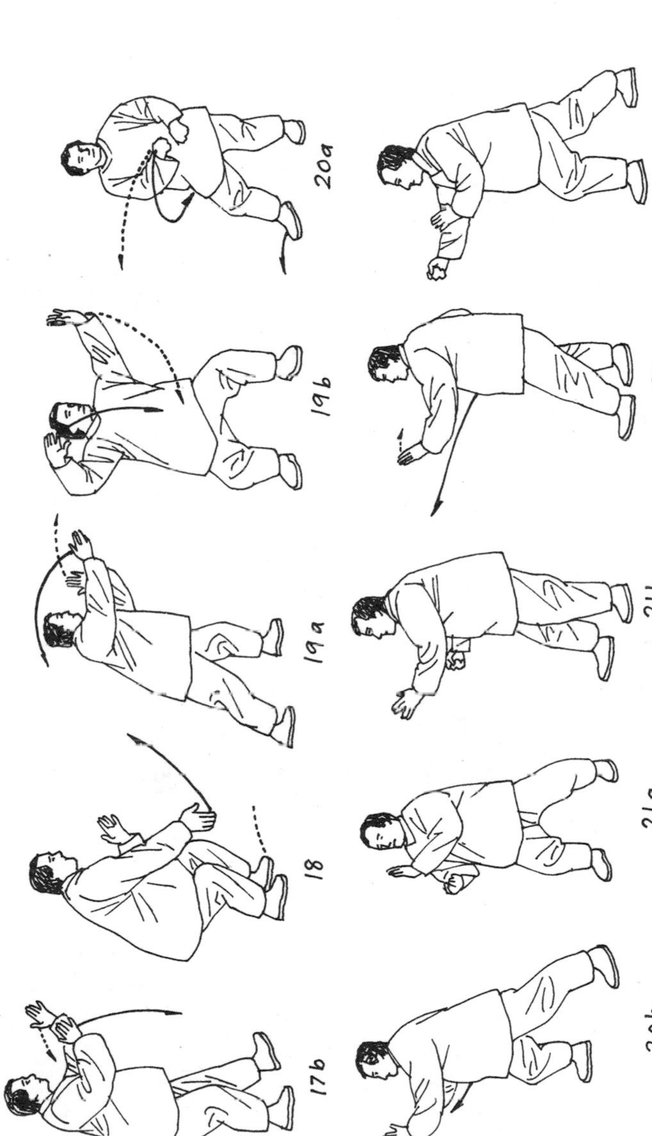

Fig 17.2 The Tai Chi Chuan style of Wu Chuan You (2)

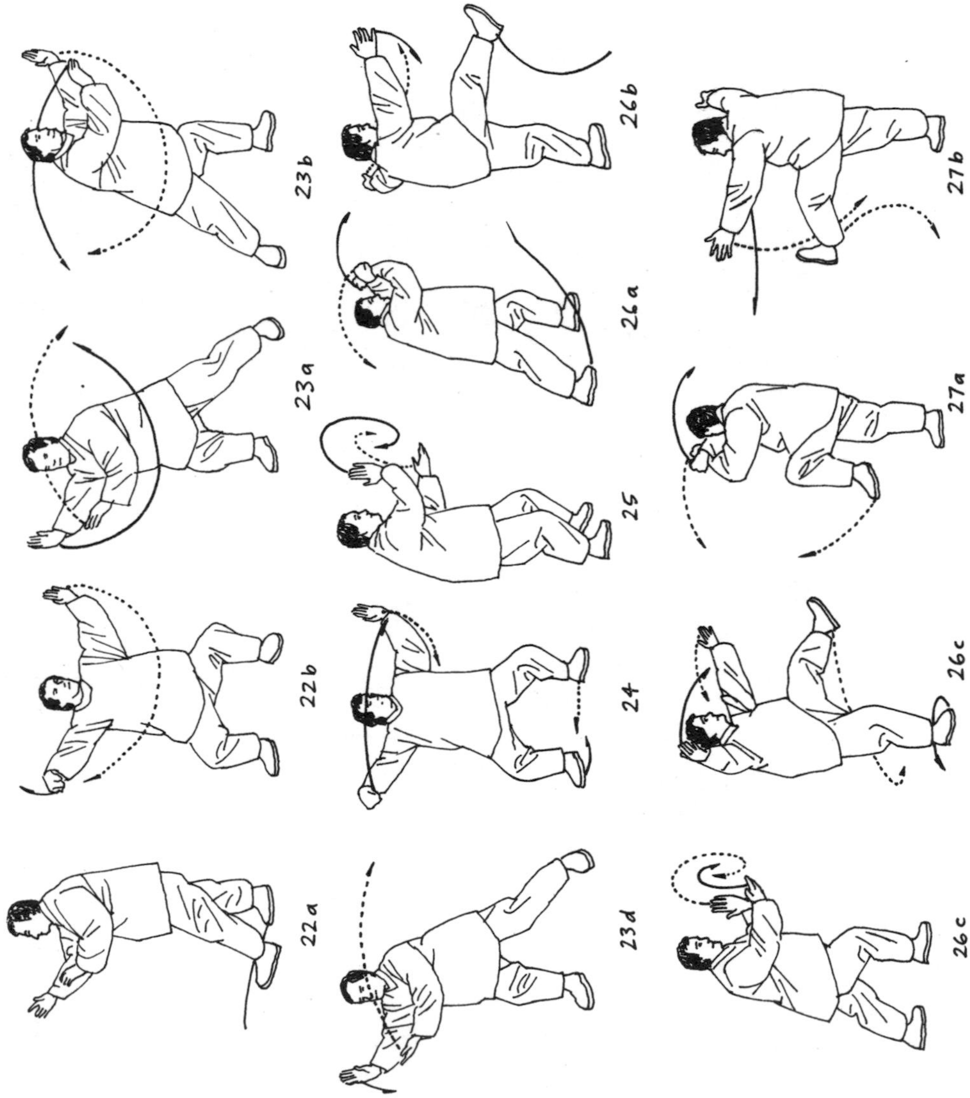

22a
22b
23a
23b
23d
24
25
26a
26b
26c
26c
27a
27b

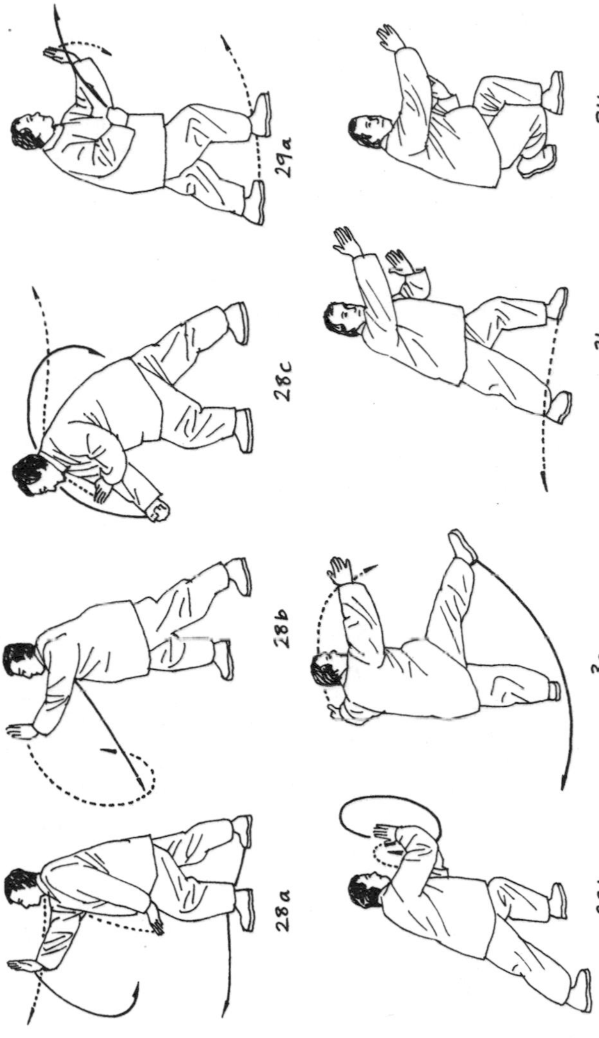

Fig 17.3 The Tai Chi Chuan style of Wu Chuan You (3)

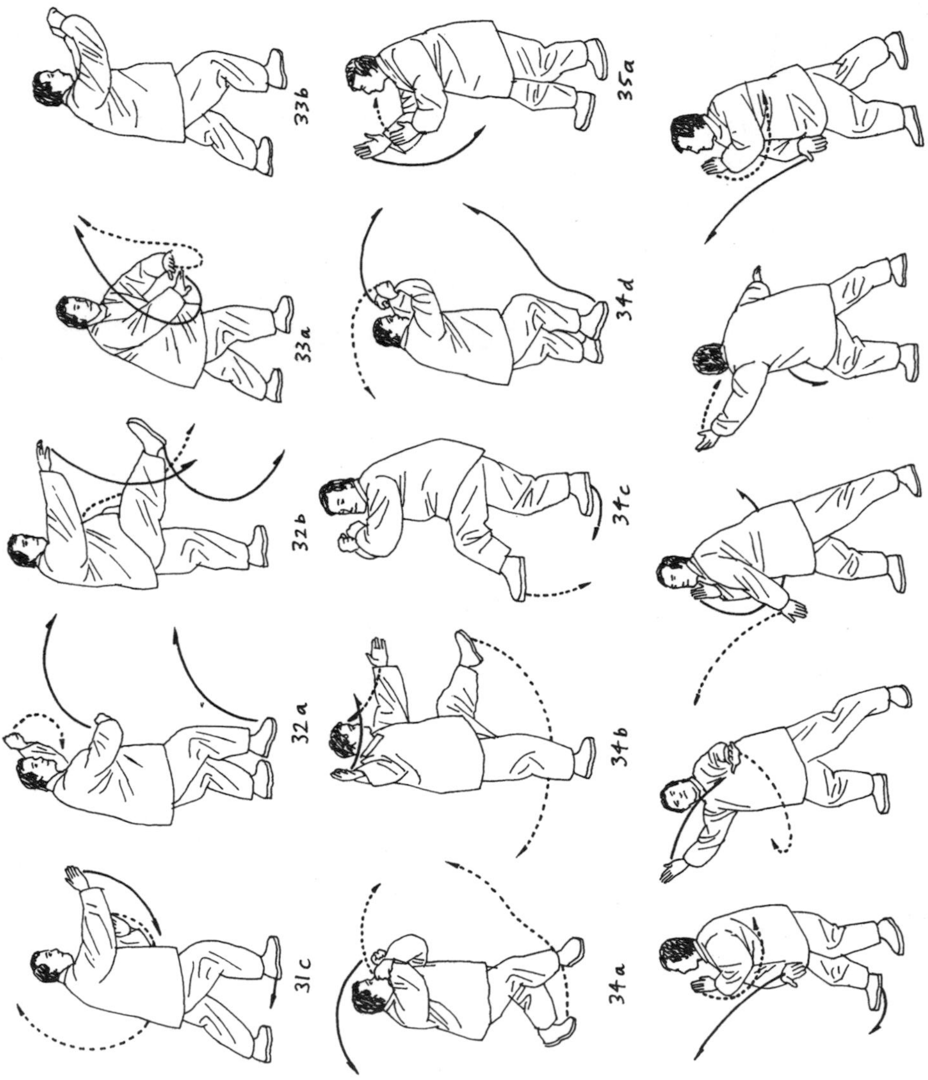

31c
32a
32b
33a
33b
34a
34b
34c
34d
35a
35b
35c
35d
35e
35f

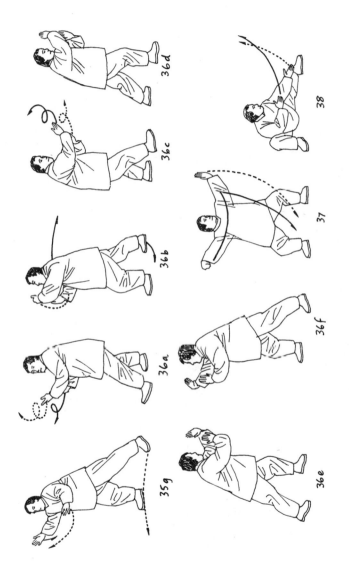

Fig 17.4 The Tai Chi Chuan style of Wu Chuan You (4)

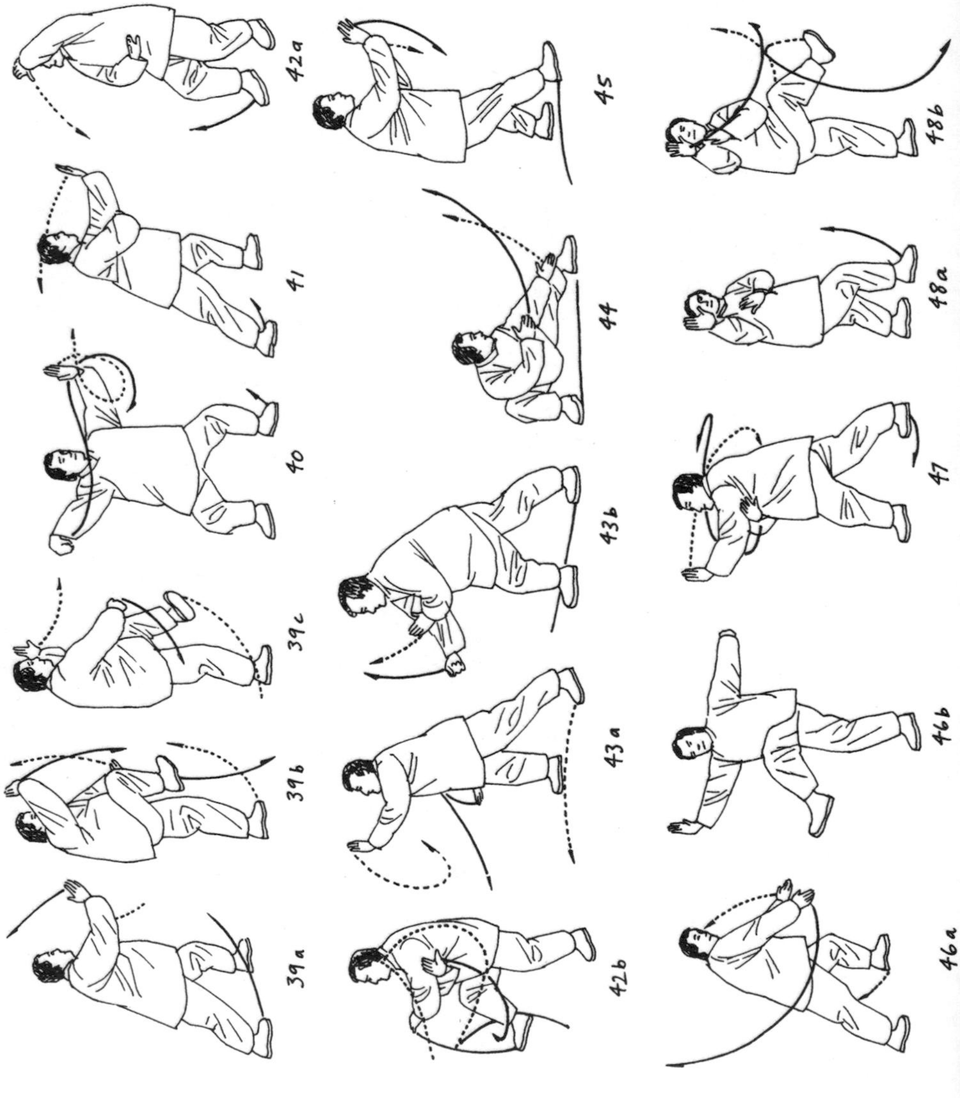
39a
39b
39c
40
41
42a
42b
43a
43b
44
45
46a
46b
47
48a
48b

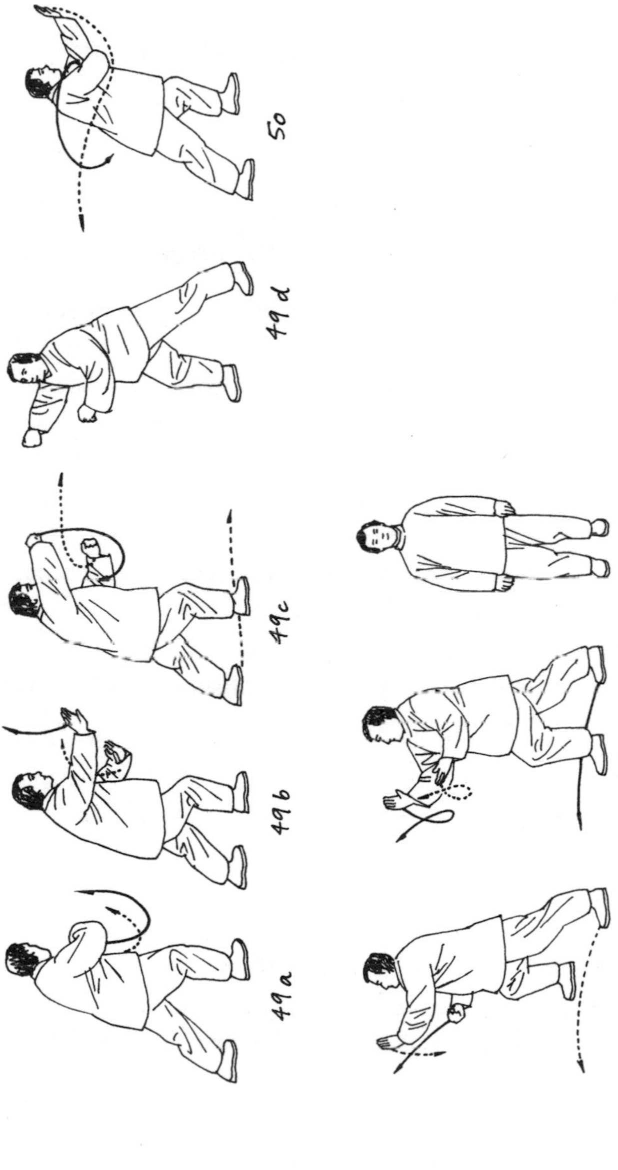

Fig 17.5 The Tai Chi Chuan style of Wu Chuan You (5)

18

Sun-style Tai Chi Chuan

High Patterns and Agile Movements

A special feature of Tai Chi Chuan is 'use will-power, don't use strength'.

Some Advice on Tai Chi Chuan Practice

Sun style Tai Chi Chuan was developed by Sun (pronouced 'Soon')Lu Tang (1861–1932), the only master who was expert in all three internal kungfu styles. When he learnt Tai Chi Chuan from Hao Wei Zhen at the age of 50, he was already an established master of Hsing Yi Kungfu and Pakua Kungfu. His example of humbly seeking knowledge when he was already an expert, is an inspiration to all of us. Not only that, he absorbed the best of the Chen, Yang and Wu Styles to develop his own style which is sometimes called High Pattern Open-Closed Agile Movement Tai Chi Chuan. His daughter, Sun Jian Yun, reported that in his later years he only practised Tai Chi Chuan.

Sun Jian Yun, who learnt Tai Chi Chuan from her father from childhood, gives the following advice:[1]

1 The head should be upright but do not use force. Let the spirit be full.
2 The mouth should be gently closed with the tongue at the upper palate. Breathe gently through the nose. (Note: Personally I prefer to have my mouth loosely open.)
3 Both shoulders should be loose and dropped. Be careful that they are not raised; raised shoulders cause *chi* to float.
4 Both elbows should be pressed down. When the elbows and shoulders are dropped, *chi* can be sunk at the *dan tian*. When the elbows are pressed down, the arms can be bent, with stored energy ready to be released.
5 The fingers should be open and loose. The wrist should be flexible.
6 The chest should be held in, not extended. An extended chest causes *chi* to float, resulting in top heaviness.

7 The waist must be flexible, as it is the commander of all the whole body's movements.
8 The legs should be bent; 'apparent' and 'solid' must be differentiated, otherwise agility is lost.
9 '*Chi* sunk at *dan tian*' means deep breathing. Deep breathing is very important in Tai Chi Chuan, but it must not be forced.
10 Meditation is seeking movement in stillness; Tai Chi Chuan is seeking stillness in movement. During practice, the heart must be calm and the mind must be focused; only then can the physical movements be smooth and agile.
11 A special feature of Tai Chi Chuan is 'use will-power, don't use strength'. The aim is to achieve force that is alive, with extreme softness yet extreme hardness, extreme heaviness yet extreme agility. When will-power arrives, power arrives. If mechanical strength is used, it becomes sluggish and clumsy, floating externally, out of place in internal arts.

The Patterns of Sun-style Tai Chi Chuan

Sun-style Tai Chi Chuan is characterized by small circular movements and high stances. It is closest to the style of Wu Xiang Yu, which is only to be expected, as Sun Lu Tang's teacher practised the Wu Style.

The pattern called 'Opening and Closing' is of particular importance in this style. It is used to develop *chi*, and is performed as follows. First focus your *chi* at your *dan tian*. With the palms facing each other, bring your hands slowly together. When your palms are quite close, you may feel a ball of energy between your palms. Gently compress the energy; then slowly let the ball expand as you gradually bring your palms apart to release the compression. Play with this ball of energy a few times; then as you perform subsequent patterns visualize energy from this ball flowing to your arms.

There are 97 patterns in the original Sun Style set, but in the one presented below based on the demonstrations of the second generation lady-master Sun Jiam Yun, some repeated patterns have been eliminated, leaving only 72.

1 Tai Chi Starting Pattern
2 Yin-yang of Cosmos
3 Lifting Up Hands
4 White Crane Flaps Wings
5 Opening and Closing

6 Twist Knee Throw Step
7 Playing the Lute
8 Move–Intercept–Punch
9 Like Sealed As If Closed
10 Opening and Closing
11 Lazy to Roll Sleeves
12 Opening and Closing
13 Single Whip
14 Playing the Lute
15 Repulse Monkey
16 Playing the Lute
17 White Crane Flaps Wings
18 Opening and Closing
19 Twist Knee Throw Step
20 Needle at Sea Bottom
21 Fan Going Through Back
22 Lazy to Roll Sleeves
23 Opening and Closing
24 Single Whip
25 Cloud-hands
26 High Patting Horse
27 Right Thrust Kick
28 Left Thrust Kick
29 Turn Round Thrust Kick
30 Move Forward Plant Fist
31 Turn Body Double Kick
32 Taming Tiger
33 Left Thrust Kick
34 Right Thrust Kick
35 Move–Intercept–Punch
36 Like Sealed As If Closed
37 Opening and Closing
38 Twist Knee Throw Step
39 Lazy to Roll Sleeves
40 Wild Horse Spreads Mane
41 Lazy to Roll Sleeves
42 Opening and Closing
43 Single Whip
44 Through the Back
45 Jade Girl Threads Shuttle

46 Lazy to Roll Sleeves
47 Opening and Closing
48 Single Whip
49 Low Stance
50 Golden Cockerel Stands Soliditary
51 Repulse Monkey
52 Playing the Lute
53 White Crane Flaps Wings
54 Opening and Closing
55 Twist Knee Throw Step
56 Needle at Sea Bottom
57 Through the Back
58 Lazy to Roll Sleeves
59 Opening and Closing
60 Single Whip
61 Cloud-hands
62 High Patting Horse
63 Cross-hands Sway Lotus
64 Lazy to Roll Sleeves
65 Opening and Closing
66 Single-whip Low Stance
67 Ride Tiger
68 Turn Around Sway Lotus
69 Shoot Tiger
70 Move Forward with Double Punches
71 Seven Stars
72 Infinite Ultimate Stance

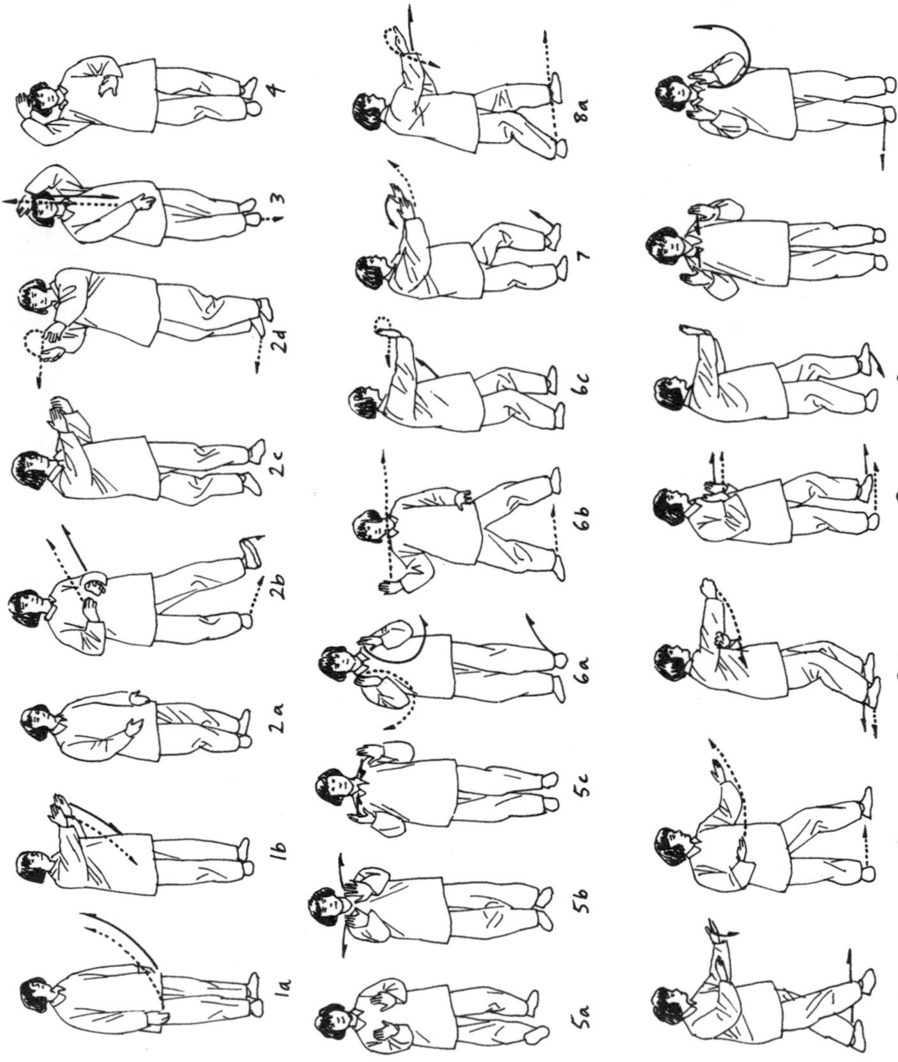
1a
1b
2a
2b
2c
2d
3
4
5a
5b
5c
6a
6b
6c
7
8a
8b
8c
8d
9a
9b
10
11a

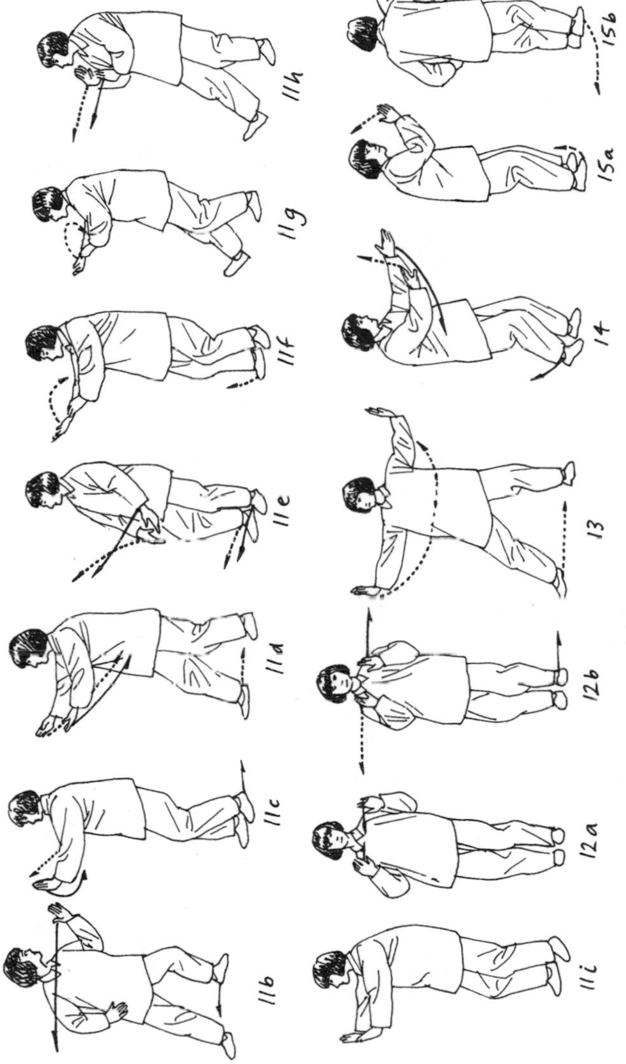

Fig 18.1 Sun-style Tai Chi Chuan (1)

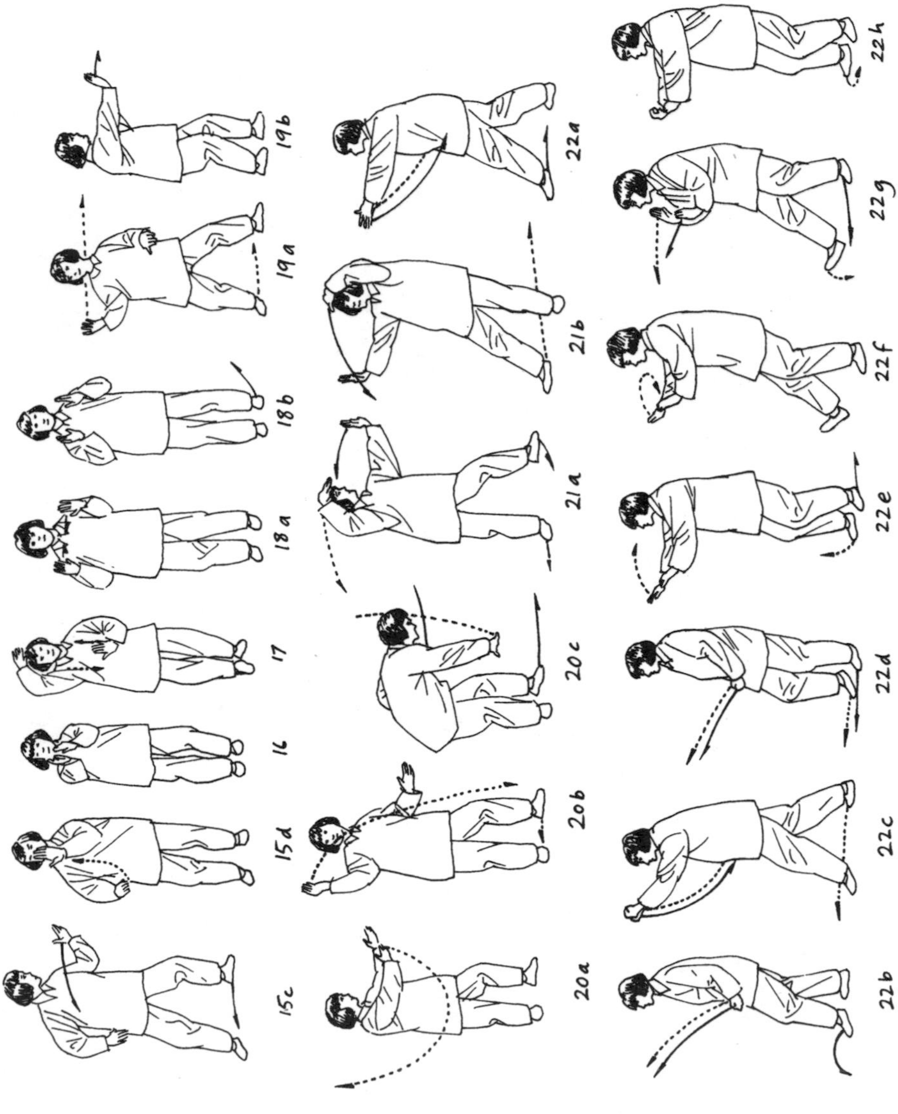
15c
15d
16
17
18a
18b
19a
19b
20a
20b
20c
21a
21b
22a
22b
22c
22d
22e
22f
22g
22h

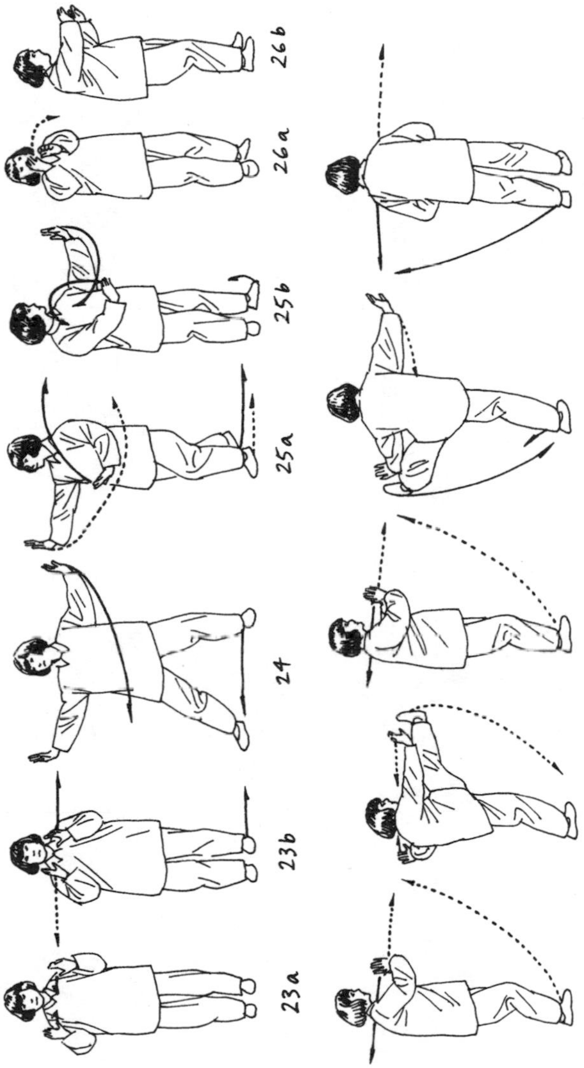

Fig 18.2 Sun-style Tai Chi Chuan (2)

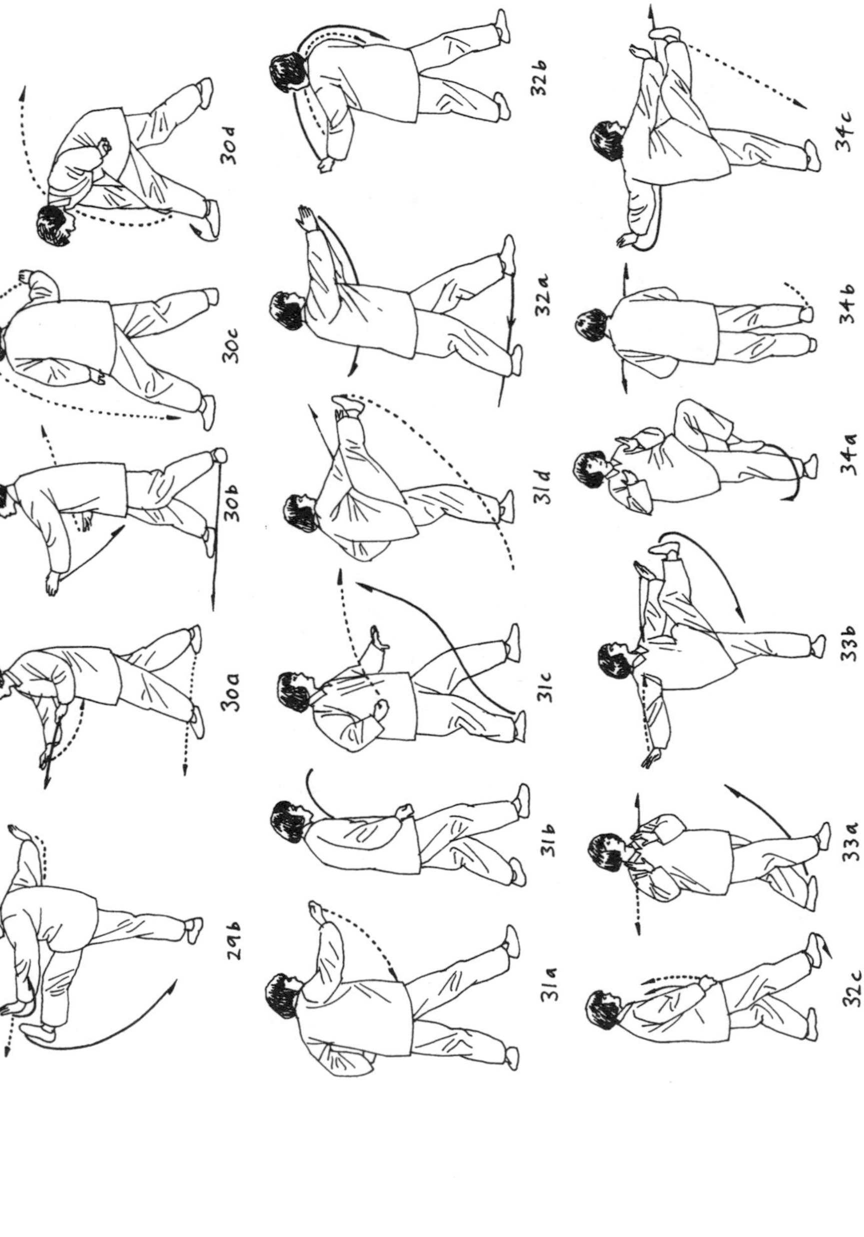
29b
30a
30b
30c
30d
31a
31b
31c
31d
32a
32b
32c
33a
33b
34a
34b
34c

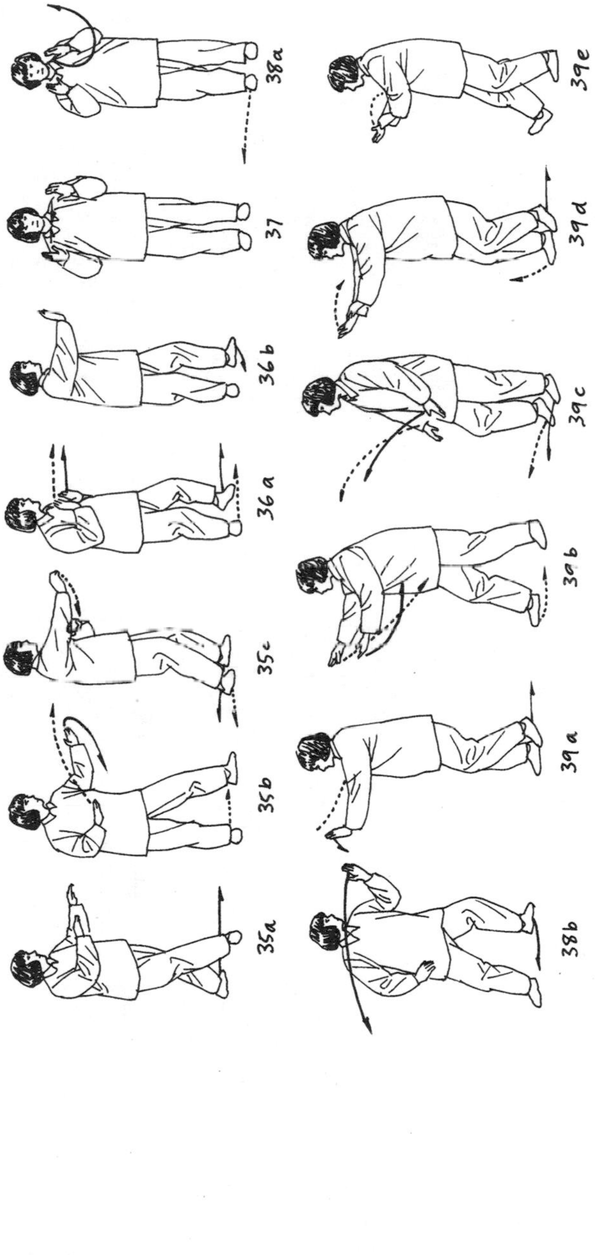

Fig 18.3 Sun-style Tai Chi Chuan (3)

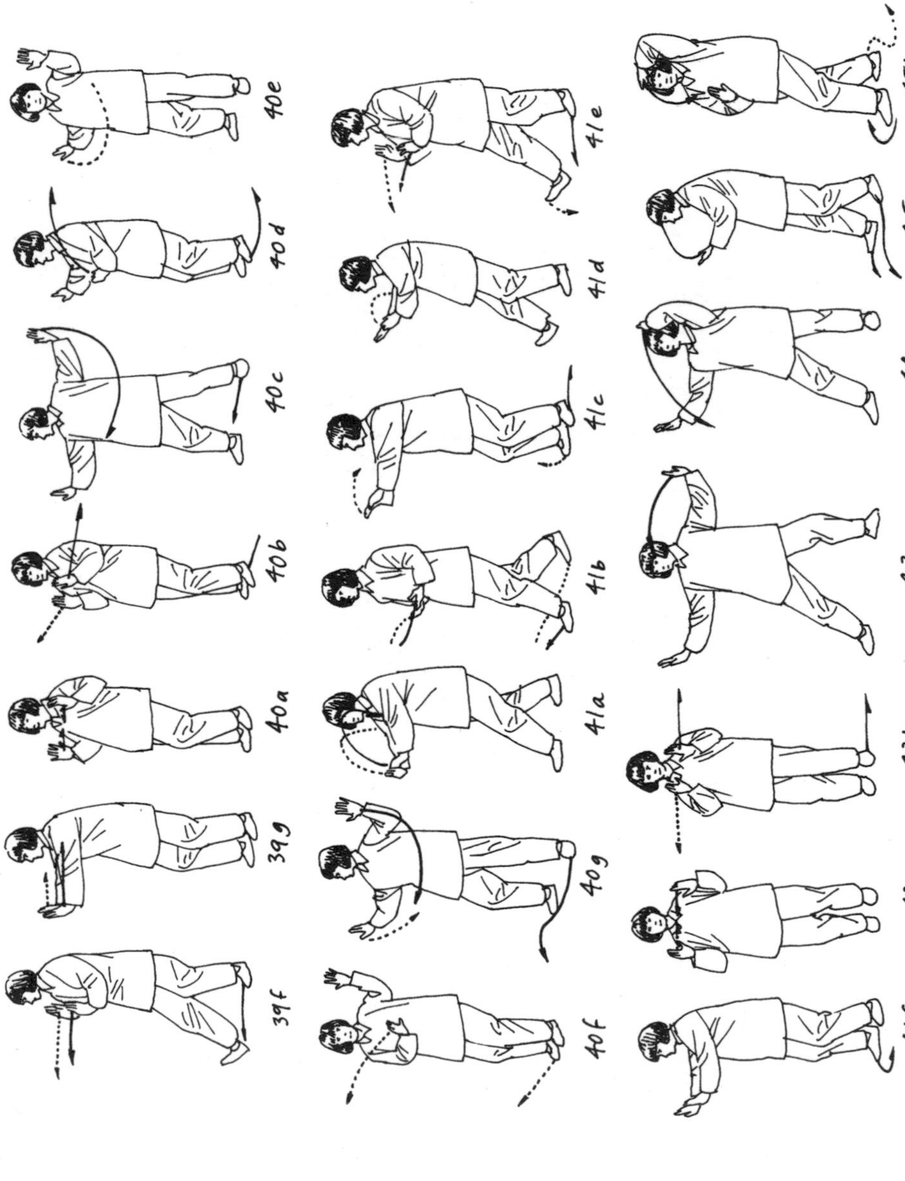
39f
39g
40a
40b
40c
40d
40e
40f
40g
41a
41b
41c
41d
41e
41f
42a
42b
43
44
45a
45b

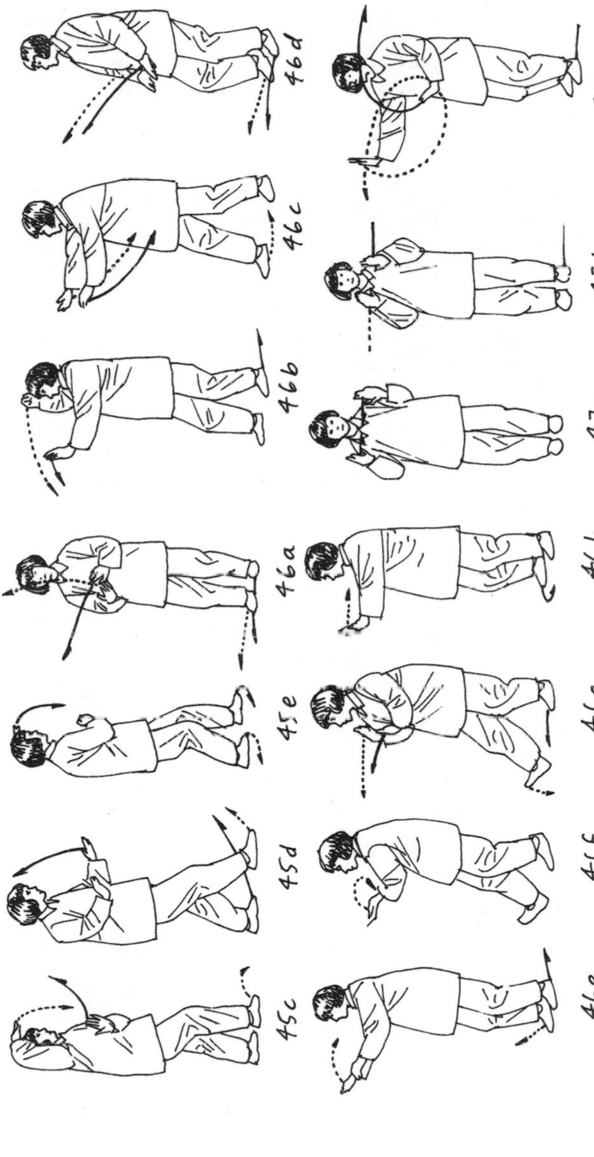

Fig 18.4 Sun-style Tai Chi Chuan (4)

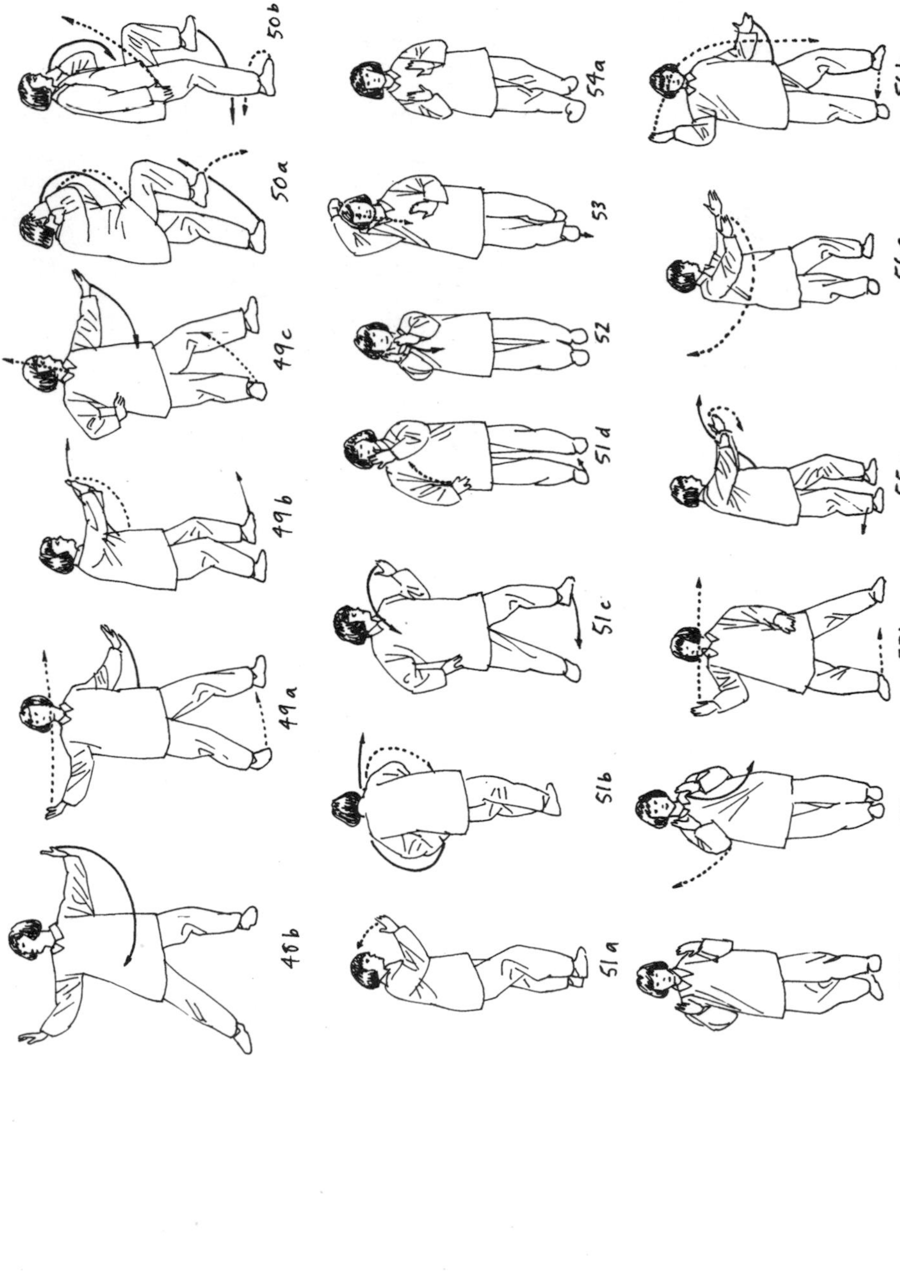
48b
49a
49b
49c
50a
50b
51a
51b
51c
51d
52
53
54a
54b
55a
55b
55c
56a
56b

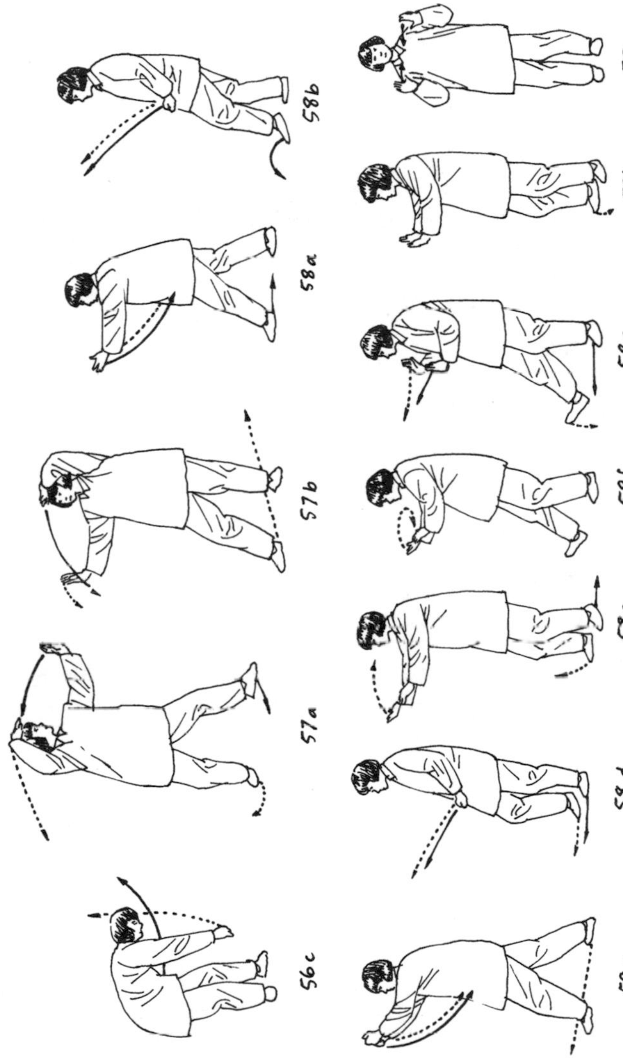

Fig 18.5 Sun-style Tai Chi Chuan (5)

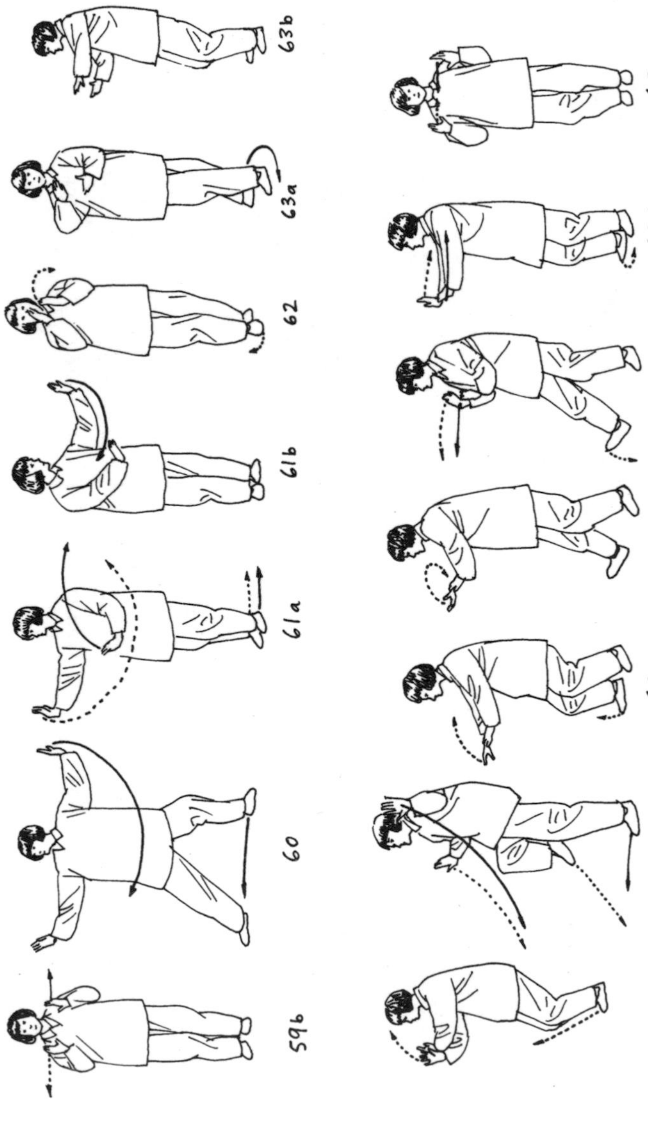
59b
60
61a
61b
62
63a
63b
63c
63d
64a
64b
64c
64d
65a

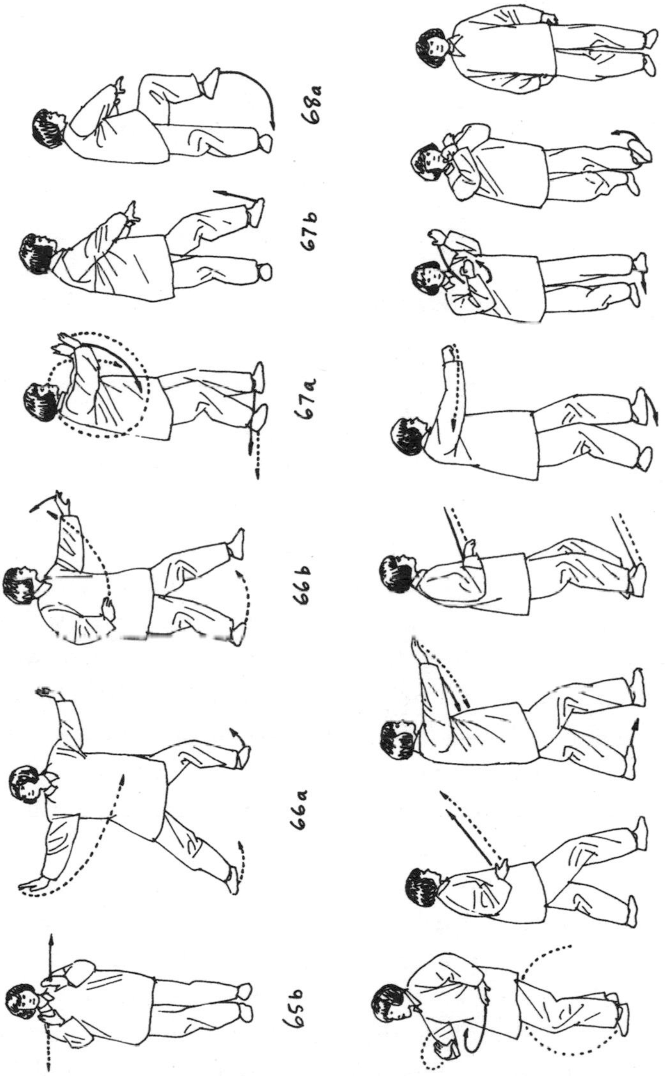

Fig 18.6 Sun-style Tai Chi Chuan (6)

19

Tai Chi Chuan Weapons

Transmitting Energy to Extended Hands

The purpose of Tai Chi Chuan weapon training, apart from using weapons for combat as in the past, is to provide a method for students to transmit their energy flow to the tips of their weapons.

Why Weapons Are Not Widely Used in Tai Chi Chuan

Unlike in Shaolin Kungfu, which uses a tremendous range of weapons including some fairly exotic ones, and in which weapons play an integral part in the training programme, weapon training is less popular in Tai Chi Chuan. I can think of four possible reasons for this. Shaolin Kungfu is much older and was established at a time when fighting with weapons rather than unarmed combat was the norm. If one could use weapons freely in fighting it was natural to emphasize weapon training rather than unarmed combat in martial arts, and this tradition has been passed down, even though most countries today do not permit the carrying of weapons in public. Tai Chi Chuan does not have this tradition, because by the time it became popular, during the Qing Dynasty, carrying a weapon in public had been prohibited for four centuries. Weapon training was part of Tai Chi Chuan training, but it never assumed the significance it had in Shaolin Kungfu.

Secondly, apart from the time when it was practised by Taoist priests at Wudang Mountain for spiritual development, and by the Chen family at Chen Jia Gou for self-defence, Tai Chi Chuan has throughout the years been practised more for health than for combat or spirituality. When Yang Lu Chan made it available to the public for the first time, he taught high-ranking officials and members of the Manchurian royal family, who neither needed nor were willing to undergo the demanding training of combat Tai Chi Chuan. Outside this exalted circle, students who were taught by other Tai Chi Chuan masters were mostly scholars and wealthy merchants. Unlike the revolutionaries and patriotic fighters who generally preferred Shaolin Kungfu, these students often considered weapons barbaric.

The third reason concerns the different approaches of the two systems. Weapons are still regularly used in Shaolin Kungfu today, despite the fact that few Shaolin students really use weapons to fight, because weapon training is a progression from unarmed training, with the weapons as weights. If you can habitually perform a weapon set well, you can generally perform an unarmed set even better, without the weight of the weapon. The Tai Chi Chuan approach to increasing power and skill is different; since it emphasizes mind control and energy flow for increasing internal force, holding a weight is an encumbrance rather than an aid.

The fourth reason is related to the third. In Shaolin Kungfu students can start weapon training after they have attained a reasonable standard in basic stances and kungfu movements, and the benefits of the weapon training in terms of increasing power and stamina can be felt in a comparatively short time. In genuine Tai Chi Chuan, students generally commence weapon training only when they have reached an advanced level. The purpose of Tai Chi Chuan weapon training, apart from using weapons for combat as in the past, is to provide a method for students to transmit their energy flow to the tips of their weapons. Such an ability enabled Wudang masters, for example, to use an ordinary stick like a sword.

But if you are not advanced enough to transmit your energy flow to your own hands, it is no use trying to do so with a weapon. Few Tai Chi students today have the opportunity to experience what internal force is, let alone to transmit it to where they want. Hence, very few Tai Chi students nowadays are ready to train with weapons meaningfully. Moreover, the time and effort needed for such training is long and exacting. To use their own hands adroitly is difficult enough for some students, who will often train only when their teacher is around; to use a weapon skilfully as an extended hand would be virtually impossible.

Some Functions of Weapon Training

Nevertheless, weapon training does serve some purpose in Tai Chi Chuan, and at various different levels. At the lowest level of Tai Chi Chuan as dance, a Tai Chi sword dance is easy to perform as well as pleasant to watch, especially if it is performed with grace and elegance. It is certainly easier to perform a Tai Chi sword dance, or any other Tai Chi dance for that matter, than most other kinds, including modern disco dancing and classical Indian dance drama – Tai Chi dancers do not need as much stamina, for example, nor do they have to do preliminary exercises like stretching the neck and legs.

At the intermediate level, where Tai Chi Chuan is treated as a martial art, weapon training serves several useful functions. For instance, it can illustrate basic principles more obviously than unarmed set practice does.

The Wudang sword is a good illustration. While Shaolin Kungfu is famous for its staff, which has become an unofficial symbol of Shaolin weapons, Wudang Tai Chi Chuan is best known for its sword. Philosophically, the Shaolin staff manifests what Shaolin Kungfu stands for: simple yet versatile, hardy yet compassionate. It is difficult to find a weapon simpler than a staff, yet the techniques for other weapons, like the spear, halberd, mace, battle axe, scimitar, sword or dagger, are all incorporated in staff training! A staff, like a Shaolin disciple, is made for all seasons. And though it is hardy, its combat application is a hallmark of compassion, since it is devoid of any sharp or pointed parts which can maim or kill an opponent. On the other hand, to use a Chinese sword well in any style of kungfu, including Shaolin and Tai Chi Chuan, one has to be gentle, graceful and flowing – qualities for which Tai Chi Chuan is famous. If one were to use a delicate sword as a staff for blocking or hacking, one would succeed in breaking it.

One does not block a heavy weapon with a dainty sword, just as in unarmed Tai Chi Chuan one does not meet a powerful attack head on. One effective way to counter such an attack is to follow its momentum and 'lead' it to failure, continuing the movement to strike before the opponent can recover. Another way is to 'swallow' the attack and 'shoot out' at the opponent as the attack passes. Both methods follow typical Tai Chi Chuan principles, and are illustrated in *figure 19.1*.

In *figure 19.1a* the attacker chops the staff, which may also represent a halberd, mace or any other heavy weapon, down onto the defender. The latter moves to the left, and using only a wrist movement, brings the sword round the attacking staff as it comes down *(figure 19.1b)*. Continuing this circular movement without a break, the defender then slashes at the attacker's right wrist *(figure 19.1c)*.

In *figure 19.1d* the attacker sweeps the staff against the defender's waist. As the staff approaches, the latter takes a small step back with the back leg and drops back into a low stance *(figure 19.1e)*. As soon as the staff has passed, and without any break in the movement, the defender shoots forward and thrusts the sword into the attacker's ribs. Alternatively to avoid causing serious injury the defender can slash the attacker's forearm *(figure 19.1f)*.

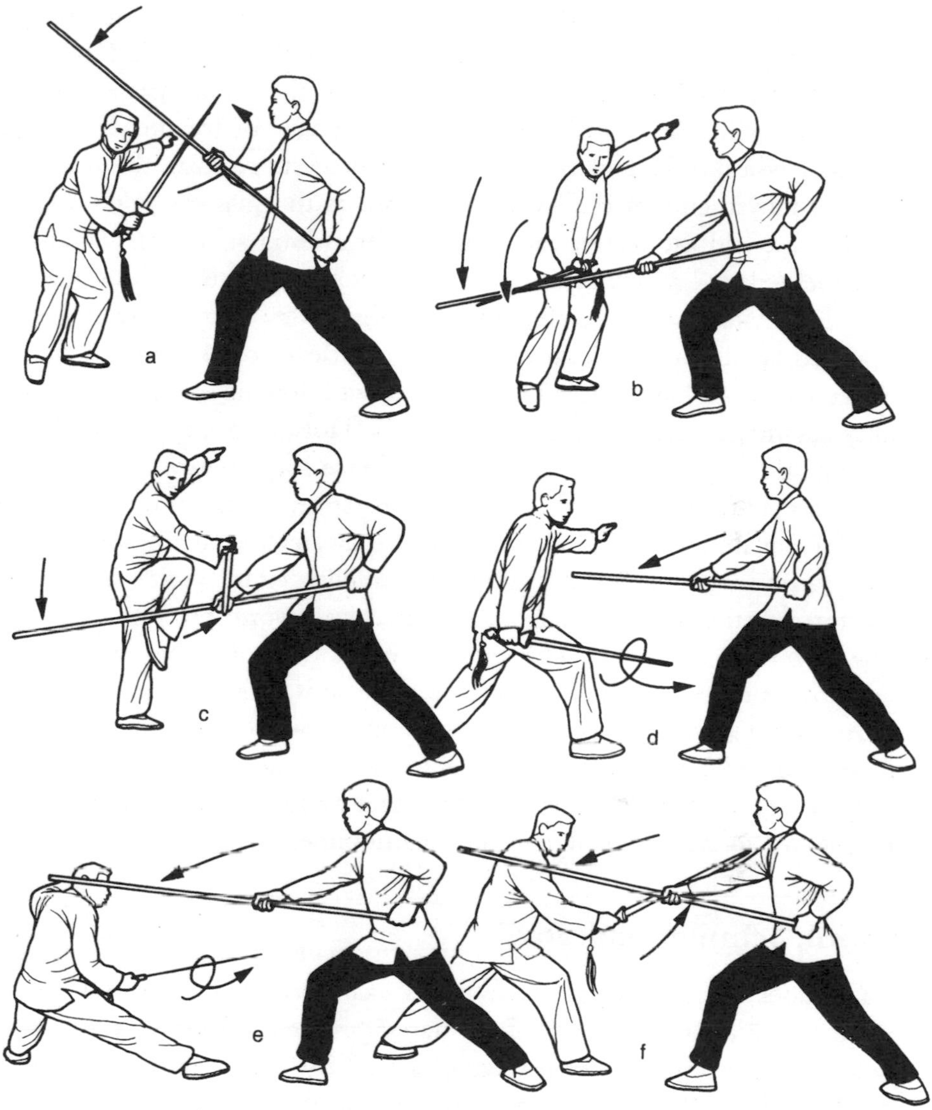

Fig 19.1 Dainty sword against hardy staff

It is obvious that a student who can successfully apply the principles of swordsmanship, which emphasizes flowing with the attack instead of going against the opponent, and dodging a powerful attack instead of meeting it directly, and which demands great agility, grace and fluidity, will better appreciate and be able to put into practice the same principles in unarmed Tai Chi Chuan.

At a very advanced level a Wudang master will train *chi* to flow to the weapon, using it as if it were an integral part of his body. The structure and techniques of the sword are such that it is the most ideal of all weapons to fulfil this advanced function. When the master has accomplished this skill, the sword flows endlessly as directed by the mind, without any physical effort and loss of stamina. Applied to combat, this means that the movements of the sword are as fast as the master's mind wills them to be, and the master can continue for as long as this mental and vital energy last – which means practically for ever, because at this level, mental and vital energy are constantly replenished by cosmic energy.

When applied to spiritual cultivation, this level of skill means that master and sword have merged into one unity of flowing energy, and this unity has merged into the infinite cosmos. In Taoist terms, the master has achieved the triple goal of transforming essence into energy, transforming energy into spirit, and returning spirit to Spirit. In terms of Wudang Tai Chi Chuan, the first stage – which is already an exceedingly advanced stage, so advanced that it is difficult for the uninitiated to credit – involves transforming the material body and the material sword into one unified flow of energy. In the second stage this unified flow of energy becomes pure consciousness. At the highest stage, pure consciousness becomes – *is* – Universal Consciousness. This is the ultimate aim of all religions and mystical disciplines, whatever different terms their adherents may use for it, however they may describe the process and whatever the methods they may choose to attain this highest spiritual fulfilment.

Sword, Scimitar and Staff

On a more down to earth level, let us examine some other Tai Chi weapon techniques. *Figure 19.2* illustrates three typical sword patterns: Yellow Dragon Emerges from Cave *(figure 19.2a)*, Yasha Testing the Sea *(figure 19.2b)* and Swallow Returns to Nest *(figure 19.2c)*.

All these patterns are graceful and beautiful, not just in their static form, but more so in their application, expressing the 'soft', flowing rhythm of Tai Chi Chuan. The following 'Song of Tai Chi Sword' sums up the essence of the Tai Chi sword:

> The art of the sword is not easily taught,
> Like dragons and rainbows it's most arcane.
> If you use a sword to chop and hew,
> San Feng will laugh till he evaporates like dew.

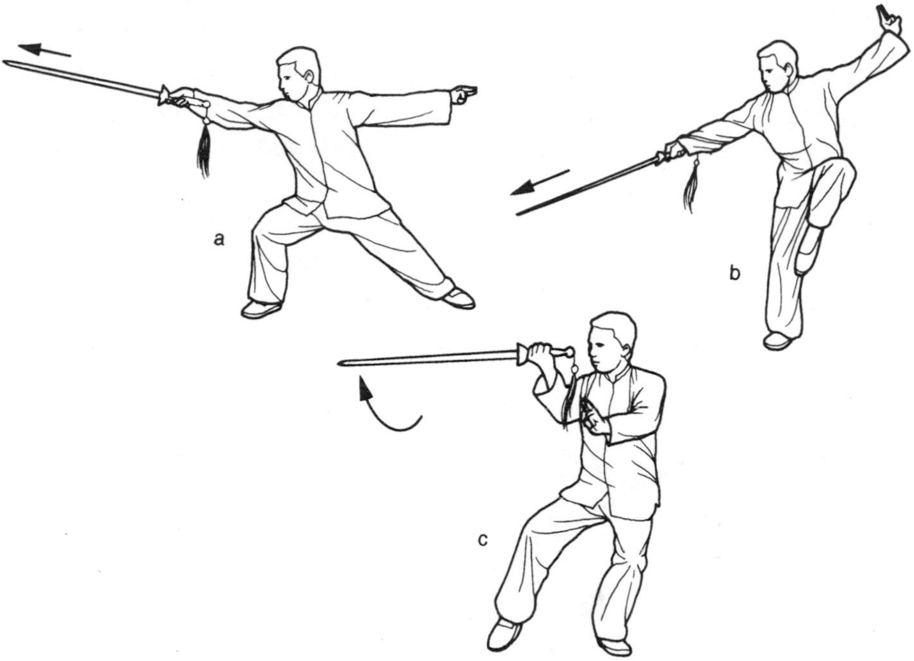

Fig 19.2 Tai Chi sword patterns

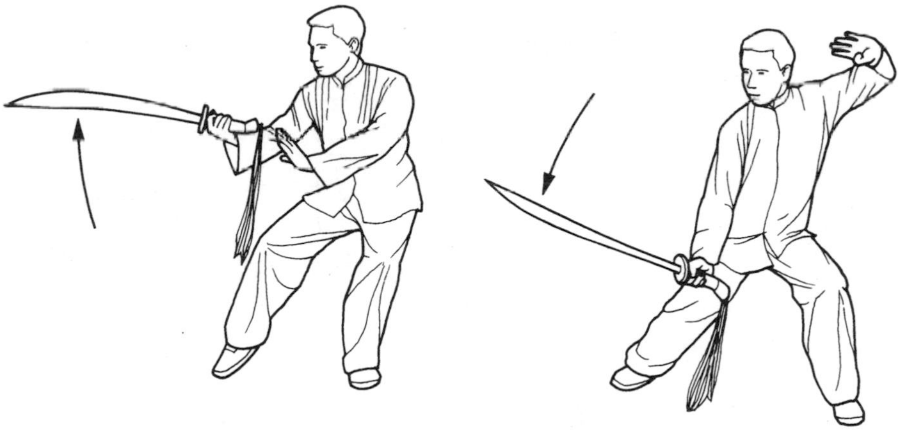

Fig 19.3 Tai Chi scimitar patterns

In Chinese weaponry, the knife or scimitar is a good contrast to the sword. While the Chinese sword is double-edged and delicate, the scimitar is single-edged and heavy. As the poem above indicates, one should not use a sword as if it were a scimitar.

Because the techniques for using a scimitar are more akin to forceful, 'external' kungfu than gentle 'internal' Tai Chi Chuan, it is not very popular. Nevertheless, when it is used in Tai Chi Chuan, its subtle and agile features are emphasized. *Figure 19.3* shows two Tai Chi scimitar patterns: White Monkey Presents Fruit *(figure 19.3a)*, and Han Emperor Kills Snake *(figure 19.3b)*.

The Tai Chi staff originated from the Tai Chi spear, which is unfortunately seldom used nowadays. And staff techniques are not usually practised in a complete set like the sword and the scimitar, but individually in the form of specific techniques. *Figure 19.4* illustrates some typical Tai

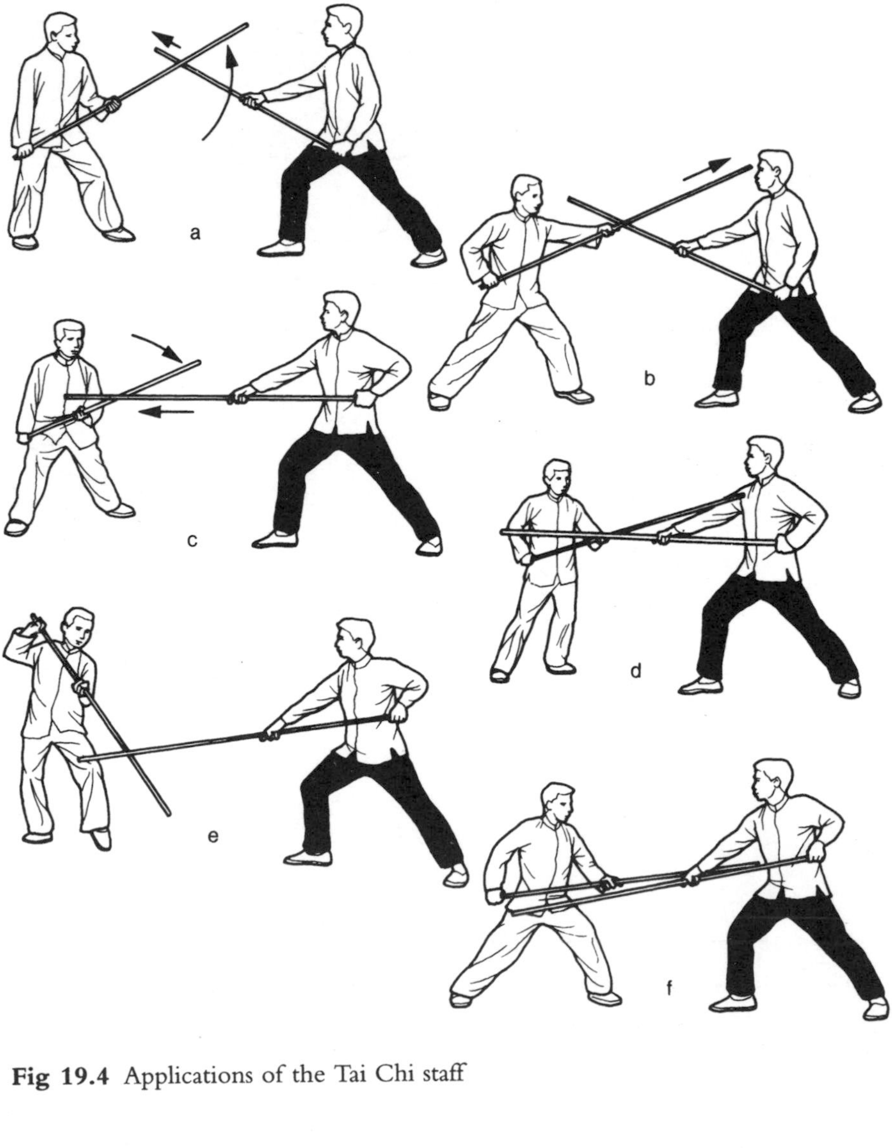

Fig 19.4 Applications of the Tai Chi staff

Chi staff techniques, which are evidently derived from the Shaolin staff techniques taught by the great Ming general Cheng Zong Dou, and which were in turn modified from his spear techniques.

As the opponent attacks the exponent's upper body, the exponent flicks away the attack *(figure 19.4a)*, and counter-attacks to the opponent's head, *(figure 19.4b)*. In *figure 19.4c* the opponent attacks the exponent's middle body. The exponent moves the front leg to the left and deflects the attack, immediately shifting the body sideways by moving to a sideways Four-six Stance and striking the opponent's body *(figure 19.4d)*. In *figure 19.4e* the opponent attacks the exponent's lower body. The exponent sweeps away the attack, then counter-attacks *(figure 19.4f)*.

Lamenting that there were no staff sets in Tai Chi Chuan, three fourth-generation masters of Wu Yu Xiang style Tai Chi Chuan, Han Qin Xian, Li Sheng Duan and Hao Zhong Tian, composed a staff set from Tai Chi spear techniques,[1] which are similar to Shaolin staff techniques. *Figure 19.5* shows three patterns from the Tai Chi staff set: Separate Grass to Seek Snake *(figure 19.5a)*, Five Flowers *(figure 19.5b)*, and Tai Mountain on Head *(figure 19.5c)*.

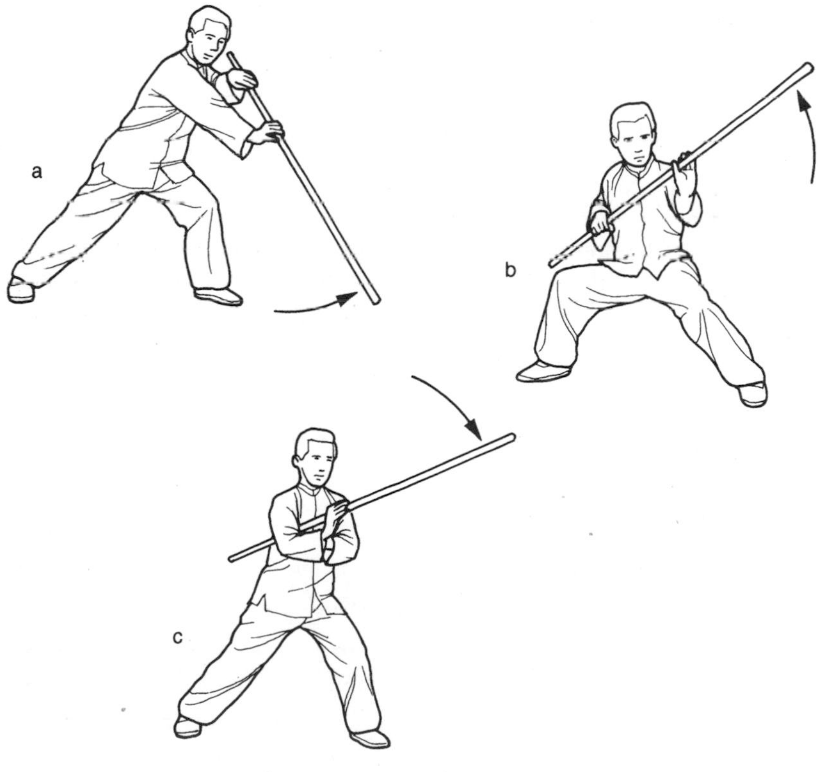

Fig 19.5 Tai Chi staff patterns

20

The Philosophy of Tai Chi Chuan

The Evergreen Classic of Wang Zong Yue

He mainly stresses the principles of 'running' and 'sticking' in Pushing Hands, and he offers very good advice on how students can master this basic skill.

The Treatise on Tai Chi Chuan

If you asked Tai Chi Chuan masters to name the one piece of writing that best explains or represents the art, many would name *The Treatise on Tai Chi Chuan* by Wang Zong Yue, who lived between 1733 and 1795. All Tai Chi Chuan styles tacitly regard this treatise as the final authority on the subject, and almost all Chinese books which touch on Tai Chi Chuan philosophy quote it. It contains the essence of Tai Chi Chuan, yet consists of only 357 words in classical Chinese.

I give below my translation of the treatise, but because of the conciseness of classical Chinese and the profundity of its concepts, it is not easy to understand. I have therefore provided a commentary which may be helpful.

The original treatise is in continuous Chinese prose; in my translation, I have divided it into convenient numbered passages to facilitate study and reference.

1 The cosmos is born of the void; is the source of motion and stillness; and the mother of yin and yang. Because of motion, there is separation; because of stillness, there is integration.

2 There is no excess for which there is no match; when there is constraint, there is stretching. When the opponent is forceful, I become gentle: this is the principle of running. When I am in a favourable position and the opponent in an adverse position, this is the principle of sticking.

3 If the movements are fast, respond with appropriate speed; if the movements are graceful, follow gracefully. Although there are countless variations, there is only one fundamental principle.

4 From dedicated practice, we develop the art of understanding force; from understanding force, we develop marvellous skills. Unless we have spent much time and effort practising it, we will not be able to apply this marvellous art naturally.

5 Keep the head upright, and keep out all irrelevant thoughts. Focus vital energy at the energy field at the abdomen. Do not slump, and do not slant. Suddenly we show, and suddenly we disappear.

6 If heavy on the left, empty the left; if heavy on the right, avoid the right. Rising, I become tall; lowering my stance, I become deep. Advancing, I become long; retreating, I become fast.

7 Not a feather can be added, nor a fly can land. The opponent does not understand me; but I understand the opponent. The great warrior is forever victorious; this is the reason.

8 There are many other arts which are different, mainly they are none other than strong against weak, fast against slow, using strength against those with less strength. All these are natural; not derived from profound art.

9 Using four *tahils* against a thousand *katies* is not dependent on mere strength. Seeing an old man handling many youths demonstrates that speed may be futile.

10 Stand with good balance, agile like a wheel. Slant sinking is clumsy, double heaviness is awkward.

11 Those who have practised many years but do not know how to neutralize the opponent's strength are still defeated by their opponents, because they have not overcome the weakness of double heaviness.

12 To overcome this weakness, we must know the principle of hard and soft. Sticking is running, running is sticking. Yin is never parted from yang, and yang never parted from yin. When yin and yang are in harmony, only then the art of understanding force is possible. Once we have accomplished the art of understanding force, we become more and more skilful as we train.

13 Understand the techniques of contacting arms so that we can advance as we wish. Originally we may wish to yield, but we often make the mistake of yielding near or attaining far. Hence, a miss of a fraction

of an inch is as good as a thousand miles. This must not be unexplained; hence this treatise.

There are two main difficulties with such writing. First, it is a convention in classical Chinese to state the bare minimum; information that readers are expected to know is often not mentioned, even though the information may be crucial to understanding the passage. For example, in the above quotation, the writer merely says 'The cosmos is born of the void', without further explanation, because those readers for whom this passage was originally intended would have had no difficulty in understanding the implied meaning. This, of course, is not the case with modern readers, who may not have the necessary background information.

Secondly, this material was written for initiates, usually students of the writer who could understand the master's concise terms perfectly. It was not meant for public consumption. Hence, it was enough for the master to say, 'There is no excess for which there is no match; when there is constraint, there is stretching'; the intended readers knew what he meant because they had been taught it before. The master's statement was meant to remind them of the importance of this principle. Modern readers, of course, do not have this advantage. Even an explicit statement like 'When the opponent is forceful, I become gentle: this is the principle of running' would present some difficulty, unless they had had some training in the application of 'hard' and 'soft' force. The explanation below will hopefully overcome these problems.

Explanation of the Treatise

1 The cosmos is born of the void, which is a Chinese term to describe the ultimate reality. The void is both nothing and everything; it is undifferentiated. When the first signs or stages of differentiation appeared (in our human concept), we called the void the cosmos. The Cosmos is therefore the source of all motion and all stillness. (If there were no motion or stillness, it would still be the void; because of the first motion or stillness, the void is called the cosmos.)

Stillness and motion represent two archetypical aspects of reality, which are termed yin and yang. Yin and yang also apply to the opposing yet complementary aspects of all other phenomena in the universe. The cosmos is therefore the mother of yin-yang.

This principle of yin-yang, which is manifested in stillness and motion, is the fundamental operative principle for the constant transformation of the universe from infinitesimal subatomic particles to the infinite stars. Because of motion, *chi* or energy, the stuff of which the whole universe is made, disperses to become nebulous; because of stillness, *chi* coalesces to form particles.

2 There is nothing too small and nothing too big for *chi* to infiltrate. When *chi* is compressed, it expands; when it expands it compresses *chi* elsewhere. Hence, there is no excess for which there is no match; when there is constraint, there is stretching, and vice versa.

Tai Chi Chuan is so named because of this philosophy of the cosmos and yin-yang, and its ever-changing nature, which applies to this style of martial art as much as to the whole universe. In Tai Chi Chuan, this yin-yang principle is found in every aspect and dimension. Some examples include its health and martial dimensions, its quiescent and dynamic movements in both force training and combat application, its internal energy flow and external techniques, and the convenient classification of its skills and patterns into 'soft' and 'hard'.

In combat, for example, when facing a strong opponent, I make use of this yin-yang principle by becoming gentle, which does not necessarily mean the absence of force. This force is termed 'soft', in contrast to the opponent's mechanical strength, which is 'hard' force. If a strong opponent throws a powerful punch at me, I do not block or meet it head on. Without moving my feet, I can shift my body backwards by lowering my stance, thereby moving my body away from the punch, and simultaneously guide it to one side with my hand following its momentum. This is the principle of 'running' or yielding.

When the punch misses and is withdrawn, I move in with my hand in contact with my opponent's hand or arm, and following the opponent's momentum I manoeuvre in such a way that I attain a favourable position. This is the principle of 'sticking'.

3 This 'sticking' technique is to be executed in accordance with yin-yang harmony: if my opponent withdraws fast, I move in with appropriate speed; if my opponent pushes forward, I follow the momentum gracefully; if my opponent tries to push my hand to either side, I follow accordingly. There may be countless variations in the opponent's reaction, but the fundamental principle is the same.

4 In order to apply the principles of 'running' and 'sticking' efficiently, we must practise conscientiously. From dedicated practice, we develop the art of understanding force, which is a Tai Chi Chuan term for spontaneous response, ie we can respond to an opponent's force or movements spontaneously according to yin-yang harmony. As we train

further, from this ability to respond spontaneously we develop marvellous skills in yielding or 'sticking' techniques. Such skills are not inborn: unless we spend a lot of time and effort on our training, they cannot become second nature to us.

5 In our training as well as in actual combat, we must keep the head upright, and keep out all irrelevant thoughts. We must focus our vital energy at the energy field at the abdomen; in this way we become balanced, and are able to use this energy when it is needed. We must not slump forward, nor slant to one side in our posture. Our stances should be such that the opponent cannot tell whether we intend to stay stationary or move in the next instant.

6 When an opponent attacks on the left, shift your weight from the left to the right and move your body accordingly, so that the attack fails. Reverse the process if the attack comes on the right. If an opponent adopts a low stance and tries to lift you up or throw you off balance, rise so that you are taller than him or her, thus following the momentum of the attack and frustrating it. If the opponent adopts a high stance and tries to press you down, lower your stance still deeper, thus neutralizing his attack.

If an opponent moves in to attack you, retreat to tempt the other person forward until he or she cannot advance any further; then strike when the forward movement is spent. When the opponent tries to retreat before your attack, move in faster and strike.

7 All your movements should be so well co-ordinated, you should be so relaxed yet alert, and your awareness should be so sharp that not a feather can be added to your body, nor a fly land on it without your knowing.

In any combat it is important to have a good understanding of your opponent and the combat situation. Great warriors win because they know their opponents, but their opponents do not know them. In Tai Chi Chuan, one principle way of knowing an opponent is to stick to him or her and move in yin-yang harmony. When the opponent moves in forcefully, we yield; when the opponent retreats, we move in. Our movements start after the opponent's, but they arrive before them. This means that we sense any moves and follow accordingly; and when an opportunity arises, we attack so fast that our attack arrives before the opponent can avoid or block it. If the opponent does not move, we do not move; once the opponent moves, we move faster.

8 Many of the other martial arts are different from Tai Chi Chuan. They are generally arts where combat victory is the result of the strong overcoming the weak, the fast overcoming the slow, and those with strength overcoming those with less strength. This happens naturally, ie victory depends on natural abilities like the strong overcoming the weak, not on abilities derived from learning a profound art.

9 Tai Chi Chuan is different: using minimum force which is gentle and graceful to overcome an opponent who is stronger and bigger indicates the depth of the art; it is not dependent on mere strength. The ability of an old man effectively to handle several youths who are faster than him demonstrates that speed alone is not the decisive factor in combat. These two examples show that in Tai Chi Chuan other factors besides mechanical strength and speed are important.

10 What are these other factors? They are good balance and spontaneous response. Our posture must be balanced, and we must be flexible like a turning wheel. For example, if an opponent pushes me on my right-hand side, I do not resist but rotate in a clockwise direction like a wheel. This is the principle of yielding. To be able to do this, our balance must be perfect. If our posture is unbalanced, for example when our centre of gravity has gone beyond the base of our feet, we will be clumsy in our movements. And if we use our weight against an opponent's weight, or force against force, our movement will be awkward.

11 There are people who have practised the art for many years but still do not know how to neutralize an opponent's strength. They are likely to be defeated, because they have not overcome this weakness of 'double heaviness', ie using strength against strength.

12 To overcome this weakness, we must know the principle of 'hard' and 'soft'. If an opponent is 'hard', for example, advancing and attacking powerfully, we must be 'soft', ie we yield. If the opponent is 'soft', for example when retreating after a failed attack, we must be 'hard', ie we strike before the opponent can recover from the previous movement. These principles of yielding and 'sticking' are in harmony; they must never be separated from each other. As we 'stick' to the opponent, we also yield; and as we yield, we also 'stick'.

This is a manifestation of the yin-yang principle. The yin aspect of Tai Chi Chuan is never separated from its yang aspect, and vice versa.

For example, if we wish to gain the maximum benefit from the health (or yin) aspect of Tai Chi Chuan, we must not neglect its martial (or yang) aspect, because many health benefits, like physical agility, emotional stability and mental freshness, are derived from the martial training. On the other hand, if we wish to be effective in its martial aspect, we must not neglect its health aspect, for example by over-stretching ourselves in training, hurting ourselves through hard conditioning, or sustaining injury in sparring.

The art of spontaneous response, which is essential for combat efficiency, is possible only when yin and yang are in harmony. For example, suppose an opponent moves forward to attack, which is symbolized by yang. If we also move forward to meet the attack with equal force, which is also symbolized as yang, we are matching force with force, or clashing yang with yang, which is not advised in Tai Chi Chuan. Or if, when the opponent withdraws after an unsuccessful attempt, we also retreat, this is meeting yin with yin. In Tai Chi Chuan, yin-yang harmony is attained when we meet yin with yang, and yang with yin. In other words, when the opponent attacks, we yield; when the opponent retreats, we move in. Once we have accomplished the art of spontaneous response in appropriate yielding or advancing, we will become more and more skilful as we continue in our training.

13 We must understand the principles and techniques involved in keeping our arms in contact with the opponent's so that we can advance or retreat as gracefully and effectively as we wish. If, for instance, we retreat to avoid an attack, but make the mistake of not withdrawing far enough, we will still be near enough for our opponent to defeat us. Similarly, if we move in to attack after the opponent's move is spent but do not advance far enough, our attack will not be effective. Hence, missing by a fraction of an inch is as good as missing by a thousand miles.

Three Levels of Attainment

Apart from the initial mention of cosmic reality, what is described by Wang Zong Yue is basically fundamental combat training of Tai Chi Chuan. He mainly stresses the principles of 'running' and 'sticking' in Pushing Hands, and he offers very good advice on how students can master this basic skill.

The classical masters have said that there are three levels of attainment in Tai Chi Chuan. At the first level, exponents can perform a Tai Chi set beautifully; they attain good health at this level. At the intermediate level, they develop internal force and can apply Tai Chi Chuan movements flawlessly for fighting; they attain combat efficiency. At the advanced level, masters are on the path to immortality; they attain spiritual fulfilment, whatever their religion or lack of it. At the first level, the emphasis in training is on *jing* or form; at the second, it is on *chi* or energy; at the highest level, it is on *shen* or mind.

21

Taoism and Spiritual Development in Tai Chi Chuan

Attaining Immortality and Returning to the Void

If aspirants aim for the highest goal, they choose to transcend even immortality and return to the void.

Tai Chi Chuan Principles in the *Tao Te Ching*

Tai Chi Chuan is called a Taoist art because its philosophy and practice are derived from Lao Tzu's *Tao Te Ching*, the most representative and authoritative of Taoist teachings. For example, typical Tai Chi Chuan principles like not struggling, not initiating an attack and non-aggression are frequently mentioned in the Taoist classic.[1]

The best thing is water.
Water benefits all things yet does not struggle.
Section 8

The wise fighters do not start an attack.
The wise warriors are not aggressive.
The wise soldiers do not meet the enemy head on.
The wise administrators care for their subordinates.
This is the virtue of non-struggle.
Section 68

In Tai Chi Chuan, meeting strength with strength is considered the worst of martial arts tactics and strategy because both the winner and the loser suffer. This philosophy is clearly seen in the *Tao Te Ching*:

Imperial advisers who know Tao
Will not use an army to force others into submission.

Its effect is reciprocal;
Land where battles were fought,
Wild grasses grow abundantly.
The time after a war
Is always a time of suffering.
The wise use the army for defence,
Dare not use for aggression.

Section 30

Another characteristic tenet of Tai Chi Chuan is its 'softness'. But how could anybody ever think of an incredible tactical or strategic principle like 'soft overcoming hard'? The originator of Tai Chi Chuan drew his inspiration from the *Tao Te Ching*:

The softest thing in the world
Overcomes the hardest thing in the world.
Nowhere can the soft not enter the hard.

Section 43

Even the techniques for implementing the tactics of 'soft overcoming hard' are inspired by the *Tao Te Ching*:

Of the softest things in the world,
Nothing is softer than water.
Any hard objects in the way
Will be defeated by water.
Water never changes.
Hence soft defeats hard,
Weak defeats strong.
Everyone knows this
But few practise it.

Section 78

As soft can overcome hard, the best thing to use to overcome something hard is the softest, and the softest thing in the world is water. In Taoist writing, the term 'water' does not merely refer to ordinary water; it is a symbol for the characteristics represented by water, which are flowing and spreading. Hence, Tai Chi Chuan movements flow and spread like water. When an opponent attacks, Tai Chi Chuan exponents let their movement flow along or over the attack instead of going against it.

Like flowing water, their movement continues gracefully without any break. An opponent may use different modes of attack, symbolized by the different elemental processes of metal, wood, fire or earth, all of which are harder than water. But Tai Chi Chuan exponents need not change their flowing movements; they follow Lao Tzu's teaching that 'any hard objects in the way will be defeated by water' – symbolized by water rusting metal, rotting wood, extinguishing fire and washing away earth – and while the other elemental processes are all changed by water, water remains intact. Thus, an opponent may make ten different moves, but a Tai Chi Chuan exponent makes only one. That movement, however, flows continuously and eventually overwhelms the opponent. This characteristic combat feature of Tai Chi Chuan draws inspiration from Lao Tzu's 'Water never changes, hence soft defeats hard, weak defeats strong.'

This idea of the flowing and spreading of water is also the fundamental principle for promoting health in Tai Chi Chuan practice, manifested as harmonious energy flow. If you are staccato in your movements, or have your vital energy locked in various parts of your body instead of spread over all of it, not only do you not gain any health benefits, but you may even suffer adverse effects. But if your Tai Chi movements flow like water, you will certainly benefit. As Lao Tzu says: 'The best thing is water; water benefits all things yet does not struggle.'

Attaining the Tao

More significant than the correlation between the *Tao Te Ching* and Tai Chi Chuan for health and combat are the principles and practice behind the highest attainment in the art, which are also derived from Lao Tzu's classic. Right at the start he says:

> Tao that can be called Tao is not the real Tao.
> The name that can be named is not the real Name.
> The nameless is the origin of the cosmos.
> The named is the mother of all things.
> Thus without desire one sees its ultimate.
> With desire one sees its minute appearances.
> The two are the same but have different names.
> This is mysticism,
> Mystical and marvellous,
> The gate to all wonders.

Tao or ultimate reality cannot be named, but for convenience Lao Tzu calls it Tao. Other people may call it by different names, such as God, Brahman, Buddha or the unified energy field.

Why can we not give a name to ultimate reality? Ultimate reality is undifferentiated. The individual, differentiated things we see are only relatively, but not ultimately, real. In other words, a tree, a car, a person or any other object appears to us according to our set of conditions, such as the way our eyes are made to perceive light, the way our mind has been trained to interpret sensory data, and the environment in which the perception is made. If the conditions are different – if the perceiver is wearing a pair of glasses with distorting lenses, for example, or is affected by psychedelic drugs, or if there is a thick mist between the perceiver and the perceived object – the object will appear differently.

Imagine then what another being, like a cow or a microbe, with a set of conditions radically different from ours, sees when it looks at what we humans would call a tree, a car or a person. It may be difficult to imagine, but it is not difficult to understand that its image would be very different from ours. Almost all the world's peoples throughout history have believed in the existence of life in other dimensions or worlds, such as fairies, spirits, gods and beings in other galaxies. Only Westerners have abandoned such beliefs, although they held them in the past. These beings, vibrating at frequencies very different from ours, will experience reality relative to their own conditions, in ways unimaginable to those of us who still cling to the belief that we, on our incredibly puny earth with our exceedingly gross sensual perception, are the only beings that can perceive reality as it really is.

Interestingly, modern science is telling us categorically that there is actually no such thing as objective reality, that the phenomena we see are just appearances – which is what the word 'phenomena' actually means. An electron, for example, is a wave or a particle according to how we choose to measure or conceptualize it; a mass of atoms, each of which is 99.999 per cent 'empty', is seen by us as a solid object because of the way our brain and senses operate.

So if the phenomena seen by us and other beings are relative, what then is ultimate reality? Teachers of all the great religious and mystical disciplines have given the same answer: that ultimate reality is inexplicable, indescribable, and has to be directly experienced. For the sake of those who have not attained the highly developed spiritual stage necessary to experience it directly, the great masters describe it as infinite, eternal and undifferentiated. But once we define ultimate reality or any part of it in any form, from the minute to the enormous, it is no longer undifferentiated or omnipresent, but conceptualized into phenomena.

For instance, if we conceptualize ultimate reality as an electron, or as

God in an anthropomorphic form, it is no longer omnipresent for it is then limited both in time and space by its form. This form, which is really a phenomenon or 'appearance', does not exist when it is not being conceptualized; when it *is* being conceptualized, what falls outside its form does not belong to it. This is why Christian and Muslim saints, like Buddhist, Hindu and Taoist masters but in different words, exclaimed in their deepest religious ecstasy that God is in them and they are in God, with no boundary between the worshipper and the worshipped, the knower and the known.

In view of this, it becomes easier to understand Lao Tzu's famous opening lines. Ultimate reality that can be given a term like Tao, God, Buddha or the Supreme Being is no longer ultimate reality, because the very act of giving it a name, any name, is the start of the process of conceptualization and differentiation. And once there is conceptualization and differentiation, reality is manifested as phenomena according to the conditions of the perceiver.

So although we must call ultimate reality something, for the sake of convenience, we must remember that whatever is denoted by the name is an imitation, not ultimate reality itself. It is an imitation because the concept denoted by the named is a reflection of what the people conceptualize according to their own set of conditions. For example, ultimate reality is called Tao by Taoists, Buddha or Tathagata by Buddhists, God by Christians, Jews and Muslims, and Brahman by Hindus. But because of the religious, linguistic and other differences between these groups, their conceptualization of the same ultimate reality may also be different.

This nameless ultimate reality is the origin of the cosmos. In other words, before there was the cosmos there was ultimate reality. How and when did the cosmos come into existence? It came into existence as soon as we, or any beings in any dimension, gave names to phenomena that arose as a result of our set of conditions. There was no one definite beginning to the cosmos, nor will there be one definite end. For different beings the cosmos began and will end at different times or aeons. On our human scale, the cosmos began billions of years ago when the infinitesimal parts of ultimate reality in our puny part of the universe which we have defined were isolated. For example, according to our set of conditions, we call one infinitesimal part a tree, others a person, a mountain, the sky and so on. But in ultimate reality, all these parts are one continuous unity; their appearance as individual parts is an illusion.

If we can eliminate the conditions which give rise to phenomena, we can transcend illusion and experience reality as it ultimately is. In Taoism these conditions are figuratively and collectively referred to as desire, because it is desire that initiates the operation of the series of conditions. Without desire, we see ultimate reality: the cosmos ends – or to put it another way, the cosmos does not begin. With desire, we set in operation a series of conditions that result in our seeing the minute appearances that make up our cosmos. In reality, ultimate reality, or the void, is the same as the phenomenal world, or the cosmos. In Tai Chi Chuan, the void is called *Wuji*, and the cosmos is called *Tai Chi*. The difference exists only in us, with our very crude sense perception which can interpret only a minute portion of the known physical reality.

The highest aim of Tai Chi Chuan is to gain glimpses of such cosmic truths, and eventually to experience ultimate reality directly. In Tai Chi Chuan and Taoist terms, it is attaining the Tao, or returning to the great void; in other terms, it is attaining enlightenment, bodhi or Buddhahood, returning to God, or union with the ultimate.

Immortality and the Great Void

Spiritual cultivation in both Tai Chi Chuan and Taoism may be divided into three stages: transforming *jing* or essence into *chi* or energy; transforming energy into *shen* or spirit, and returning spirit to the great void. The first two stages are primarily accomplished through Chi Kung, and the highest stage through meditation. Taoism is rich in Chi Kung and meditation literature, but even those who understand classical Chinese often still have difficulty understanding the content because it is usually written in arcane, symbolic language. Moreover, such advanced training must be performed only under the personal supervision of a master. The description which follows, therefore, which presents some of these teachings in a highly condensed form, is provided for interest, not for use as a teaching aid.

The most important arts of Taoist Chi Kung for spiritual cultivation are the Small Universe and the Big Universe. The Small Universe, also called the Microcosmic Flow, circulates vital energy round the body along the *ren* or conceptual meridian, and the *du* or governing meridian. The constant flow of energy around these two important meridians brings tremendous benefits for health as well as in combat. Masters have summarized the health benefits in the saying 'If one attains the breakthrough of energy flow along the *ren* and *du* meridians, one will eliminate hundreds of illness.' For martial artists, this endless flow of vital energy supplies a tremendous source of internal power. For spiritualists, the Small Universe provides an effective means of transforming essence into energy, and energy into spirit.

The Big Universe, also known as Macrocosmic Flow, is of two types. Health-care specialists and martial artists generally refer to it as the art that channels vital energy through all the 12 primary meridians of the lungs, colon, stomach, spleen, heart, intestines, bladder, kidneys, pericardium, triple warmer, gall bladder and liver in that order. Spiritualists often refer to the Big Universe as the art in which energy from the *dan tian* or any other energy field is diffused throughout the body without having first to flow through the 12 primary meridians. But whatever type it is, it is effective for transforming energy into spirit, and for returning spirit to the great void.

It is often the Small Universe rather than the Big Universe that is emphasized for attaining the highest goal in Tai Chi Chuan or Taoist cultivation. This does not mean that the Big Universe is seldom used. However, much of the training is in the Small Universe, and when that is achieved, with great amounts of energy stored at various energy fields, the transition to the Big Universe, where energy is diffused throughout the body, is comparatively quick – so quick in fact that the term Big Universe is often not mentioned.

People who aim to become immortals rather than merging with the void can even by-pass the Big Universe. After accomplishing the Small Universe, they build a pearl of energy at the lower *dan tian*, usually at the *guanyuan* ('gate of original *chi*') energy field at the abdomen. They usually adopt the double-lotus or single-lotus position with their hands on their knees *(figure 21.1a)* or held together in front on their laps *(figure 21.1b)*. Taoist meditation is called *jing-zuo* or silent sitting.

After nourishing this pearl of energy in *jing-zuo* for some time – usually a few years – they transport it to the middle *dan tian*, usually at the *huangting* ('yellow palace') or *zhongting* ('central palace'), the stomach or heart respectively. Here they infuse their consciousness with this pearl of energy and figuratively call it their 'divine foetus'.

After some years, they transport this 'divine foetus' to the upper *dan tian*, usually at the *niyuan* ('mud-pill') energy centre at the pineal gland. Here the pearl of energy is transformed into spirit, representing the spiritual replica of the aspirant. When the spirit has been nurtured by many years of cultivation, the *baihui* ('meeting of 100 meridians') energy field at the crown of the head opens, and the spirit is emancipated from the physical body as an immortal.

Those who aim for the highest goal choose to transcend even immortality and return to the void. It is a higher goal because to be an immortal is still existence in the phenomenal realm, still limited by time and space, even though for an immortal these are measured on scales that are astronomical. To return to the void, however, is to be transcendental, infinite and eternal.

Returning to the great void is not extinguishing oneself, as is sometimes believed. So where do Tai Chi Chuan or Taoist masters go when they return to the great void? They go nowhere; indeed their physical bodies can still be seen by the unenlightened. In attaining the void, these masters overcome the limitations of their physical bodies and personal spirits, and realize that they actually are the cosmos and the universal spirit.

This highest attainment is accomplished through the Small Universe and silent sitting or *jing-zuo*. Aspirants focus the pearl of energy at a suitable energy field, such as the *zhongting, huangting* or *niyuan*. They let it glow and grow until it covers the whole body; meanwhile they transform their energy into spirit. As their spirits expand, and when the time is right, they attain the blissful, wonderful realization that they themselves are actually the great void.

True to the concept of yin-yang harmony in Tai Chi Chuan, spiritual fulfilment can be accomplished not only by quiescent methods like those described above, but also by dynamic means. Performing a set of Wudang Tai Chi Chuan (see Chapter 13) or Wudang sword techniques (see Chapter 19) until we become a continuous flow of energy and merge with the universal energy of the cosmos is a way of returning to the great void.

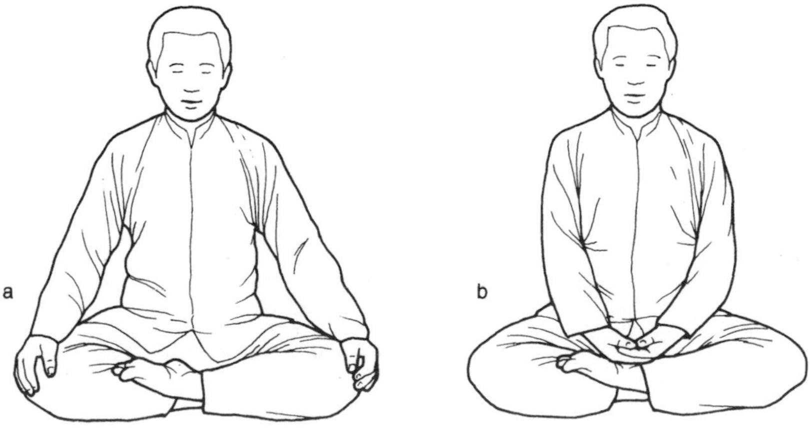

Fig 21.1 Lotus positions for silent sitting

Understandably, not many people believe in or are ready for cosmic realization. But whether you believe in it or not, it is obvious that Tai Chi Chuan is much more than mere dance, as this guide has shown. Even at its lowest level, if it is practised properly, it promotes good health, while at its intermediate level it is excellent for self-defence. And at its highest level it can lead us to the greatest achievement anyone can ever attain.

Notes

Chapter 3

[1] Zhang San Feng, *The Secret of Training the Internal Elixir in the Tai Chi Art*, preserved by Taiyi Shanren, reprinted from an ancient text by Anhua Publications, Hong Kong, undated, pp 68–9. In Chinese.

[2] Cited in Pei Xi Rong and Li Chun Sheng (ed), *Wudang Martial Arts*, Hunan Science and Technology Publications, Changsa City, 1984, p 2. In Chinese.

[3] Quoted in Li Wen Tao, *Introduction to Tai Chi Chuan and Tai Chi Chi Kung*, Guang Quing Publications, Kowloon, 1986, pp 21–2. In Chinese.

Chapter 4

[1] Quoted in Li Wen Tao, op. cit, pp 37–8. In Chinese.

[2] Ibid, pp 39–40.

[3] Yeng Deng Fu, *Yang-style Tai Chi Chuan* (a record of the master's teaching by his disciples), Taiping Book Company, Hong Kong, 1968, pp 4–6. In Chinese.

[4] *Cheng Man Ching's Advanced T'ai-Chi Form Instructions*, compiled and translated by Douglas Wile, Sweet Ch'i Press, New York, 1986, p 20.

Chapter 6

[1] For a comprehensive and in-depth study of Chi Kung, please refer to my book, *The Art of Chi Kung*, Element Books, 1993.

[2] Please see my book, *The Art of Shaolin Kungfu*, Element Books, 1996.

Chapter 10

[1] Please see my book, *The Art of Shaolin Kungfu*, Element Books, 1996, for a substantiation of this claim.

Chapter 12

[1] Please see my book, *The Art of Shaolin Kungfu*, Element Books, 1996.

[2] James MacRitchie, *Chi Kung: Cultivating Personal Energy*, Element Books, 1993, pp.14–5.

[3] Please see my book *The Art of Chi Kung*, Element Books, 1993.

Chapter 13

[1] Pei Xi Rong and Li Chun Sheng, op cit, p6.

Chapter 14

[1] Gu Liu Xiang and Shen Jia Zhen, *Chen-style Taijiquan*, People's Physical Education Publications, China, 1994, pp 5–64. In Chinese.

Chapter 15

[1] Zhao Bin, Zhao You Bin and Lu Di Min, *The True Art of Yang Style Taijiquan*, San Qin Publications, Sian, China, 1994, p 275. In Chinese.

Chapter 16

[1] Hao Shao Ru, *Wu-style Taijiquan*, Taiping Book Company, Hong Kong, 1971, pp 8–9. In Chinese.

[2] Guo Fu Hou, *Commentary and Explanation on Taijiquan Secrets*, Tianjin Science and Technology Publications, Tianjin, China, 1994, p 92. In Chinese.

Chapter 17

[1] Xu Zhi Yi, *Taijiquan Style of Wu Jian Quan*, Qing San Books Company, Hong Kong, 1958, pp 1–7. In Chinese.

Chapter 18

[1] Sun Jian Yun, *Sun-style Tai Chi Chuan*, Taiping Book Company, Hong Kong, 1969, pp 2–3. In Chinese.

Chapter 19

[1] Chen Gu An, *Tai Chi Staff*, Henan Science and Technology Publications, China, 1988, p 1. In Chinese.

Chapter 21

[1] The quotations in this chapter are taken from *Tao Te Ching*, Sheng Tian Tang Publications, Taizhong, Taiwan, undated. In Chinese.

Further Reading

In English

1 Klein Bob, *Movements of Magic: The Spirit of Tai Chi Chuan*, Aquarian Press, Wellingborough, 1987.

2 Wile Douglas, *Cheng Man Ching's Advanced T'ai-Chi Form Instructions*, Sweet Chi Press, New York, 1986.

3 General Tao Hanzhang, *Sun Tzu's Art of War*, trans. from the Chinese by Yuan Shibing, Eastern Dragon Books, Kuala Lumpur, 1991.

4 MacRitchie James, *Chi Kung: Cultivating Personal Energy*, Element, Shaftesbury, 1993.

5 Blofeld John, *Taoism: the Quest for Immortality*, Unwin Hyman, London, 1989, (first published 1979).

6 Palmer Martin, *The Elements of Taoism*, Element, Shaftesbury, 1991.

7 Crompton Paul, *The Elements of Tai Chi*, Element, Shaftesbury, 1990.

8 Wong Kiew Kit, *The Art of Chi Kung*, Element, Shaftesbury, 1993.

9 Wong Kiew Kit, *The Art of Shaolin Kung Fu*, Element, Shaftesbury, 1996.

In Chinese

1 Chen Gong, *Tai Chi Chuan Fist, Knife, Sword and Staff*, Health Publishing House, Hong Kong, Undated.

2 Chen Gu An, *Tai Chi Staff*, Henan Science and Technology Publication, Chengdu, 1988.

3 Chen Xiao Wang, *The 38-Pattern Chen-style Tai Chi Chuan*, Shanghai Book Shop, Hong Kong, 1987.

4 Deng Mong Hen, *Tai Chi Chuan for Self Defence and Health*, Bailing Publishing House, Hong Kong, Undated.

5 Editorial Committee, *Martial Artists and Martial Arts*, Shanghai Educational Publications, Shanghai, 1985.

6 Fang Jin Hui and others (ed), *Encyclopedia of Chinese Martial Arts*, Anwei People's Publications, Anwei, 1987.

7 Gu Liu Xiang and Shen Jia Zhen, *Chen-style Tai Chi Chuan*, People's Physical Education Publication, Beijing, 1994.

8 Guo Fu Hou, *Commentary and Explanation on Tai Chi Chuan Secrets*, Tianjin Science and Technology Publications, Tianjin, China, 1994.

9 Hao Shao Ru, *Wu-style Tai Chi Chuan*, People's Physical Education Publications, Beijing, 1984.

10 Huang Zhao and others (ed), *History of Taoist Thoughts*, Hunan Teachers' Training University Press, 1991.

11 Lao Tzu, *Tao Te Ching*, Sheng Tian Tang Publications, Taizhong, Taiwan, Undated.

12 Li Tian Ji, *The Art of Wudang Sword*, People's Physical Education Publishing House, Beijing, 1988.

13 Li Wen Tao, *Introduction to Taiji Chi Kung*, Guang Qing Publishing House, Kowloon, 1986.

14 Lian Yang the Recluse, *Taoist Immortality and Zen Meditation*, Wuling Publishing House, Taipei, 1988.

15 Pei Xi Rong and Feng Guo Dong, *Principles of Tai Chi Chuan Pushing Hands*, 1983.

16 Pei Xi Rong and Li Chun Sheng (ed), *Wudang Martial Arts*, Hunan Science and Technology Publications, Changsa City, 1984.

17 Pei Xi Rong (ed), *Discourse on Wudang Chi Kung*, Sanlian Books, Shanghai, 1989.

18 Qui Ling (ed), *Selection of Ancient Chinese Chi Kung*, Guangdong Science and Technology Publications, Guangzhou, 1988,

19 Sun Jian Yun, *Sun-style Tai Chi Chuan*, Taiping Book Company, Hong Kong, 1969.

20 Sun Yau Zhong, *Practice of Simplified Wu-style Tai Chi Chuan*, Beijing College of Physical Education Press, Beijing, 1993.

21 Shen Shou, *Questions on Tai Chi Chuan Pushing Hands*, People's Physical Education Publications, 1986.

22 Tang Hao, *A Study on Internal Kungfu*, Unicorn Press, Hong Kong, 1969.

23 Wang Jian Dong, *Military Strategies of Sun Tzu*, Zhi Yang Publications, Taiwan, 1994.

24 Wang Zi Zhang and Li Wen Zhen, *Tai Chi 13-Technique Sword*, People's Physical Education Publications, Beijing, 1983.

25 Xi Yun Tai, *History of Chinese Martial Arts*, People's Physical Education Publications, Beijing, 1985.

26 Xu Dao Yi, *Yi Jing and Modern Natural Sciences*, Guangdong Educational Publications, Guangzhou, 1995.

27 Xu Tao Ren (ed), *The Way of Immortality*, People's University Press, Beijing, 1992.

28 Xu Zhi Yi, *Tai Chi Chuan Style of Wu Jian Quan*, Qing San Books Company, Hong Kong, 1958.

29 Xue Nai Yin, *True Art of Wu-style Tai Chi Chuan*, Beijing College of Physical Education Press, 1993.

30 Yang Deng Fu, *Yang-style Tai Chi Chuan* (recorded by his disciples), Taiping Book Company, Hong Kong, 1976.

31 Zhang San Feng, *The Secret of Training the Internal Elixir in the Taiji Art*, preserved by Taiyi Shanren. Reprinted from ancient text by Anhua Publications, Hong Kong. Undated.

32 Zhao Bin, Zhao You Bin and Lu Di Min, *The True Art of Yang-style Taijiquan*, San Qin Publications, Sian, China, 1994.

33 Zhu Yue Li, *Questions on Taoism*, Cultural Publications, Beijing, 1989.

34 Zou Xue Xi, *Essence of Yi Jing Studies*, Sichuan Science and Technology Publications, 1992.

Useful Addresses

Australia

Master Selina Griffin,
Shaolin Wahnam Chi Kung and Taijiquan,
RSD Strathfieldsaye Road,
Strathfieldsaye, Bendigo,
Victoria 3551, Australia.
Tel (61-54) 393257.

Master John Trevor,
Shaolin Wahnam Chi Kung and Taijiquan,
PO Box 2088, Murraybridge,
SA 5253, Australia.
Tel (61-8) 2988659; (61-85) 321940.

Europe

Master Reimer Buerkner,
Shaolin Wahnam Chi Kung,
Eichendorffstrasse 23,
D-63 303 Dreieich (near Frankfurt),
Germany.
Tel (49) 6103-84451.

Masters Deolinda and Jose Ferro,
College of Chinese Traditional Medicine,
(Shaolin Kungfu, Chi Kung and Taijiquan),
Praca Ilha do Faial, 13-cv,
1000 Lisboa, Portugal.
Tel and Fax (351-1) 315 8388.

Master Douglas Wiesenthal,
Shaolin Wahnam Chi Kung and Kungfu,
Crta de Humera, 87, 3-3B,
Pozuelo de Alarcon,
28224 Madrid, Spain.
Tel (34-1) 3512115;
Fax (34-1) 3512163.

British Tai Chi Chuan & Shaolin Kung Fu Association,
28 Linden Farm Drive,
Countesthorpe,
Leicester LE8 3SX

Malaysia and Singapore

Master Wong Kiew Kit,
Shaolin Wahnam Chi Kung and Kungfu,
81 Taman Intan B/5,
08000 Sungai Petani,
Kedah, Malaysia.
Tel (60-4) 422 2353.
Fax (60-4) 421 7645

Master Ng Kowi Beng,
Shaolin Wahnam Chi Kung and Kungfu,
c/o H & P Plastic Pte Ltd,
Plot 935, Lorong Makmur 13/1,
Taman Makmur, Mk. Sg. Seluang,
Daerah Kulim, Malaysia.
Tel (60-4) 484 1159;
Fax (60-4) 484 1425.

Master Chan Chee Kong,
Shaolin Wahnam Chi Kung and Kungfu,
301 Block A, Manara Megah,
Jalan Kolam Air, Off Jalan Ipon,
Kuala Lumpur, Malaysia.
Tel (60-3) 444 2150; 010 211 6036.

Master Cheong Huat Seng,
Shaolin Wahnam Chi Kung and Kungfu,
22 Taman Mutiara, 08000 Sungai Petani,
Kedah, Malaysia.
Tel (60-4) 421 0634.

Master Goh Kok Hin,
86 Jalan Sungai Emas,
08500 Kota Kuala Muda,
Kedah, Malaysia.
Tel (60-4) 437 4301.

Master Yong Peng Wah,
Shaolin Wahnam Chi Kung,
181 Taman Kota Jaya,
34700 Simpang, Taiping,
Perak, Malaysia.
Tel (60-5) 847 1431.

Master Mike Yap,
Shaolin Chi Kung and Freestyle Fighting,
35 Jalan 14/34, Petaling Jaya 46100,
Selangnor, Malaysia.
Tel (60-3) 756 0743.

Master Lawrence Leong Swee Lun,
Hapkung-do International,
(Bagua, Shaolin and Taijiquan),
17 Jalan 67 (Jalan Belipas),
Kepong Baru,
52100 Kuala Lumpur, Malaysia.
Tel (60-3) 636 3033; 018-829 6229.

Master Yap Soon Yeong,
(Shaolin One-Finger Zen Chi Kung),
Yap Chi Kung Institute,
1B Jalan Fetees,
11200 Penang, Malaysia.

Master Chin Chee Ching,
Shaolin Damo Chi Kung,
Block 929, 13-447 Tampines St 91,
Singapore 520929.
Tel (65) 7829958;
Fax (65) 7873969.

USA

Master Richard Mooney,
Sarasota Shaolin Academy,
4655 Flatbush Avenue,
Sarasota, FL 34233-1920,
USA.

Dr Yang Jwing Ming,
Yang's Martial Arts Association,
38 Hyde Park Avenue, Jamaica Plain,
MA 02130-4132, USA.
Tel (1-617) 5248892;
Fax (1-617) 5244184.

Master Paul Hannah, M.D.
Tai Chi Chuan, Baguaquan and
Xingyiquan,
2200 Grant Street, Suite 109,
Gary, IN 46404, USA.
Tel (1-219) 9449300;
Fax (1-219) 9448735.

Index